Controversies in Severe Traumatic Brain Injury Management

Shelly D. Timmons

Editor

Controversies in Severe Traumatic Brain Injury Management

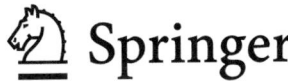 Springer

Editor
Shelly D. Timmons
Department of Neurosurgery
Penn State University Milton S. Hershey Medical Center
Hershey, PA
USA

ISBN 978-3-030-07781-5   ISBN 978-3-319-89477-5   (eBook)
https://doi.org/10.1007/978-3-319-89477-5

Printed on acid-free paper

This Springer imprint is published by the registered company Springer Nature Switzerland AG
The registered company address is: Gewerbestrasse 11, 6330 Cham, Switzerland

Preface

Management of severe traumatic brain injury (TBI) remains one of the most complicated and controversial areas of neurosurgery, trauma care, and critical care medicine. The human, social, and financial toll of severe traumatic brain injury is astronomical, and management is aimed at mitigating the long-term effects on each individual suffering from this malady.

While major improvements in mortality from severe TBI have been achieved in the last few decades, optimization of outcome in survivors depends on a host of prognostic variables and treatment paradigms. While the implementation of treatment guidelines and protocols has led to some standardized therapeutic approaches, much remains to be understood about the impact of almost all potential therapeutic interventions. Care is often complicated by the involvement of multiple medical disciplines, the presence of polytrauma, and our aging population with a variety of pre-injury comorbidities. Decision-making must at once be based on evidence from population medicine but tailored to the individual patient's injury patterns, comorbid conditions, pre-injury value systems, and evolving and changing cerebral physiology also. Longer term treatment strategies must encompass multifactorial approaches aimed at the many different patterns of complications and deficits that may be seen post-injury.

This book aims to address the current levels of evidence for management of a variety of critical parameters after severe TBI, as well as to provide the reader with practical approaches to care based upon existing evidence and anatomical and physiological principles. A range of topics are included, from specific critical care approaches to TBI to broader questions of prognostication and philosophies of treatment. Critical care topics will include, for example, the type, timing, and safety of deep vein thrombosis (DVT) prophylaxis; the choice of sedative agents in brain-injured patients; the practical application of multimodality neuromonitoring for prevention of secondary insults and injury; and the optimal treatment of dysautonomia. Broad approaches to treatment include concepts such as organization of trauma systems to maximize outcomes end-of-life decision-making with incomplete data on prognosis the use of medications to enhance recovery in the post-acute phase and utilization of functional neurosurgical approaches for the restoration of function after injury.

Written by subject matter experts in the field, topics include commonly encountered clinical questions in TBI management. The current evidence for a variety of treatments is addressed, and relevant questions that have not been adequately addressed in the literature are outlined. Options for treatment are reviewed and suggestions for future research directions proposed. Such approaches to this subject matter are often requested by a variety of health-care professionals in all disciplines, yet resources are lacking that not only emphasize a critical appraisal of the existing literature but also highlight the gamut of available treatment options and the rationale for using them even in the absence of strong research data.

This text aims to fill some of those gaps and will be of practical utility to neurosurgeons, neurointensivists, trauma surgeons, anesthesiologists, neurologists, physiatrists, nutritionists, and clinical pharmacologists, as well as physical, occupational, and speech therapists who treat TBI patients. It can also serve as a comprehensive educational reference for medical students, residents, and fellows with an interest in traumatic brain injury, as well as researchers seeking clarification of important clinical questions yet to be answered.

It is clear that evidence-based medicine is an important tool in the clinical armamentarium for fighting injury and illness. The role of well-designed laboratory, clinical, and registry science trials is pivotal, and as further data become available, they will continue to inform our decision-making processes and refine our understanding of the impact of various interventions. Meanwhile, we are faced with making myriad decisions every day on critically ill TBI patients and must formulate our best treatment plans upon what evidence exists, our understanding of cerebral and medical physiology, sound medical and surgical principles, and the wealth of experience gained as TBI treatment has evolved over the past several years.

Hershey, PA, USA   Shelly D. Timmons

Contents

Contributors

Justice O. Agyei, MD Department of Neurological Surgery, Jacobs School of Medicine and Biomedical Sciences, Buffalo, NY, USA

Beth M. Ansel, PhD, CCC-SLP The Eunice Kennedy Shriver National Institute of Child Health and Human Development, The National Institutes of Health, Spencerville, MD, USA

Rocco Armonda, MD Department of Neurosurgery, Georgetown University Hospital, Washington Hospital Center, Washington, DC, USA

Randy Bell, MD Department of Neurosurgery, Walter Reed National Military Medical Center, Bethesda, MD, USA

Bradley A. Boucher, PharmD, FCCP, FNAP, MCCM, BCPS Department of Clinical Pharmacy and Translational Science, College of Pharmacy, University of Tennessee Health Science Center, Memphis, TN, USA

Gretchen M. Brophy, PharmD, BCPS, FCCP, FCCM, FNCS Department of Pharmacotherapy and Outcomes Science and Neurosurgery, Virginia Commonwealth University, Richmond, VA, USA

M. Ross Bullock, MD, PhD Department of Neurosurgery, University of Miami-Miller School of Medicine, Miami, FL, USA

William R. Y. Carlton Jr., MD Department of Neurosurgery, Shands Hospital of the University of Florida, Gainesville, FL, USA

Anthony Conte, MD Department of Neurosurgery, Georgetown University Hospital, Washington Hospital Center, Washington, DC, USA

Justin R. Davanzo, MD Department of Neurosurgery, Penn State University Milton S. Hershey Medical Center, Hershey, PA, USA

Jonathan H. DeAntonio, MD Department of Surgery, Virginia Commonwealth University Health System, VCU School of Medicine, Richmond, VA, USA

James Ecklund, MD, FACS Inova Neuroscience and Spine Institute, Falls Church, VA, USA

Howard M. Eisenberg, MD Department of Neurosurgery, University of Maryland, Baltimore, MD, USA

Ilyas Eli, MD Department of Neurosurgery, University of Utah, Clinical Neurosciences Center, Salt Lake City, UT, USA

Rocky Felbaum, MD Department of Neurosurgery, Georgetown University Hospital, Washington, DC, USA

Gabriel N. Friedman, BA Department of Neurosurgery, Harvard Medical School, Massachusetts General Hospital, Boston, MA, USA

Kevin J. Gibbons, MD Department of Neurological Surgery, Jacobs School of Medicine and Biomedical Sciences, Buffalo, NY, USA

William B. Gormley, MD, MPH, MBA Department of Neurosurgery, Brigham and Women's Hospital, Boston, MA, USA

Gregory W. J. Hawryluk, MD, PhD Department of Neurosurgery, University of Utah, Clinical Neurosciences Center, Salt Lake City, UT, USA

David S. Hersh, MD Department of Neurosurgery, University of Maryland, Baltimore, MD, USA

Michael Huang, MD Department of Neurological Surgery, Brain and Spinal Injury Center, Zuckerberg San Francisco General Hospital, University of California, San Francisco, CA, USA

Jack Jallo, MD, PhD, FACS Department of Neurological Surgery, Thomas Jefferson University, Philadelphia, PA, USA

Sudha Jayaraman, MD, MSc, FACS Division of Acute Care Surgical Services, Virginia Commonwealth University Health System, Richmond, VA, USA

Evan Joyce, MD, MS Department of Neurosurgery, University of Utah, Clinical Neurosciences Center, Salt Lake City, UT, USA

Sanjay Konakondla, MD Department of Neurosurgery, Geisinger Health System, Danville, PA, USA

Timothy J. Kovanda, MD Department of Neurological Surgery, Indiana University School of Medicine, Indianapolis, IN, USA

Young Lee, MD Department of Neurological Surgery, University of California San Francisco, San Francisco, CA, USA

James Leiphart, MD, PhD, FACS Inova Neuroscience and Spine Institute, Falls Church, VA, USA

Peter Le Roux, MD, FACS Department of Neurosurgery, The Brain and Spine Center, Lankenau Medical Center, Wynnewood, PA, USA

Geoffrey T. Manley, MD, PhD Department of Neurological Surgery, University of California San Francisco, San Francisco, CA, USA

Department of Neurosurgery, Zuckerberg San Francisco General Hospital and Trauma Center, Brain and Spinal Injury Center (BASIC), San Francisco, CA, USA

Kimberly N. Means, PharmD, BSN, RN Department of Pharmacy Services, Medical College of Virginia, Richmond, VA, USA

John F. Morrison, MD Department of Neurological Surgery, Jacobs School of Medicine and Biomedical Sciences, Buffalo, NY, USA

Ziev B. Moses, MD Department of Neurosurgery, Brigham and Women's Hospital, Boston, MA, USA

Kyle Mueller, MD Department of Neurosurgery, Georgetown University Hospital, Washington, DC, USA

Gregory J. A. Murad, MD, FAANS Department of Neurosurgery, Shands Hospital of the University of Florida, Gainesville, FL, USA

David O. Okonkwo, MD, PhD Department of Neurological Surgery, University of Pittsburgh, Pittsburgh, PA, USA

Angel Ordaz, BS Department of Neurological Surgery, University of California San Francisco, San Francisco, CA, USA

Rani Patal, MD Department of Neurosurgery, Hadassah-Hebrew University Medical Center, Jerusalem, Israel

Courtney Pendleton, MD Department of Neurological Surgery, Thomas Jefferson University, Philadelphia, PA, USA

P. B. Raksin, MD Department of Neurosurgery, Rush University Medical Center, Chicago, IL, USA

Division of Neurosurgery, John H. Stroger Jr. Hospital of Cook County, (formerly Cook County Hospital), Chicago, IL, USA

Ashley Ralston, MD Department of Neurosurgery, University of Miami-Miller School of Medicine, Miami, FL, USA

Christian B. Ricks, MD, MS Department of Neurological Surgery, University of Pittsburgh, Pittsburgh, PA, USA

Richard B. Rodgers, MD, FAANS, FACS Department of Neurological Surgery, Indiana University School of Medicine, Goodman Campbell Brain and Spine, Indianapolis, IN, USA

Guy Rosenthal, MD Department of Neurosurgery, Hadassah-Hebrew University Medical Center, Jerusalem, Israel

Hussain Shallwani, MD Department of Neurological Surgery, Jacobs School of Medicine and Biomedical Sciences, Buffalo, NY, USA

Emily P. Sieg, BS, MS, MD Department of Neurosurgery, Penn State Health Milton S. Hershey Medical Center, Hershey, PA, USA

Ian Tafel, MD Department of Neurosurgery, Brigham and Women's Hospital, Boston, MA, USA

Shelly D. Timmons, MD, PhD, FACS, FAANS Department of Neurosurgery, Penn State University Milton S. Hershey Medical Center, Hershey, PA, USA

J. Christopher Zacko, MS, MD Department of Neurosurgery, Penn State University Health Milton S. Hershey Medical Center, Hershey, PA, USA

Prehospital Transportation and Optimal Utilization of Resources

Sanjay Konakondla and Shelly D. Timmons

Introduction

Prehospital guidelines for the management of severe traumatic brain injury (sTBI) have been published since 2008 [1]. These guidelines, published by the Brain Trauma Foundation, outline issues of injury prevention, initial evaluation, early treatment goals, and triage concerns and call for specific resuscitative efforts and neurologic assessments. Recommendations to avoid hypotension (systolic blood pressure [SBP] <90), to avoid hypoxemia (arterial O_2 saturation <90%), and to use the Glasgow Coma Scale (GCS) post-resuscitation to establish neurological status and guide clinical progression are also included. Endotracheal intubation is generally recommended for patients with a GCS 3-8, for patients who are unable to maintain an airway, or for patients with hypoxemia not corrected by noninvasive methods. With the advent and common usage of portable oxygen saturation monitoring and end-tidal CO_2 monitoring during transport, refinements in recommendations have now become possible. For example, hyperventilation, once a mainstay during transportation of sTBI patients, is now reserved for patients showing signs of cerebral herniation with the goal of $ETCO_2$ of 30–35 mmHg.

All of these measures are aimed at the avoidance of secondary insults contributing to secondary injury cascades in the brain following TBI. Secondary insults include episodes of hypotension and cerebral hypoperfusion, hypoxemia and hypercarbia, hyper- or hypoglycemia, hyperthermia, acidosis, anemia, arterial or fat thromboemboli to the brain, seizures, etc., all of which must be minimized during the initial assessment and treatment of brain-injured patients in the field. Secondary injury cascades may result from the trauma but may also be exacerbated by these events. These include cerebral tissue ischemia, cellular metabolic crisis and mitochondrial failure, ion fluxes resulting in hyperexcitability and calcium-mediated cellular damage, lipid peroxidation and membrane failure, oxygen-free radical production, inflammatory processes, and neurochemical, neurotransmitter, and receptor changes. Care beginning at the scene of injury from the moment a brain-injured patient is identified and, extending through all of the acute care phases into the rehabilitative phase, must be focused on avoiding these types of insults and

S. Konakondla, MD
Department of Neurosurgery,
Geisinger Health System, Danville, PA, USA
e-mail: skonakondla@geisinger.edu

S. D. Timmons, MD, PhD, FACS, FAANS (✉)
Department of Neurosurgery, Penn State University
Milton S. Hershey Medical Center,
Hershey, PA, USA
e-mail: stimmons@mac.com

© Springer International Publishing AG, part of Springer Nature 2018
S. D. Timmons (ed.), *Controversies in Severe Traumatic Brain Injury Management*,
https://doi.org/10.1007/978-3-319-89477-5_1

mitigating secondary injury cascades in order to optimize functional outcome.

While specific treatments in the field, such as intubation practices, fluid resuscitation, and even administration of neuroprotective agents, have been the subject of significant study, idealized patterns of field triage, transport, and trauma systems organization play just as important a role in sTBI outcomes. There is an undeniably broad spectrum of environments in which injured patients are discovered and treated, not to mention regional variations in access to care and available resources. Considerable diversity in outcome from sTBI has been documented worldwide, with low-income countries having the highest mortality rates [2], presumably related to resource availability and intensity of treatment. Even in the United States, there is variability in outcome, with center differences in outcome having been documented even in clinical trials utilizing rigid treatment protocols [3]. The goals of specific prehospital protocols are to decrease this variability, by supporting the patient physiologically and achieving the most rapid transport times to definitive care possible.

Several factors including regional geography, topography, weather patterns, available modes of transportation, and the locales of health-care institutions and trauma centers must all be taken into account when devising transportation and prehospital treatment strategies to improve patient outcomes by getting the "right patient to the right place for the right care at the right time."

Closest Hospital Versus Trauma Center

Because time is of the essence not only to reach a neurosurgical center for those who require surgery to alleviate brain compression or herniation but also to stabilize conditions resulting in secondary insults, efforts to develop triage strategies in the field are critically important. A considerable amount of controversy exists over how best to achieve rapid and definitive care. For instance, some regionalized systems of ambulance transport have mandated that traumatically injured patients be taken to the closest hospital rather

than the closest trauma center or neurosurgical hospital, even when injuries are identified that could reasonably be anticipated to require these higher levels of care. A close look at the available data can inform policies and lead to higher-quality research in this area.

Longstanding guidelines on the "Resources for Optimal Care of the Injured Patient" have been propagated by the American College of Surgeons Committee on Trauma and used both to verify trauma center readiness and inform trauma systems development [4]. Requirements for optimal trauma systems and descriptions of trauma center levels and their roles within the system are delineated, as well as optimal prehospital care paradigms, criteria for inter-hospital transfer, and important hospital organizational features needed to provide high-quality care to trauma patients.

A further joint effort by the Centers of Disease Control (CDC) and the American College of Surgeons Committee on Trauma (ACS-COT) assists first responders by providing a decision-making triage scheme for transferring critically injured patients directly to trauma centers [5]. Similar schema exist in other countries. Factors considered in the ACS-CDC document include physiologic criteria (GCS, SBP, respiratory rate [RR]), anatomic criteria (type of injury and area affected), mechanism of injury, and special considerations (age-related SBP, anticoagulation status). According to these guidelines, patients with GCS 3-12, penetrating injuries to the head and neck, open or depressed skull fractures, or paralysis, should be transported preferentially to a trauma center with the highest level of care within a defined trauma system. Patients with head injury on anticoagulants or with bleeding disorders should be transported to "a trauma center or hospital capable of timely and thorough evaluation and initial management of potentially serious injuries" with likely transfer to a higher level of care. Further study of this growing problem in our aging population is needed [6].

While triage practices fall under the umbrella of trauma systems development, organization of trauma care varies state to state in the United States and country to country, and systems exist at different levels of maturity. Therefore, it is often up to designated regional trauma authorities and even Emergency Medical Services (EMS) providers to decide which practices and transfer criteria to employ. This is, on the one hand, a benefit, because regional authorities understand best the practice patterns, geographical and weather issues affecting transport, population needs, and social cultures of their area. On the other hand, this leads to variations in care.

Multiple studies in the United States and abroad have demonstrated that mortality is improved when suspected TBI patients are transported directly to Level I or II trauma centers, unless life-saving stabilization at a non-trauma center is required [7–9]. Indeed, one large cohort study of English National Trauma Registry TBI patients revealed that deterioration in prehospital vital signs did not vary significantly with duration of EMS transport, lending support to the strategy of direct transfer to a trauma center [10]. Field dwell-time questions remain and may differ from region to region and country to country where qualifications and training of first responders vary from basic emergency medical technicians to emergency care physicians. Long dwell times in non-trauma centers have been documented as the greatest proportion of time spent prior to arrival to a trauma center for TBI patients [11]. It is clear that excessive time spent prior to definitive care may result in secondary insults and poorer outcome, and if patients are taken to non-trauma facilities for hemodynamic stabilization, efforts to rapidly assess, treat, and move the patient to a higher level of trauma care should be employed.

However, differences in patient characteristics (both clinical and nonclinical) have been shown between those with sTBI taken directly to a trauma center and those transferred from another facility, and further study of this issue is warranted [12]. For example, the impact of neurological deterioration while en route, which occurs in up to 9% of patients with TBI [13] on long-term outcome and hospital disposition choices, needs further characterization. In the short term, deterioration during transport results in worse in-hospital outcomes and higher resource utilization [12].

Additionally, triage criteria may underestimate the degree of TBI, particularly among those trauma patients who are older, sustain low-level falls, have less severe Abbreviated Injury Scale (AIS) head injury scores, or are female, according to one study of English patients [14].

Mode of Transportation

Decisions regarding mode of transportation must be made based upon the patient's overall injury pattern and condition, as well as the care resources available both for transport and at the destination. Ground ambulance transport versus air transport by helicopter for patients with traumatic brain injuries has been studied. While early investigation in the Resuscitation Outcomes Consortium demonstrated that no differences in adjusted clinical outcomes existed, helicopters were more commonly used to transport more severely injured patients, while using more advanced life support procedures with longer per-hospital durations [15]. Similarly, a study of pediatric trauma patients found no differences except in hospital length of stay (LOS) when adjusting for injuries, scene distance, and time to hospital arrival [16]. They too noted that helicopters were used for more severely injured patients, as well as those being transported from farther distances. However, in patients with TBI specifically, air transport *has* been shown to have increased chances of survival compared to those transported by ground [17, 18]. Conclusions regarding type of transport must take into account a variety of confounders and region-specific factors. Transport decisions must be made based not only distance and time but also terrain and weather and most importantly the patient's condition.

Regionalization of Neurosurgical Care

Mortality increases as high as 26% for patients with severe TBI treated in non-neurosurgical centers versus those treated in neurosurgical centers have been reported [19]. Furthermore, sTBI patients treated in centers with protocol-driven neurocritical care had better outcomes, even when no neurosurgical operations were required [20]. Furthermore, this group found that characteristics at presentation could not predict the need for neurosurgical intervention in the sTBI patients. These findings taken together support arguments for transfer of sTBI to regionalized centers specializing in neurosurgery and neurocritical care as early as possible.

Impact of Non-transfer

As noted, the American College of Surgeons outlines specific definitions and criteria regarding transfer to a Level I or Level II trauma center [4]. The organization also recommends ongoing monitoring for both under-triage and over-triage in order to continually improve systems of care. Unfortunately, when trauma patients are taken to non-tertiary trauma centers (Levels III, IV, or V) and non-trauma centers, and should be transferred to higher levels of care according to criteria, this does not always occur. In one study using the ACS-COT inter-hospital transfer criteria, more than 95,000 patients were identified as eligible for transfer, but just under 20,000 patients were actually transferred. Patient factors associated with failure to transfer trauma patients to higher-level facilities, despite meeting transfer criteria, included older age, chest injuries, and commercial insurance, accounting for approximately one-third (36%) of transfer failures [21]. However, notably, hospital and systems factors accounted for 58% of failures to transfer. Non-trauma centers, larger hospitals (by bed number), university affiliation (versus community hospital), and those hospitals with more trauma surgeons and neurosurgeons were more likely not to transfer patients meeting criteria. Factors for non-transfer differed depending on whether the originating facility was a trauma center or not. In non-trauma centers, for-profit status was more likely to be associated with non-transfer than at trauma centers. In Level III, IV, and IV trauma centers, patient-level factors were more often

responsible for this variation (44%) than in non-trauma centers (13%).

With respect to outcomes, mortality for patients was found to be significantly higher for patients not transferred to a tertiary center compared to those transferred to a Level I or II trauma center, raising concern that economic and other factors may drive decision-making that is not in patients' best interest; however, more analysis would be needed to understand this complex issue. Interestingly, traumatic brain injury patients were among the groups that were most likely to get transferred in this study. However, lack of established follow-up for sTBI patients who should have been transferred, but were not, has been noted in other reports [22]. This is especially problematic in sTBI patients who require long-term follow-up assessments, multiple modalities of treatments and care coordination, and in whom it takes months to years to see ultimate improvements in outcome.

Telemedicine

Certainly, decisions to transfer must take into account the resources required both to transfer and to provide care in specialized centers that are sometimes far from the patient's origin. Telemedical support services and consultation with specialty centers are increasingly being used in an attempt to keep those patients with low likelihood of deterioration or need of specialized services in hospitals closer to their communities, with varying degrees of success. While it is critical to get the most severely injured high-risk patients to Level I and Level II trauma centers or similar specialty hospitals, it is equally important to devise strategies to keep low-risk patients in hospitals of origin where quality care is available. This is so that high-acuity and high-risk patients have access to the specialty centers, overall cost to the system is reduced, and patients with less severe injuries are not subjected to the stresses of transfer.

Systems of consultation between "peripheral" hospitals and neurosurgical or trauma hospitals have been described [22–25]. These systems have highlighted several issues that must be addressed, including resource utilization in the peripheral hospital, the need for more specific radiographic and clinical criteria for non-transfer, the impact of transfer delays (and the deteriorations that prompt them) on ultimate outcome, and challenges in information sharing.

Using advanced communication technologies, such as Web-based imaging review systems, may be beneficial. A reported 44% avoidance of potential neurosurgery transfers to a higher care facility from rural facilities after imaging was reviewed remotely by neurosurgeons was achieved in one study [25], and patients with mild TBI requiring surgery typically have a surgical lesion initially [26]. With these data in mind, decisions about transfer can be better informed but must still involve the neurosurgical center to help organize a system of transfer triage. However, neurosurgeons, who are already in a high demand-low supply situation in most countries, cannot be expected to provide radiological readings for all TBI patients in a large network of centers. Therefore, not only do better predictive criteria for deterioration of the less severely injured need to be developed, but formal arrangements and agreements must be in place to specify what services will be supplied by whom.

Future improvements in telemedicine using rapidly advancing computer technologies to achieve real-time patient evaluations, continuous inter-institutional communications, instantaneous image transfer, subspecialty consultations, and automatic feedback are achievable [27]. Similar technologies have been implemented for distance learning [28], which will no doubt inform future training modules in injury management. The feasibility and cost of transferring large amounts of potentially sensitive patient protected data in a timely fashion, while guaranteeing security and interoperability, remain major challenges [29, 30], as do issues of cost recovery for services provided remotely (which are not reimbursed by most payors). A system that shares telephonic and videographic communications, as well as shared imaging and physiological data, will best guide patients to their ideal destinations and in turn should lead to even better outcomes

for even more patients. The advancement of such "tele-cooperation" will link data from multiple sources starting at the initial field resuscitation and extending to emergency consultation with subspecialty input. These data will inform appropriate transfers in the short timeframes required to achieve good outcomes by limiting secondary insults. Furthermore, resources will be utilized where, when, and how they can help the greatest number of patients.

Conclusions

In summary, the ultimate goal of prehospital care for sTBI patients is to prevent secondary insults leading to poorer outcomes. By lessening the duration of prehospital time for severely brain-injured patients, as long as no hemodynamic instability requiring emergency department stabilization exists, secondary insults will be minimized. Stops at non-neurosurgical hospitals simply because they are closest to the scene of the injury should be avoided for those meeting sTBI field triage criteria. However, those with hemodynamic instability may benefit from treatment and evaluation at more proximate hospital locations, thereby avoiding secondary brain injury by improving blood pressure, oxygenation, and intracranial pressure prior to transfer to a neurosurgical hospital or higher-level trauma center. Telecommunications strategies and trauma systems organizational approaches hold promise for improving systems of care to provide optimal care for patients suffering brain injuries of all severities.

References

1. Badjatia N, Carney N, Crocco TJ, Fallat ME, Hennes HMA, Jagoda AS, et al; BTF Center for Guidelines Management. Guidelines for prehospital management of traumatic brain injury 2nd edition. Prehosp Emerg Care. 2008;12 Suppl 1:S1–52.
2. Georgoff P, Meghan S, Mirza K, Stein S. Geographic variation in outcomes from severe traumatic brain injury. World Neurosurg. 2010;74(2–3):331–45.
3. Timmons SD, Bee T, Webb S, Diaz-Arrastia RR, Hesdorffer D. Using the abbreviated injury severity and Glasgow coma scale scores to predict 2-week mortality after traumatic brain injury. J Trauma. 2011 Nov;71(5):1172–8.

4. Chapter 4. Interhospital transfer. In: Rotondo MF, Cribari C, Smith RS, editors. Resources for optimal care of the injured patient. Committee on Trauma American College of Surgeons; 2014. pp. 30–34. https://www.facs.org/~/media/files/quality%20programs/trauma/vrc%20resources/resources%20for%20optimal%20care.ashx.

5. Sasser SM, Hunt RC, Faul M, Sugerman D, Pearson WS, Dulski T, et al; Centers for Disease Control and Prevention (CDC). Guidelines for field triage of injured patients: recommendations of the National Expert Panel on Field Triage, 2011. MMWR Recomm Rep. 2012;61(RR-1):1–20.

6. Wasserman EB, Shah MN, Jones CM, Cushman JT, Caterino JM, Bazarian JJ, et al. Identification of a neurologic scale that optimizes EMS detection of older adult traumatic brain injury patients who require transport to a trauma center. Prehosp Emerg Care. 2015;19(2):202–12.

7. Härtl R, Gerber LM, Iacono L, Ni Q, Lyons K, Ghajar J. Direct transport within an organized state trauma system reduces mortality in patients with severe traumatic brain injury. J Trauma. 2006;60(6):1250–6; discussion 1256.

8. Mans S, Reinders Folmer E, de Jongh MA, Lansink KW. Direct transport versus inter hospital transfer of severely injured trauma patients. Injury. 2016;47(1):26–31.

9. Prabhakaran K, Petrone P, Lombardo G, Stoller C, Policastro A, Marini CP. Mortality rates of severe traumatic brain injury patients: impact of direct versus nondirect transfers. J Surg Res. 2017 Nov;219:66–71.

10. Fuller G, Woodford M, Lawrence T, Coats T, Lecky F. Do prolonged primary transport times for traumatic brain injury patients result in deteriorating physiology? A cohort study. Prehosp Emerg Care. 2014;18(1):60–7.

11. Dunn LT. Secondary insults during the interhospital transfer of head-injured patients: an audit of transfers in the Mersey Region. Injury. 1997;28:427–31.

12. Sugerman DE, Xu L, Pearson WS, Faul M. Patients with severe traumatic brain injury transferred to a Level I or II trauma center: United States, 2007 to 2009. J Trauma Acute Care Surg. 2012;73(6):1491–9.

13. Majidi S, Siddiq F, Qureshi AI. Prehospital neurologic deterioration is independent predictor of outcome in traumatic brain injury: analysis from National Trauma Data Bank. Am J Emerg Med. 2013;31(8):1215–9.

14. Fuller G, Lawrence T, Woodford M, Lecky F. The accuracy of alternative triage rules for identification of significant traumatic brain injury: a diagnostic cohort study. Emerg Med J. 2014;31(11):914–9.

15. Bulger EM, Guffey D, Guyette FX, MacDonald RD, Brasel K, Kerby JD, et al; Resuscitation Outcomes Consortium Investigators. Impact of prehospital mode of transport after severe injury: a multicenter evaluation from the Resuscitation Outcomes Consortium. J Trauma Acute Care Surg. 2012;72(3):567–73; discussion 573–5; quiz 803.

16. Farach SM, Walford NE, Bendure L, Amankwah EK, Danielson PD, Chandler NM. Helicopter transport from the scene of injury: are there improved outcomes for pediatric trauma patients? Pediatr Emerg Care. 2018;34(5):344–8.

17. Sun H, Samra NS, Kalakoti P, Sharma K, Patra DP, Dossani RH, et al. Impact of prehospital transportation on survival in skiers and snowboarders with traumatic brain injury. World Neurosurg. 2017;104:909–918.e8.

18. Aiolfi A, Benjamin E, Recinos G, De Leon CA, Inaba K, Demetriades D. Air versus ground transportation in isolated severe head trauma: a National Trauma Data Bank study. J Emerg Med. 2017;54(3):328–34. pii: S0736-4679(17)31094-6.

19. Patel HC, Bouamra O, Woodford M, King AT, Yates DW, Lecky FE, Trauma Audit and Research Network. Trends in head injury outcome from 1989 to 2003 and the effect of neurosurgical care: an observational study. Lancet. 2005;366(9496):1538–44.

20. Patel HC, Menon DK, Tebbs S, Hawker R, Hutchinson PJ, Kirkpatrick PJ. Specialist neurocritical care and outcome from head injury. Intensive Care Med. 2002;28(5):547–53.

21. Zhou Q, Rosengart MR, Billiar TR, Peitzman AB, Sperry JL, Brown JB. Factors associated with nontransfer in trauma patients meeting American College of Surgeons' Criteria for transfer at nontertiary centers. JAMA Surg. 2017;152(4):369–76.

22. Zulu BMW, Mulaudzi TV, Madiba TE, Muckart DJJ. Outcome of head injuries in general surgical units with an off-site neurosurgical service. Injury. 2007;38:576–83.

23. Fabbri A, Servadei F, Marchesini G, Stein SC, Vandelli A. Observational approach to subjects with mild-to-moderate head injury and initial non-neurosurgical lesions. J Neurol Neurosurg Psychiatry. 2008;79:1180–5.

24. Moya M, Valdez J, Yonas H, Alverson DC. The impact of a telehealth web-based solution on neurosurgery triage and consultation. Telemed J E Health. 2010;16:945–9.

25. Hassan R, Siregar JA, A Rahman Mohd NA. The implementation of teleneurosurgery in the management of referrals to a neurosurgical department in hospital sultanah amninah johor bahru. Malays J Med Sci. 2014;21:54–62.

26. Carlson AP, Ramirez P, Kennedy G, McLean AR, Murray-Krezan C, Stippler M. Low rate of delayed deterioration requiring surgical treatment in patients transferred to a tertiary care center for mild traumatic brain injury. Neurosurg Focus. 2010;29(5):E3.

27. Breen G-M, Matusitz J. An evolutionary examination of telemedicine: a health and computer-mediated communication perspective. Soc Work Public Health. 2010;25:59–71.

28. Jacobs J, Caudell T, Wilks D, Keep MF, Mitchell S, Buchanan H, et al. Integration of advanced technologies to enhance problem-based learning over distance: project TOUCH. Anat Rec B New Anat. 2003;270((1):16–22.

29. Staemmler M, Walz M, Weisser G, Engelmann U, Weininger R, Ernstberger A, Sturm J. Establishing end-to-end security in a nationwide network for telecooperation. Stud Health Technol Inform. 2012;180:512–6.

30. Neuhaus P, Weber T, Dugas M, Juhra C, Breil B. Characterization of image transfer patterns in a regional trauma network. J Med Syst. 2014;38(11):137.

To Treat or Not to Treat: Early Withdrawal of Therapy and the Limits of Prognostic Ability

Young Lee, Angel Ordaz, Michael Huang, and Geoffrey T. Manley

Introduction

Traumatic brain injury (TBI) has had a ubiquitous presence in human history, even pre-dating the understanding of the brain as the central organ of the nervous system. It remains the main cause of death and disability in young adults worldwide. In more recent history, the development of computed tomography (CT), simple classifications of the severity of traumatic brain injury such as the Glasgow Coma Scale (GCS), monitoring of intracranial pressure, and the concept of prevention of secondary brain injury have helped advance the ability to prognosticate and improve outcomes after traumatic brain injury [1]. However, the art of determining prognosis after severe traumatic brain injury remains imprecise in many situations, leading to controversy over which patients may benefit from aggressive treatment and which patients may suffer futile outcomes despite intervention. A 2005 survey found that 80% of physicians thought that an accurate prognostic assessment was required for decisions on whether or not to withdraw treatment, but only around a third felt that they could accurately assess prognosis [2].

Early Prognostic Factors for Mortality and Unfavorable Outcome After Severe Traumatic Brain Injury

There have been multiple attempts to develop models for prognostication of mortality and unfavorable outcome (death or severe disability on the Glasgow Outcome Scale) after traumatic brain injury. Certain cases may have a straightforward prognosis, such as a comatose patient with cerebral herniation and complete loss of all brainstem reflexes or a neurologically intact patient with isolated epidural hemorrhage without mass effect, whereas intermediate examples between these two extremes yield an unclear prognosis. To address these uncertainties, large trials have been per-

Y. Lee, MD · A. Ordaz, BS
Department of Neurological Surgery, University of California San Francisco, San Francisco, CA, USA
e-mail: young.lee@ucsf.edu; Angel.ordaz@ucsf.edu

M. Huang, MD
Department of Neurological Surgery, Brain and Spinal Injury Center, Zuckerberg San Francisco General Hospital, University of California, San Francisco, CA, USA
e-mail: Michael.Huang@ucsf.edu

G. T. Manley, MD, PhD (✉)
Department of Neurological Surgery, University of California San Francisco, San Francisco, CA, USA

Department of Neurological Surgery, Brain and Spinal Injury Center, Zuckerberg San Francisco General Hospital, University of California, San Francisco, CA, USA
e-mail: manleyg@ucsf.edu; manleyg@neurosurg.ucsf.edu

© Springer International Publishing AG, part of Springer Nature 2018
S. D. Timmons (ed.), *Controversies in Severe Traumatic Brain Injury Management*,
https://doi.org/10.1007/978-3-319-89477-5_2

formed to provide data, including the International Mission on Prognosis and Analysis of Clinical Trials (IMPACT) and Corticoid Randomization After Significant Head Injury (CRASH) prognostic models. Both models were based on large numbers of patients, with IMPACT produced from 8509 patients over 11 studies and CRASH based on a total of 10,008 patients. Common factors identified as affecting mortality and unfavorable outcome after traumatic brain injury included age, Glasgow Coma Score at presentation, pupil reactivity to light, presence of major extracranial injury, and classification of hemorrhagic findings on CT scan. These models have been externally validated in multiple studies [3]. Additional factors identified in the IMPACT model included the presence of secondary insults such as hypotension and hypoxia and laboratory parameters such as serum glucose and hemoglobin. Strong prognostic factors included age, which predicted an approximate doubling of poor outcome for each increase in age of around 25 years in both IMPACT and CRASH. In the IMPACT model, CT findings consistent with increased intracranial pressure (ICP) or mass lesion (Marshall CT classes III to VI) also approximately doubled the odds of poor outcome, as did the presence of traumatic subarachnoid hemorrhage. The CRASH model found that obliteration of the third ventricle and midline shift were the strongest predictors of mortality at 2 weeks, while non-evacuated hematoma was the strongest predictor of unfavorable outcomes at 6 months. Non-CT predictors of especially poor outcomes at 6 months were GCS motor scores of 1 or 2. Statistically significant but more moderate predictors of poor outcome included higher glucose levels and lower hemoglobin levels.

Despite the large numbers of patients in these studies, in practice, the IMPACT and CRASH models only account for approximately one-third of outcome variability at 6 months. This makes absolute prognostication quite difficult, and it is often up to the treating physician to make a "gestalt" prediction of outcome. This is not made any easier by widely publicized yet rare cases of patients in minimally conscious states who have lived on to demonstrate recovery up to 10 years after initial brain injury [4]. Families may also

struggle to hold realistic expectations even in cases of near predictive certainty, as anecdotal cases of the recovery of so-called "brain dead" patients in the press may lead many to believe in the possibility of miraculous recoveries regardless of medical prognosis [5].

Clinical Nihilism and Traumatic Brain Injury

There are significant differences in the practices of withdrawal of life-sustaining therapy around the world. This is of great importance, as the withdrawal of life support in patients with severe traumatic brain injury will almost invariably lead to death. Turgeon et al. discovered that within Canada there was wide variability in mortality after severe traumatic brain injury (from 10.8 to 44.2%). Additionally, over two-thirds of deaths involved the withdrawal of life-sustaining therapy, with this ranging from 45 to 87% [6, 7]. Similar findings have been reported in the United States. More than three-quarters of mortality was related to the withdrawal of support at one medical center [8]. Approximately two-thirds of withdrawal of care were related to injuries thought incompatible with survival, while the rest were related to expectation of survival but with poor neurologic function unacceptable to the patient's wishes [9]. The medical center was found to be an independent predictor of withdrawal of life-sustaining therapy, and the variability of mortality between centers was affected by the rate and timing of withdrawal of life-sustaining therapy. Even the type of medical center, whether academic or community, may affect the decision to initially withhold or withdraw support [10]. Factors related to the attitude and culture of treating physicians and medical centers toward withdrawal of care in severe traumatic brain injury appear to overshadow clinical and radiographic factors in the decision to withdraw support [8]. Although there is some indirect evidence that the timing of withdrawal of care may not affect mortality [11], early withdrawal of care may be a self-fulfilling prophecy that reduces the chances of survival and could increase the mortality in patients who may have recovered, if only given more time.

There is also evidence that the initial attitude of the treating physician may have a dominant influence on the continued care of the patient, despite changing clinical and radiographic data over the patient's course of care. Multiple studies have found that a craniotomy procedure and/or other non-neurosurgical procedures are less associated with death related to withdrawal of care. When controlled for other clinical and radiographic factors, these studies support the assertion that the initial attitude of the treating physician may play a dominant role [7]. Evidence that physician bias may affect patient outcome include findings that in younger patients some physicians prognosticate with disproportionate pessimism, leading to withdrawal of care that may increase mortality. Likewise, older patients are less likely to undergo surgery and thus have a higher likelihood of withdrawal of support [8]. When compared with patient surrogates' prediction of patient prognosis, physicians tend to be both more accurate and more pessimistic, although the self-fulfilling prophecy of withdrawal of care may tend to reinforce the physician's attitude toward clinical nihilism, which is defined as a lack of belief in attempting therapy due to its perceived futility in improving the outcome of the patient [12]. In case of vignette studies of physician decisions, physicians tended to make decisions on withdrawal of care based solely on limited information related to admission [13]. In a study of intensivists, nonclinical and nonradiographic factors such as physicians' beliefs, specialty perspective, and workload were found to explain a significant proportion of the variability in the decision to recommend withdrawal of care in the intensive care unit (ICU) [13]. This finding, and the presence of inter- and intra-center variation of physician prognostication and withdrawal of care, raises the issue of clinical nihilism.

Long-Term Outcome After Severe Traumatic Brain Injury

There are important differences between patients with brain injury and general patients who are critically ill. Traumatic brain injury occurs in patients suddenly, and many may have been previously healthy without an explicit discussion of end-of-life decisions. In many cases, severe traumatic brain injury (sTBI) without death results in poor functional outcome and inability to make decisions. In these cases, the decision to withdraw support is what leads to death. Therefore, the accurate determination of long-term outcome after severe traumatic brain injury plays a pivotal role in the one-third of patients who have withdrawal of support performed because patients' surrogates deem the predicted outcome to be incompatible with patient wishes. Although imperfect, the most commonly utilized measurements of functional outcome include the Glasgow Outcome Scale Extended (GOS-E) and the modified Rankin Scale (mRS), which are similar measurements. Both separate patients into functional categories. The GOS-E has eight categories, death, vegetative state, severe disability (lower and upper), moderate disability (lower and upper), and good recovery (lower and upper), while the modified Rankin Scale has seven categories: death, severe disability, moderate severe disability, moderate disability, slight disability, no significant disability, and no symptoms. Although physicians may accurately predict survival (with or without the presence of self-fulfilling prophecies), they struggle in predicting poor functional outcome after sTBI [12]. Both IMPACT and CRASH models were better than clinician judgment alone in the determination of functional outcome [14]. Accurate determination of outcomes following sTBI can help guide not only how aggressive interventions are but also provide patient surrogates with important data with respect to decisions for the continuation or withdrawal of care.

Prospective studies of children and adolescents have found that while there is a substantial decrease in overall functional outcome 3 months after severe injury, they tended to improve at 12 and 24 months, despite remaining significantly impaired [15]. Regarding communication and ability for self-care specifically, functional outcome remained unimproved at 24 months. Children with sTBI were found to have a quality of life worse than that of children undergoing active treatment for cancer. Better results were observed in a cohort of children in the United States at 10 years, with 81% of survivors returning to school and 18% with disability and reliance on caregivers [16].

In adults, Andelic et al. [17, 18] found significant variation in 12-month functional outcome in a Norwegian cohort of survivors after sTBI, ranging from 71% of patients with favorable outcome (GOS-E 6-8) with early rehabilitation, compared to 37% in those with no early rehabilitation. A German study found significant mortality and disability in patients undergoing decompressive craniectomy for sTBI, with 68% of patients either dead or in a vegetative state 4 years after surgery. Predictors of worsened outcome include increased age, increased midline shift, presence of anisocoria, and intradural hemorrhage (compared to epidural hemorrhage). In a separate smaller cohort of patients ($n = 33$) in Germany with sTBI and decompressive craniectomy due to massive brain swelling, Morgalla et al. [19] found that although 40% of patients remained dead or in a vegetative state, 18% of patients suffered from only mild deficits and 39.4% of patients experienced full rehabilitation, with 15% of patients resuming their former jobs and 12% remaining employed in a different job. Patients who could be fully rehabilitated were significantly younger (mean age 32.3 years) than those who had death or vegetative outcome (mean age 45 years). A study of 1-year clinical outcome after moderate and severe TBI in Hong Kong found age, GCS, coma duration, and baseline functional status at the initiation of rehabilitation in survivors to be the best predictors of 1-year functional outcome [20]. A study from the University of Maryland Shock Trauma Center in Baltimore, Maryland, found both CRASH and IMPACT to be better objective predictive models for patient poor functional outcome at 6 months, with accuracy of predictions made within the first 7 days for 6-month poor functional outcome ranging from 24 to 37%. Importantly, physicians were likely to be overly pessimistic in determining patient's ultimate functional recovery and were wrong more than 70% of the time. Less information is available for even longer-term prognostic factors in the context

of sTBI. One study in Norway found that the majority of patients surviving to 10 years with moderate to severe TBI had good recovery (48%) or moderate disability (44%) with an employment rate of 58%, although when compared with the general population, they had lower scores in general health as measured by the Short Form 36 [17]. Both IMPACT and CRASH were found to be significantly better than clinician judgment alone when predicting 6-month outcome [14]. Various studies of outcome have identified predictors of poorer functional outcome at 6–12 months, which include increased age [21, 22], lower initial GCS [23], increased intracranial pressure [24], increased length of unconsciousness, and poor baseline functional status [17, 25, 26].

The inability of clinician judgment to predict long-term functional outcome, and the near absence of prognostic models for even longer-term outcome (up to 10 years), highlights the importance of research to identify prognostic factors and models to help guide clinicians and families with respect to decision-making. Physicians should rely on a combination of clinical judgment, prognostic models, and prospectively identified predictors of functional outcome in their discussions with patient surrogates.

Modalities for Prognostication After Severe Traumatic Brain Injury

Our best models for prognosis after sTBI remain the models derived from the large CRASH and IMPACT studies, which consider clinical and radiographic factors. Despite the integration of clinical findings and radiographic imaging, however, these models fail to account for two-thirds of the variability in outcomes after sTBI. There is a need for alternate prognostic modalities to complement our current methods for predicting outcome after sTBI. In the United States, examples of alternate prognostic modalities in clinical use today include advanced neuroimaging and electrophysiological tests (electroencephalography, electrocorticography, and evoked potentials). The development of these methods may advance our ability to prognosticate after sTBI.

Neuroimaging: Computed Tomography and Magnetic Resonance Imaging

Since the advent of the CT scan, physicians have had the ability to quickly determine most types of clinically important life-threatening intracranial lesions, allowing for the diagnosis of different types of hemorrhages (subdural, epidural, intraparenchymal, subarachnoid, and intraventricular). This has helped place patients into broad prognostic groups and direct patients toward timely surgical intervention. Easily identifiable findings on head CT scan that strongly help prognosticate include midline shift, effacement of basal cisterns, cerebral infarction, subarachnoid hemorrhage, intraventricular hemorrhage, diffuse injury, and the presence of extra-axial hematomas [27–29].

In patients with neurologic deficit or altered mental status not explained by findings on a CT scan, magnetic resonance imaging (MRI) can offer prognostic power. Specific MRI sequences, including the diffusion-weighted (DTI) and susceptibility-weighted image sequences, increase the accuracy of outcome predictions and are also more sensitive for the detection of diffuse axonal injury [30–32]. Galanaud et al. found in a prospective study of 105 patients with TBI that the use of DTI MRI in combination with the IMPACT model provided significantly better long-term outcome prediction than IMPACT alone. The further development of advanced MRI imaging modalities and the use of more powerful MRI scanners may contribute to our understanding of the relationship between structural lesions and prognosis after sTBI.

Electroencephalography

Electroencephalography (EEG) involves the placement of electrodes on the surface of the head to measure electrical activity in different parts of the brain and is a commonly used modality in the monitoring of patients for ictal and inter-ictal activity. Its use in the prognosis of outcome after traumatic brain injury, however, is less studied. In a retrospective study of 64 patients undergoing continuous EEG monitoring after severe traumatic brain injury, status epilepticus or electrographic seizures were found to be associated with poorer outcome, which was defined as death or discharge to a skilled nursing facility [33]. Additionally, only one-third of patients had characteristic EEG findings of sleep, the lack of which was correlated with a poor outcome at the time of discharge. Even in those patients requiring discharge to a skilled nursing facility, the presence of sleep features predicted shorter inpatient hospital stay and earlier participation in rehabilitation therapy, when controlled for GCS. For patients that make it to rehabilitation with a diagnosis of impaired consciousness following traumatic brain injury, EEG has been shown to be correlated with the level of basal cognitive functioning at admission and at 3 months after admission [34]. It is clear that unfavorable EEG patterns such as burst suppression, nonreactive, or flat line are strongly predictive of poor outcome in anoxic coma, as they reflect harmful brain activity or the absence of brain activity [35–37]. Their prognostic utility in conjunction with current models such as IMPACT merits further study in the context of sTBI.

Electrocorticography

Like electroencephalography, electrocorticography involves the placement of electrodes; only this time they are placed directly on the human cortex during surgery to measure electrical activity. Once placed in the context of a craniectomy for sTBI, they allow the monitoring of spreading depolarizations, which are slowly propagating cortical electrical waves characterized by near-complete sustained depolarization of neurons and astrocytes. These electrical findings are associated with increased metabolic demands that may cause neuronal injury, mitochondrial damage, and excitotoxicity. The presence of spontaneous spreading depolarizations has been postulated as a mechanism for the penumbral spread of cerebral infarcts [38]. The presence of spreading depolarizations has been associated with unfavorable 6-month outcomes after sTBI [39]. A multicenter study reported by Hartings et al. enrolled adult patients who underwent craniotomy within 7 days of sTBI [38]. Electrode strips were placed during surgery on damaged but viable-appearing cortex, and electrocorticography was performed in the ICU for up to 7 days. Multivariate analysis revealed that the presence of isoelectric spreading depolarizations portended an odds ratio of 7.58 (95% CI 2.64–21.8, $p = 0.0002$) for unfavorable 6-month outcome (GOS-E 1-4) when controlled for age, GCS, and pupillary reactivity, while the presence of cortical spreading depolarization alone was not predictive [38]. While electrocorticography may yield potentially valuable prognostic information, it cannot be used in patients who do not undergo a neurosurgical procedure and therefore is of limited use to a subset of sTBI patients.

Somatosensory and Auditory Evoked Potentials

Evoked potential, also known as an evoked response, is a modality in which electrical activity from the nervous system is recorded from a sensor after the presentation of a stimulus, giving information about the integrity of pathways within the nervous system. There are several types of evoked potentials, including somatosensory evoked potentials (SSEPs), motor evoked potentials, and auditory evoked potentials (AEPs). These have frequently been used during neurosurgical procedures to avoid damage to eloquent areas of the brain and spinal cord. While auditory evoked potentials may give a good indication of the degrees of consciousness of a patient under anesthesia, they have also been studied for the prediction of functional outcome after brain injury. A study in Japan of 17 TBI and 15 acute stroke patients requiring emergency craniotomy found, using a mobile AEP monitor, that patients with favorable outcome (using a cerebral performance category) had a significantly greater increase in AEPs on postoperative day 5 when compared to those with unfavorable outcome [40].

Likewise, somatosensory evoked potentials have been used in the prognosis of patients after acute TBI. In one study, the use of SSEPs in combination with CT scan findings significantly increased the outcome prediction power as measured by GOS [41]. SSEPs may also have greater predictive strength for the likelihood of awakening from a prolonged posttraumatic coma compared to an EEG [42–44]. The advantages of evoked potentials include the ability to demonstrate abnormal sensory system conductions when the neurological exam is equivocal and the ability to define the anatomic distribution of injury and its potential functional implication in the disease process of sTBI.

Conclusions

The question "to treat or not to treat?" in the context of severe traumatic brain injury is one that is asked daily in neurological intensive care units around the world. Physicians rely on a combination of clinical judgment and established outcome models to determine both the survivability and likely functional outcome after severe traumatic brain injury. When making the decision on whether to withdraw or continue life support, patients' surrogates rely heavily on physicians' ability to accurately prognosticate outcome in the context of their sociocultural beliefs and on what is compatible with the patient's wishes. The decision to withdraw care is the single most predictive factor for mortality, and the awareness of clinical nihilism is important as there is evidence of a "self-fulfilling prophecy" in which mortality associated with withdrawal of care can reinforce a pessimistic bias and worsen outcomes. Physician judgment alone is a relatively poor predictor of functional outcome, and objective models such as IMPACT and CRASH, which consider objective factors, should be a routine part of functional outcome prognostication. Emerging modalities of mortality and functional outcome prognostication are being developed and may improve our ability to make accurate decisions on whether "to treat or not to treat."

References

1. Marshall LF. Head injury: recent past, present, and future. Neurosurgery. 2000;47(3):546–61.
2. Perel P, Wasserberg J, Ravi RR, Shakur H, Edwards P, Roberts I. Prognosis following head injury: a survey of doctors from developing and developed countries. J Eval Clin Pract. 2007;13(3):464–5.
3. Roozenbeek B, Lingsma HF, Lecky FE, Lu J, Weir J, Butcher I, et al. Prediction of outcome after moderate and severe traumatic brain injury: external validation of the international mission on prognosis and analysis of clinical trials (impact) and corticoid randomisation after significant head injury (crash) prognostic models. Crit Care Med. 2012;40(5):1609–17.
4. McMillan TM, Herbert CM. Further recovery in a potential treatment withdrawal case 10 years after brain injury. Brain Inj. 2004;18(9):935–40.
5. Jacobs LM, Burns K, Bennett Jacobs B. Trauma death: views of the public and trauma professionals on death and dying from injuries. Arch Surg. 2008;143(8):730–5.
6. Turgeon AF, Lauzier F, Simard JF, Scales DC, Burns KE, Moore L, et al. Mortality associated with withdrawal of life-sustaining therapy for patients with severe traumatic brain injury: a Canadian multicentre cohort study. CMAJ. 2011;183(14):1581–8.
7. Cote N, Turgeon AF, Lauzier F, Moore L, Scales DC, Bernard F, et al. Factors associated with the withdrawal of life-sustaining therapies in patients with severe traumatic brain injury: a multicenter cohort study. Neurocrit Care. 2013;18(1):154–60.
8. Becker KJ, Baxter AB, Cohen WA, Bybee HM, Tirschwell DL, Newell DW, et al. Withdrawal of support in intracerebral hemorrhage may lead to self-fulfilling prophecies. Neurology. 2001;56(6):766–72.
9. Livingston DH, Mosenthal AC. Withdrawing life-sustaining therapy for patients with severe traumatic brain injury. CMAJ. 2011;183(14):1570–1.
10. Keenan SP, Busche KD, Chen LM, Esmail R, Inman KJ, Sibbald WJ. Withdrawal and withholding of life support in the intensive care unit: a comparison of teaching and community hospitals. The southwestern ontario critical care research network. Crit Care Med. 1998;26(2):245–51.
11. McCredie VA, Alali AS, Xiong W, Rubenfeld GD, Cuthbertson BH, Scales DC, et al. Timing of withdrawal of life-sustaining therapies in severe traumatic brain injury: impact on overall mortality. J Trauma Acute Care Surg. 2016;80(3):484–91.
12. White DB, Ernecoff N, Buddadhumaruk P, Hong S, Weissfeld L, Curtis R, et al. Prognosis Between Physicians and Surrogate Decision Makers of Critically Ill Patients. JAMA. 2016;315(19):2086–94.
13. Izzy S, Compton R, Carandang R, Hall W, Muehlschlegel S. Self-fulfilling prophecies through withdrawal of care: do they exist in traumatic brain injury, too? Neurocrit Care. 2013;19(3):347–63.
14. Bonds BW, Dhanda A, Wade C, Massetti J, Diaz C, Stein DM. Prognostication of Mortality and Long term Functional Outcomes Following Traumatic Brain Injury: Can We Do Better? J Neurotrauma. 2015. EPublication ahead of print.
15. Rivara FP, Koepsell TD, Wang J, Temkin N, Dorsch A, Vavilala MS, et al. Disability 3, 12, and 24 months after traumatic brain injury among children and adolescents. Pediatrics. 2011;128(5):e1129–38.
16. Jagannathan J, Okonkwo DO, Dumont AS, Ahmed H, Bahari A, Prevedello DM, et al. Outcome following decompressive craniectomy in children with severe traumatic brain injury: a 10-year single-center experience with long-term follow up. J Neurosurg. 2007;106(4 Suppl):268–75.
17. Andelic N, Hammergren N, Bautz-Holter E, Sveen U, Brunborg C, Roe C. Functional outcome and health-related quality of life 10 years after moderate-to-severe traumatic brain injury. Acta Neurol Scand. 2009;120(1):16–23.
18. Andelic N, Bautz-Holter E, Ronning P, Olafsen K, Sigurdardottir S, Schanke AK, et al. Does an early onset and continuous chain of rehabilitation improve the long-term functional outcome of patients with severe traumatic brain injury? J Neurotrauma. 2012;29(1):66–74.
19. Morgalla MH, Will BE, Roser F, Tatagiba M. Do long-term results justify decompressive craniectomy after severe traumatic brain injury? J Neurosurg. 2008;109(4):685–90.
20. Poon WS, Zhu XL, Ng SC, Wong GK. Predicting one year clinical outcome in traumatic brain injury (TBI) at the beginning of rehabilitation. Acta Neurochir Suppl. 2005;93:207–8.
21. Scholten AC, Haagsma JA, Andriessen TM, Vos PE, Steyerberg EW, van Beeck EF, et al. Health-related quality of life after mild, moderate and severe traumatic brain injury: patterns and predictors of suboptimal functioning during the first year after injury. Injury. 2015;46(4):616–24.
22. LeBlanc J, de Guise E, Gosselin N, Feyz M. Comparison of functional outcome following acute care in young, middle-aged and elderly patients with traumatic brain injury. Brain Inj. 2006;20(8):779–90.
23. Kouloulas EJ, Papadeas AG, Michail X, Sakas DE, Boviatsis EJ. Prognostic value of time-related Glasgow coma scale components in severe traumatic brain injury: a prospective evaluation with respect to 1-year survival and functional outcome. Int J Rehabil Res. 2013;36(3):260–7.
24. Badri S, Chen J, Barber J, Temkin NR, Dikmen SS, Chesnut RM, et al. Mortality and long-term functional outcome associated with intracranial pressure after traumatic brain injury. Intensive Care Med. 2012;38(11):1800–9.
25. King JT Jr, Carlier PM, Marion DW. Early Glasgow outcome scale scores predict long-term functional outcome in patients with severe traumatic brain injury. J Neurotrauma. 2005;22(9):947–54.
26. Whitlock JA Jr, Hamilton BB. Functional outcome after rehabilitation for severe traumatic brain injury. Arch Phys Med Rehabil. 1995;76(12):1103–12.

27. Maas AI, Steyerberg EW, Butcher I, Dammers R, Lu J, Marmarou A, et al. Prognostic value of computerized tomography scan characteristics in traumatic brain injury: results from the impact study. J Neurotrauma. 2007;24(2):303–14.

28. Maas AI, Hukkelhoven CW, Marshall LF, Steyerberg EW. Prediction of outcome in traumatic brain injury with computed tomographic characteristics: a comparison between the computed tomographic classification and combinations of computed tomographic predictors. Neurosurgery. 2005;57(6):1173–82; discussion 1173–1182.

29. Marshall LF, Toole BM, Bowers SA. The national traumatic coma data bank. Part 2: patients who talk and deteriorate: implications for treatment. J Neurosurg. 1983;59(2):285–8.

30. Huisman TA, Schwamm LH, Schaefer PW, Koroshetz WJ, Shetty-Alva N, Ozsunar Y, et al. Diffusion tensor imaging as potential biomarker of white matter injury in diffuse axonal injury. AJNR Am J Neuroradiol. 2004;25(3):370–6.

31. Tong KA, Ashwal S, Holshouser BA, Nickerson JP, Wall CJ, Shutter LA, et al. Diffuse axonal injury in children: clinical correlation with hemorrhagic lesions. Ann Neurol. 2004;56(1):36–50.

32. Schaefer PW, Huisman TA, Sorensen AG, Gonzalez RG, Schwamm LH. Diffusion-weighted MR imaging in closed head injury: high correlation with initial Glasgow coma scale score and score on modified Rankin scale at discharge. Radiology. 2004;233(1):58–66.

33. Sandsmark DK, Kumar MA, Woodward CS, Schmitt SE, Park S, Lim MM. Sleep features on continuous electroencephalography predict rehabilitation outcomes after severe traumatic brain injury. J Head Trauma Rehabil. 2016;31(2):101–7.

34. Bagnato S, Boccagni C, Prestandrea C, Sant'Angelo A, Castiglione A, Galardi G. Prognostic value of standard EEG in traumatic and non-traumatic disorders of consciousness following coma. Clin Neurophysiol. 2010;121(3):274–80.

35. Chen R, Bolton CF, Young B. Prediction of outcome in patients with anoxic coma: a clinical and electrophysiologic study. Crit Care Med. 1996;24(4):672–8.

36. Freeman WD, Barrett KM, Freeman ML, Johnson M, Divertie G, Rossetti AO, et al. Predictors of awakening from postanoxic status epilepticus after therapeutic hypothermia. Neurology. 2009;73(18):1512; author reply 1512–3.

37. Geocadin RG, Buitrago MM, Torbey MT, Chandra-Strobos N, Williams MA, Kaplan PW. Neurologic prognosis and withdrawal of life support after resuscitation from cardiac arrest. Neurology. 2006;67(1):105–8.

38. Hartings JA, Bullock MR, Okonkwo DO, Murray LS, Murray GD, Fabricius M, et al. Spreading depolarisations and outcome after traumatic brain injury: a prospective observational study. Lancet Neurol. 2011;10(12):1058–64.

39. Hartings JA, Watanabe T, Bullock MR, Okonkwo DO, Fabricius M, Woitzik J, et al. Spreading depolarizations have prolonged direct current shifts and are associated with poor outcome in brain trauma. Brain. 2011;134(Pt 5):1529–40.

40. Tsurukiri J, Nagata K, Hoshiai A, Oomura T, Jimbo H, Ikeda Y. Middle latency auditory-evoked potential index monitoring of cerebral function to predict functional outcome after emergency craniotomy in patients with brain damage. Scand J Trauma Resusc Emerg Med. 2015;23:80.

41. Bosco E, Zanatta P, Ponzin D, Marton E, Feletti A, Scarpa B, et al. Prognostic value of somatosensory-evoked potentials and CT scan evaluation in acute traumatic brain injury. J Neurosurg Anesthesiol. 2014;26(4):299–305.

42. Amantini A, Grippo A, Fossi S, Cesaretti C, Piccioli A, Peris A, et al. Prediction of 'awakening' and outcome in prolonged acute coma from severe traumatic brain injury: evidence for validity of short latency seps. Clin Neurophysiol. 2005;116(1):229–35.

43. Gutling E, Gonser A, Imhof HG, Landis T. EEG reactivity in the prognosis of severe head injury. Neurology. 1995;45(5):915–8.

44. Fischer C, Mutschler V. [Traumatic brain injuries in adults: from coma to wakefulness. Neurophysiological data]. Ann Readapt Med Phys. 2002;45(8):448–55.

Use of Multimodality Neuromonitoring in the Management of Traumatic Brain Injury

Justin R. Davanzo, Emily P. Sieg,
J. Christopher Zacko, and Shelly D. Timmons

Introduction

Multimodality neuromonitoring has become an essential part of neurocritical care over the past several decades. Until the 1980s, electronic monitoring in the intensive care unit (ICU) was limited to typical cardiopulmonary vital signs to augment the neurologic examination and older techniques of monitoring intracranial pressure (ICP) via cerebrospinal fluid (CSF) drainage and fluid-coupled mechanisms. Prior to this, clinicians did not have the consistent ability to directly measure and manage physiologic parameters specific to the nervous system. The first brain-specific phys-iologic monitoring technology to emerge was intracranial pressure. Beginning in the 1980s, ICP parenchymal monitoring became available, and the technique became widespread in the United States. Monitoring was used to study the impact of ICP on outcome and with the clinical goal of reducing intracranial pressure to prevent secondary neurologic injury. Imputed cerebral perfusion pressure (CPP) values were now possible to obtain in continuous fashion, and attention was also placed on identifying optimal CPP to reduce secondary injury, which was the focus of a good deal of research in the 1990s. Since that time, cerebral monitoring has become more common as well as more diverse. Physiologic parameters that can now be measured include cerebral blood flow (CBF), partial pressure of oxygen in brain tissue or oxygen saturation (pB_tO_2), brain temperature, and various measures of cerebral metabolism via microdialysis.

Despite these advances in neuromonitoring techniques, crucial questions persist regarding their use in routine traumatic brain injury (TBI) management and impact on outcomes. These monitoring techniques are often costly, and that cost must be justified by the value conferred to patients, based upon the potential for outcomes improvement that they may facilitate. Ideally, the

J. R. Davanzo, MD · E. P. Sieg, BS, MS, MD
J. C. Zacko, MS, MD (✉)
Department of Neurosurgery, Penn State Health
Milton S. Hershey Medical Center,
Hershey, PA, USA
e-mail: jdavanzo@pennstatehealth.psu.edu;
esieg@hmc.psu.edu; jzacko@pennstatehealth.psu.edu

S. D. Timmons, MD, PhD, FACS, FAANS
Department of Neurosurgery, Penn State University
Milton S. Hershey Medical Center,
Hershey, PA, USA
e-mail: stimmons@mac.com

© Springer International Publishing AG, part of Springer Nature 2018
S. D. Timmons (ed.), *Controversies in Severe Traumatic Brain Injury Management*,
https://doi.org/10.1007/978-3-319-89477-5_3

management strategies employed based on the information provided by multimodality monitoring should minimize secondary injury and not instigate deleterious effects. The aim of this chapter is to discuss available advanced neuro-monitoring techniques, to review evidence for patient outcomes in the setting of multimodality monitoring, and to discuss in brief the logistical implications of implementing these techniques in the neurocritical care unit (NCCU).

Neurocritical Care

Dr. Walter E. Dandy is credited with opening a three-bed unit for postoperative neurosurgical patients at the Johns Hopkins Hospital in 1932 as the earliest known example of a neurocritical care unit. Creating a unit specifically for patients with neurological disease allows for the care team to be more adept at noticing the subtle neu-rologic changes in patients that are often harbin-gers of disaster as well as to tailor the patient's systemic care to achieve the best neurologic out-comes [1]. A number of observational studies have demonstrated that neurologic diseases are better cared for in a neurocritical care unit, including a retrospective study of intracerebral hemorrhage (ICH) patients admitted to NCCU versus a general intensive care unit (ICU) show-ing reduced mortality rates [2]. A similar study of patients with severe brain injuries in which an NCCU protocol for ICP and cerebral perfusion pressure (CPP) therapy was implemented by neu-rointensivists demonstrated significant improve-ments in patient outcomes compared to the control group [3]. A cohort study using historical controls to study length of stay and mortality rates with the introduction of a neurointensive care team showed improved in-hospital mortality rates and decreased length of stay, while no change was seen in readmission rates or long-term mortality [4]. Multiple studies examining the effect of a neurocritical care team on patients with neurologic disease performed by one center demonstrated improved outcomes and shortened

lengths of stay for these patients when compared to patients cared for in a standard ICU [5–7].

Creating specialty ICUs in the hospital setting can be costly, requiring dedicated physical space, recruitment, ongoing training, and retention of appropriately trained staff and attainment of the necessary equipment to run such a unit. While overall expenses may vary and are sometimes difficult to quantify, multiple data demonstrate improved patient outcomes, lower mortality rates, and decreased lengths of stay when patients with neurologic disease are cared for in an NCCU, suggesting that the benefits gained in patient care and outcomes outweigh the costs.

Multimodality Neuromonitoring

While simply creating a neurocritical care unit may improve outcomes in patients with neuro-logic disease based upon nursing and physician expertise and other organizational advantages, there are likely specific interventions and moni-toring techniques that contribute further to improvement in patient outcomes. Understanding that the ideal "neuromonitor" has yet to be achieved, the concept of multimodality neuro-monitoring utilizing multiple parameters for physiological management has emerged. Patients who have an acute insult to the brain, such as ischemic cerebral infarction, subarachnoid hem-orrhage (SAH), ICH, and particularly TBI, sus-tain both primary and secondary brain injury. The purpose of multimodality neuromonitoring is to (1) help prevent secondary insults that lead to fur-ther secondary injury and (2) to detect secondary injury markers early so as to guide treatment strategies to correct and attenuate deleterious pathophysiologic trends. While none of the tech-niques available can directly measure secondary injury directly, they indirectly provide measure-ments that can be used to make reasonable cor-relations. By using multiple measures, an overall picture of cerebral physiologic status can be obtained for specific time points, and treatment can be individualized to best prevent secondary brain injury in real time and ultimately to maximize outcomes [1].

Multimodality monitoring includes the ongoing measurement and synthesis of data from a variety of physiological parameters, linkage to events with time-stamped correlations, and ideally incorporation of calculations and algorithms to help make rapid bedside decisions. "Head's up" video displays correlating multiple waveforms and numerical data are an important means of accomplishing this. Clinicians must synthesize a great deal of second-to-second and minute-to-minute data, including neuromonitoring values, ventilator parameters, laboratory values, imaging data, and clinical examination findings, in order to make the best decisions. These tools aid in that synthesis, in addition to storing continuous physiological data for trending and tracking and later review, as well as for research when warranted. See Fig. 1.

Intracranial Monitoring

There are several types of monitors that may be placed intracranially, including those for intracranial pressure (and by calculation cerebral perfusion pressure), brain tissue oxygenation, brain temperature, cerebral blood flow, and microdialysis to assess various metabolic states.

Intracranial Pressure and Cerebral Perfusion Pressure

Intracranial pressure can either be measured by a fluid-coupled ventricular catheter (with or without transduction to a numeric digital displayed value) or an intraparenchymal fiber-optic catheter. Monitoring ICP has long been used by clinicians to tailor therapy for patients with cerebral edema and space-occupying lesions [8]. The basis for monitoring intracranial pressure comes

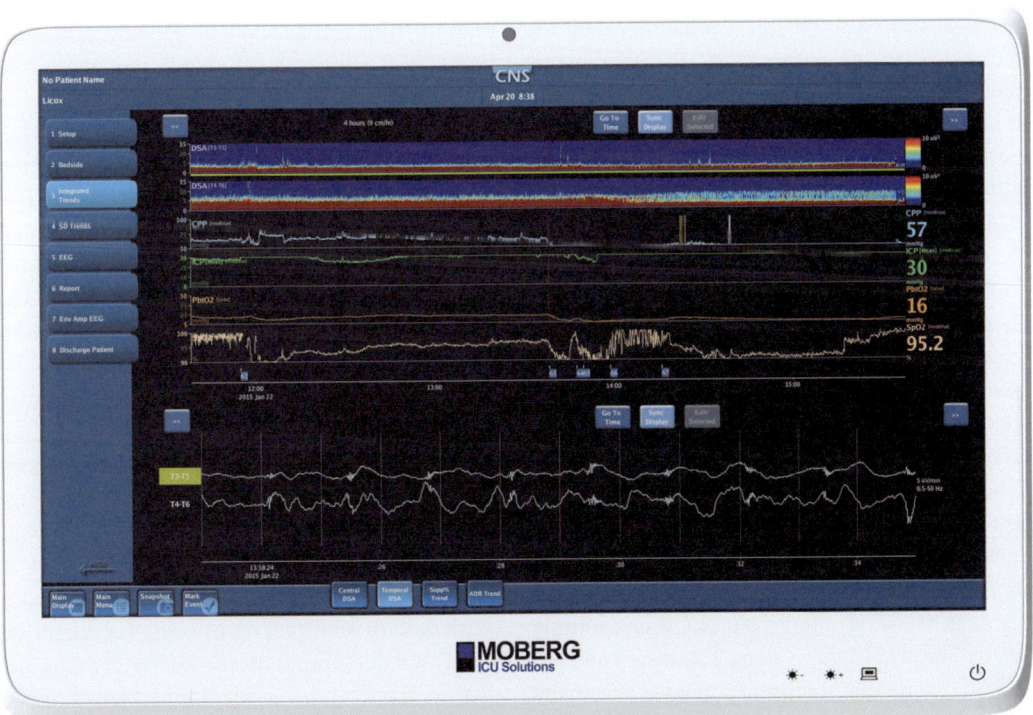

Fig. 1 Example of multimodality neuromonitoring display screen demonstrating a variety of neuromonitoring parameters in a single display, time-locked to one another, and with touch-screen capability to access additional data. Image courtesy of Moberg ICU Solutions, Moberg Research Inc., Ambler, PA

from the Monro-Kellie hypothesis, which states that the skull contains a fixed volume and therefore, as the volume of each compartment (brain, blood, and CSF) increases, so does the intracranial pressure unless the volume of one or more components is decreased in a compensatory manner. Further, when mass lesions are present, the additional volume may increase ICP [9]. Measuring intracranial pressure is thus an important component of treatment of mass lesions and cerebral edema after TBI. ICP may also be considered to be an indirect surrogate for cerebral blood flow, the prevailing concept being that if ICP is elevated, achieving adequate CBF may be impaired—particularly problematic when CBF is inadequate to meet the increased metabolic demands of the injured brain.

Both measurement options can reliably provide accurate data, and each has advantages and disadvantages. The main advantages of external ventricular drainage (EVD) catheters include low-cost materials, accuracy, reliability, and the ability to use the catheter for the therapeutic maneuver of draining CSF to lower the ICP. Even in austere environments, this technique can be employed by using a fluid column to measure ICP. If basic cardiopulmonary monitors are available, the EVD can be pressure transduced to an electronic monitor via a relatively inexpensive arterial line transducer. Disadvantages include having to close the system to drainage to obtain an accurate measurement, thereby limiting the ability to obtain continuous ICP measurements if continuous drainage is employed or limiting CSF volume drainage if continuous measurements are to be employed. To address this conflict, there are now combined products available with a transducer in the tip of the ventricular catheter that is capable of measuring ICP while continuous drainage is being employed, but this naturally adds to the cost of the system. The disadvantages of EVD include difficulty in accurate placement in settings of severe cerebral edema, mass effect, and tissue shifts, all of which make accessing the ventricle challenging. Further disadvantages include higher hemorrhage and infection rates and frequency of dysfunction/occlusion from blood products.

Benefits of parenchymal monitors include relative ease of placement and lower complication rates for infection and hemorrhage. Disadvantages include potential for drift over time, although clinically this is easily surmountable. An oft-cited disadvantage is that the catheter cannot be re-zeroed once placed, but this is seldom necessary, and if it is, a new catheter can simply be placed, albeit at a cost for a new catheter. Cost of monitoring via parenchymal techniques also includes purchase or lease of the monitor box itself, as well as transducer cables that are sometimes used to marry the displayed ICP data and waveforms to the overhead cardiopulmonary monitors for simultaneous display and interpretation or to a multimodality neuromonitoring display and analytics system.

Early TBI studies have shown that the amount of time with ICP above 20–25 mmHg correlated with poor outcomes [10]. Furthermore, patients, who died from TBI, most often died from herniation from refractory ICP. Several retrospective cohort studies have shown that the use of ICP monitoring to guide therapy was associated with decreased mortality rates [11–14]. A recent randomized controlled trial compared patients with traumatic brain injury undergoing either ICP-guided treatment or treatment guided by frequent serial clinical and radiographic examinations. Both groups underwent aggressive treatment of elevated ICP according to evidence-based guidelines, regardless of the method in which ICP elevation was diagnosed (i.e., with a monitor or based upon clinical and radiographic signs). In the settings in which the trial was conducted, no differences in functional outcomes or mortality rates at 6 months were noted between the two groups [15]. The authors highlighted that aggressive management of ICP (with or without direct monitoring for numerical value) was the important parameter, lending further credence to the concept that the use of ICP monitoring with numerical and waveform data should be utilized as part of an overall multimodality monitoring and management scheme. In other words, monitoring and treating ICP are important, but other factors besides ICP must also be used to guide treatment, including clinical examination, radiographic studies, and even other neuromonitoring modalities.

Reduction of ICP from dangerously elevated levels can be achieved by a variety of mechanisms, all of which are predicated on understanding the relative contributions of cerebral tissue edema, obstructive hydrocephalus, obstructed venous return, increased cerebral blood flow or hyperemia, or space-occupying mass lesions. The choice of therapeutic maneuver varies dramatically with each, and continuous ICP monitoring is the mechanism by which treatment effects can best be judged. Continuous ICP monitoring is thus a critical aspect of management of severe TBI (sTBI).

Sound critical care management decisions should not, however, be solely driven by measurement and normalization of only one clinical parameter. A good example of how treating a single parameter may result in detrimental outcomes is focusing only on maintaining cerebral perfusion pressure (CPP) at a specific range. CPP is a calculated value defined as ICP minus mean arterial pressure (MAP). Studies in the late 1980s led to a paradigm shift in the 1990s focusing on not only keeping ICP <20–25 mmHg but also maintaining CPP at a target range above 70 mmHg. Doing so resulted in a mortality rate of 21% and good recovery rate of 68% [16] and drew necessary attention to the need for adequate perfusion of the brain in an era when volume depletion was commonly employed as a mechanism to treat ICP. However, in the ensuing years, it became apparent that artificially elevating CPP to very high target ranges was also associated with adverse outcomes, namely, pulmonary complications and acute respiratory distress syndrome (ARDS), when large volume fluid resuscitation and pressors were used [17, 18]. Subsequent evidence-based reviews resulted in amended recommendations for a CPP range, rather than a single-digit numerical threshold, and acknowledged that each patient may require a different target CPP depending upon other factors [19–21]. So, while CPP plays a key role in the management of patients with severe TBI, its management does not come without systemic risks that can have significant effects on both patient outcomes (including mortality) and surrogate markers of outcome (such as length of ICU stay).

Despite general consensus that sTBI management should incorporate multiple parameters, studies have continued to emerge comparing "ICP-driven" vs. "CPP-driven" therapy [20]. Critical to the management of sTBI (and the understanding of how such variable results may be obtained in the ICP- vs. CPP-focused studies) is the discernment of whether cerebral autoregulation remains intact. Cerebral autoregulation is the maintenance of consistent cerebral blood flow (CBF) in the face of changing systemic blood pressure. Determination of autoregulatory status may be performed at the bedside, by observing whether steadily increasing the systemic blood pressure results in a commensurate steady increase in ICP. Maintaining adequate cerebral perfusion (and therefore oxygenation) in the initial days after sTBI when CBF is at its nadir [22] is especially important. When autoregulation is impaired, artificial methods of increasing MAP and CPP may need to be avoided, as they may result in a concomitant increase in ICP. Indeed, improved outcomes with lower CPP in the face of impaired autoregulation after TBI have been demonstrated [21]. Management of individual patients should consider BOTH ICP and CPP, the patient's autoregulatory status, and ideally other parameters of brain function to tailor therapy to the patient's cerebral demands in a continuous and oft-changing fashion. What is efficacious for one patient will not necessarily be efficacious for the next, and patient needs often change over the course of hours or days.

Cerebral Blood Flow

Ultimately, cerebral blood flow measurement is a more direct measure of cerebral demand than CPP. To date, widespread use of direct monitoring for CBF has not been adopted, although parenchymal catheters are now available that use thermal diffusion probes to measure CBF in a focal region. Traditional methods of measuring CBF have largely been employed in research settings and suffer from being largely limited to imaging techniques, logistically challenging, expensive, having significant regulatory requirements, and/ or providing only one temporal measurement for a parameter that is best understood over longer epochs of time. These methods include xenon-computed tomography (xenon-CT), positron-emission tomography (PET), single-photon emission computed tomography (SPECT), CT perfusion (CT-P), and even transcranial Doppler ultrasonography (TCD) and near-infrared spectroscopy have been used to estimate CBF. The ideal CBF monitoring system would be noninvasive, be continuous, and provide information on multiple regions of the brain. Other efforts have focused on more downstream measurements of substrate supply to the brain, namely, brain tissue oxygenation.

Brain Tissue Oxygenation

Oxygen delivery is critical to brain tissue survival, and cellular oxygen demands go up in the face of TBI. Without appropriate delivery of oxygen, metabolism fails and neuron loss occurs. Monitoring techniques can only estimate oxygen delivery and/or consumption in cerebral tissue in humans at present. Such techniques include jugular bulb oximetry to measure jugular venous oxygen saturation ($SjvO_2$) and intraparenchymal tissue oximetry to measure partial pressure of oxygen in focal brain tissue (pB_tO_2). Use of one or both of these monitoring techniques to guide therapy in patients with cerebral insults may be employed, but understanding the potential pitfalls of each is important to interpretation of available data and utilization in management strategies.

Jugular bulb oximetry provides a more global picture of cerebral oxygenation (and consumption), while the intraparenchymal catheters provide information about regional oxygen saturation in a small volume of brain tissue. While a low $SjvO_2$ value suggests (but does not prove) that cerebral oxygen demand is exceeding supply, a value that is too high can suggest relative hyperemia or a failure in oxygen consumption. Older observational studies have shown consistently improved outcomes with $SjvO_2$ monitoring and active management of desaturation episodes [23–26].

Two studies are available that have shown good correlation between pB_tO_2 and $SjvO_2$ in their assessment of global brain oxygenation [27, 28]. However, if the brain tissue oxygenation monitor is placed adjacent to pathology, results and correlations with $SjvO_2$ may be affected. Such localization leads to decreased pB_tO_2 values, which last longer than those obtained from more normal-appearing tissue [29–31].

Furthermore, altered cerebral oxygen metabolism states can alter jugular bulb oxygenation. For example, if brain tissue is globally ischemic, or past the point of recoverable metabolic failure, brain oxygen extraction drops dramatically, leading to high $SjvO_2$, which can be misinterpreted as normal. Likewise, cerebral tissue that requires increased oxygen extraction due to oxygen demand from injury, seizures, or other phenomena may produce relatively lower $SjvO_2$ readings; the situation is not necessarily deleterious but a marker of injury. Finally, $SjvO_2$ values may not reflect cerebral metabolism at all, but rather systemic problems such as low arterial oxygenation related to pulmonary problems, or even catheter malfunction for which these catheters are somewhat notorious. Therefore, it is important when using jugular venous sampling, which can be a valuable adjunct, to interpret $SjvO_2$ values in the context of other data, including ICP, CPP, CBF when available, and even pB_tO_2 to accurately interpret their meaning.

Most recent TBI research addressing brain oxygenation has utilized pB_tO_2. However, once again, study design has often been comparative in nature. For example, in one retrospective cohort study, TBI patients who underwent only ICP monitoring were compared to those who underwent both ICP and pB_tO_2 monitoring, with no significant differences in mortality seen. However, the two groups were not clinically comparable, and those who received a pB_tO_2 monitor to guide treatment in addition to an ICP monitor were more severely injured and received more intensive care. The equivalent outcomes suggest that they may have received a clinical benefit from the additional neuromonitoring used to direct treatment [32]. In one small single-center randomized controlled trial, three patient groups were compared, (1) ICP/CPP management alone, (2) ICP/CPP management with hypothermia, and (3) pB_tO_2 and CPP management with hypothermia, again with no differences in mortality seen, but notably, improved outcomes were seen in survivors from the pB_tO_2/CPP group [33]. Other studies have had methodological limitations, comprising cohort studies, prospective studies with comparison to historical controls, or retrospective studies, so it is not surprising that the data from these studies are inconsistent. While some studies have shown improved mortality and outcomes with pB_tO_2-guided treatment, others have shown no significant differences [34–38]. A systematic review of four studies yielded an odds ratio for overall favorable outcome of 2.1 (95% CI 1.4–3.1) for patients who underwent pB_tO_2-guided therapy but with admittedly heterogeneous study groups and data sets [39]. Again, it is important that this technique is not considered strictly "in comparison to" other techniques. The information gained from pB_tO_2 monitoring should be synthesized with data from other monitoring parameters to make clinical decisions, not in isolation or "instead of" other values.

There have been many attempts to determine treatment thresholds for pB_tO_2 and $SjvO_2$—mostly in small studies. Time below certain thresholds appears to be important, with poor functional outcomes and mortality increasing significantly with pB_tO_2 below 20 mmHg for more than 12 min [40], total time below 15 mmHg [41], and for incidents more than 30 min in duration with a $pB_tO_2 < 10$ mmHg [42]. Time along a continuum of values is likely most important with documented mortality risks of 50% for $pB_tO_2 < 5$ mmHg for 30 min, <10 mmHg for 1 h, or <15 mmHg for 4 h [43]. Taking these data together, the most widely accepted treatment "threshold" for pB_tO_2 is to keep values above 20 mmHg [29, 40]; however, this value like all neurophysiological parameters should be considered in the context of other values and over time. Regression analysis in one trial suggested a higher threshold of 30 mmHg, since mortality rates were significantly higher in patients in whom pB_tO_2 remained below 29 mmHg in the first 72 h [44]. Certainly prolonged low saturations below 20 mmHg should be avoided in severe TBI patients, and even higher values may be beneficial.

Treatment thresholds for $SjvO_2$ are more complicated than those for pB_tO_2. Much larger observational studies have been performed to determine optimal treatment thresholds for $SjvO_2$. Values <50% have been associated with increased mortality and worse functional outcomes, as have the number of desaturation episodes experienced by a given patient [23, 24]. Upper limits >75% have also been recommended as a treatment threshold based on worse outcomes than in those with $SjvO_2$ 50–74% [41]. Arteriovenous difference in oxygen saturation ($AVDO_2$) has been advocated as a more relevant treatment value and is calculated using SaO_2, $SjvO_2$, and hemoglobin values and targeted values generally between 5 and 7.5%. A high $AVDO_2$ value suggests that demand exceeds supply, while a low value is typically indicative of hyperemia. Higher mean $AVDO_2$ values have been associated with favorable outcomes at 6 months compared with patients who died or remained in a vegetative state [45]. Use of $AVDO_2$ can aid in the interpretation of both $SjvO_2$ and pB_tO_2. As noted with regard to ICP and CPP, isolated values should not drive therapeutic decisions but rather all available data taken together to assess clinical needs.

Treatment options for patients with inappropriate $SjvO_2$, pB_tO_2, or $AVDO_2$ center around either increasing oxygen supply or decreasing oxygen demand. On the supply side, options include increasing perfusion and cerebral blood flow through the use of vasopressors and fluid management, increasing oxygen content and saturation through ventilator management or blood transfusion, and reducing ICP and increasing CPP with the aim of improving CBF. Improving oxygen diffusion through injured tissue and hemorrhage for ultimate delivery to neurons and glia is a crucial step for which no proven therapies yet exist. On the demand side, however, decreasing cerebral metabolism with sedative and paralytic medications may be of benefit, as well as prevention of seizure activity and other complications that increase demand.

As with any treatment, these interventions may be associated with risk. For example, using pressors to increase blood pressure carries an increased risk of ARDS as previously noted [17, 18]. Blood transfusions also carry risks, including but not limited to blood-borne infection, hemolytic and non-hemolytic transfusion reactions, and transfusion-related acute lung injury (TRALI) [46–50]. Any therapy to be employed must take into account the relative risk-to-benefit ratio, even as study data are lacking or incomplete, and best clinical judgment must be employed. This is one benefit of having multimodality neuromonitoring parameters available—to avoid unnecessary and potentially harmful empiric therapies and to promote the use of targeted therapies whose potential risk can be better justified based upon physiological parameters.

Microdialysis

Cerebral microdialysis is a well-established research tool to measure the concentration of substances in fluid—in this case cerebral extracellular fluid or "microdialysate." This technique is beginning to be used more commonly clinically outside of research settings. Substances including glucose, lactate, pyruvate, glutamate, aspartate, glycerol, and drug levels [51] can be measured via implanted catheters and extraction for microdialysate concentration measurements. These measurements, when performed serially, reflect changes at the cellular level to test for ischemia, hypoxia, energy/metabolic failure, or other cellular dysfunction [1], such as membrane damage and tissue inflammation.

Most studies to date have focused on delineating normal values for different markers that can be obtained via cerebral microdialysis [52, 53], such as glutamate [54], a marker of excitotoxicity. Lactate-pyruvate ratios, signifying relative tissue ischemia or mitochondrial distress when elevated, have been measured in a number of observational TBI studies and together with pB_tO_2 may be more sensitive markers than

ICP, CPP, or $SjvO_2$ [55], especially as injuries evolve over time. Again, though, the utilization of all available measurement parameters yields a more detailed physiological picture to guide decision-making.

Some have also suggested that derangements in microdialysis values may be helpful in prognostication of long-term outcomes. A few studies have shown that worsening cerebral metabolism is predictive of poor outcomes in brain-injured patients and have suggested a role for cerebral microdialysis in predicting secondary injury [56, 57]. It is hypothesized that metabolic changes at the cellular level will precede global responses such as intracranial hypertension, and early clinical evidence confirms this phenomenon in both TBI [58] and delayed ischemic neurologic deficit (DIND) after aneurysmal subarachnoid hemorrhage (SAH) [59].

Cerebral microdialysis monitoring is a fairly labor-intensive monitoring technique for the bedside staff. Not only must samples be obtained at regular time intervals, but they must be analyzed in real time. The equipment involved is also relatively expensive compared to other neuromonitoring modalities. However, microdialysis has significant potential to change clinical management of TBI. This monitoring technique is the best candidate for measuring cellular health, and future research should target integration of its use into treatment paradigms.

Electrophysiology

In addition to invasive intracranial monitoring, electrophysiological techniques can be used in the neurocritical care unit to guide therapy. Such techniques include electroencephalography (EEG) and less commonly somatosensory evoked potentials (SSEP) or brainstem auditory evoked responses (BSAER) or potentials (BAEP). Particularly in the absence of a credible neurologic examination due to coma or sedation, these electrophysiological monitoring tests can detect subclinical status epilepticus, encephalopathy, or other dysfunctional states.

Electroencephalography

A significant proportion of severe TBI patients experience seizures, which are often subclinical, highlighting the need for EEG services in the ICU care of TBI, especially continuous EEG (cEEG) [60]. In one study of TBI patients who underwent continuous EEG for 14 days while receiving prophylactic antiepileptic drugs (AED), 22% were noted to have electrographic seizures, 52% of which were nonconvulsive and only diagnosed with EEG [61]. Six of the 94 patients in this study experienced status epilepticus with 100% mortality. In another study of TBI patients who underwent cEEG but were not receiving AEDs, 28% were found to have seizure activity and 11% were found to have been in nonconvulsive status epilepticus (NCSE) [62].

Use of EEG for prognostication in TBI patients has demonstrated failure rates of up to 20% [63–66], and EEG is not typically used for this indication. In contrast, EEG has been used fairly extensively in the setting of hypoxic-ischemic encephalopathy for prognostication. Dichotomized EEG patterns into "malignant" and "benign" patterns may be predictive of poor and better outcomes, respectively, after profound hypoxia [67]. Absence of EEG background activity has been associated with in-hospital mortality [68, 69]. To the extent that hypoxic-ischemic encephalopathy can complicate sTBI, it may be more useful for prognostication in this small subset of sTBI patients.

The cost of performing EEG, especially cEEG in the ICU, is not insignificant, requiring technical recording equipment and specialized personnel, such as an EEG technician and experienced clinicians (typically neurologists specializing in epileptology) to interpret results in real time [70]. Use of cEEG may reduce the need for other imaging modalities, ultimately leading to cost savings [61]. Certainly, posttraumatic seizures and nonconvulsive or subclinical seizures can contribute to poor outcomes and high mortality, and the use of EEG monitoring in the comatose TBI patient may prevent significant secondary injury. Coupling of EEG data with cerebral microdialysis (and other parameters) may con-

fer additional clinical, diagnostic, and prognostic benefit [71].

Evoked Potentials

The two most commonly used types of evoked potentials (EP) in the neurocritical care setting are SSEPs and BSAERs, although they are infrequently used overall. They have some limited utility as noninvasive, relatively inexpensive diagnostic and prognostic tools [72], such as after cardiopulmonary resuscitation (CPR) [73], after TBI [74], and for confirmation of brain death [75]. While certain patterns have been seen in the median nerve SSEP in the diagnosis of brain death [76, 77], no specific patterns have been noted with BSAER [78, 79]. The accuracy of SSEPs and BSAERs is improved for brain death confirmation when they are used together [80].

Conclusions: Multimodality Monitoring Integration

Critical to the management of severe TBI patients in the ICU is a thorough understanding of cerebral physiology in general, but also the specific events and trends in a given patient's physiology, which may dramatically vacillate in the hours and days following injury. Therefore, multimodality monitoring data are utilized to assess the current physiological needs as well as to initiate treatment targeted to those needs.

Use of evidence-based guidelines providing general therapeutic recommendations and therapeutic ranges (see also chapter "Use of Guidelines in the Management of Traumatic Brain Injury") has been shown to improve outcomes when systematic implementation is employed [13]. However, strict adherence to evidence-based guidelines and "optimal parameters" may be misguided when making decisions at the individual patient's bedside, and thought should be given instead to the incorporation of multiple modalities of cerebral monitoring to guide treatment strategies.

References

1. Le Roux PD, Levine JM, Kofke WA. Monitoring in neurocritical care. Philadelphia, PA: Elsevier/Saunders; 2013.
2. Diringer MN, Edwards DF. Admission to a neurologic/neurosurgical intensive care unit is associated with reduced mortality rate after intracerebral hemorrhage. Crit Care Med. 2001;29(3):635–40.
3. Patel HC, Menon DK, Tebbs S, Hawker R, Hutchinson PJ, Kirkpatrick PJ. Specialist neurocritical care and outcome from head injury. Intensive Care Med. 2002;28(5):547–53.
4. Suarez JI, Zaidat OO, Suri MF, Feen ES, Lynch G, Hickman J, et al. Length of stay and mortality in neurocritically ill patients: impact of a specialized neurocritical care team. Crit Care Med. 2004;32(11):2311–7.
5. Varelas PN, Conti MM, Spanaki MV, Potts E, Bradford D, Sunstrom C, et al. The impact of a neurointensivist-led team on a semiclosed neurosciences intensive care unit. Crit Care Med. 2004;32(11):2191–8.
6. Varelas PN, Eastwood D, Yun HJ, Spanaki MV, Hacein Bey L, Kessaris C, et al. Impact of a neurointensivist on outcomes in patients with head trauma treated in a neurosciences intensive care unit. J Neurosurg. 2006;104(5):713–9.
7. Varelas PN, Schultz L, Conti M, Spanaki M, Genarrelli T, Hacein-Bey L. The impact of a neuro-intensivist on patients with stroke admitted to a neurosciences intensive care unit. Neurocrit Care. 2008;9(3):293–9.
8. Lundberg N, Troupp H, Lorin H. Continuous recording of the ventricular-fluid pressure in patients with severe acute traumatic brain injury. A preliminary report. J Neurosurg. 1965;22(6):581–90.
9. Monro A. Observations on the structure and functions of the nervous system. London; 1783.
10. Marmarou A, Anderson RL, Ward JD, Choi SC, Young HF, Eisenberg HM, et al. Impact of ICP instability and hypotension on outcome in patients with severe head trauma. J Neurosurg. 1991;75(1):S59–66.
11. Alali AS, Fowler RA, Mainprize TG, Scales DC, Kiss A, de Mestral C, et al. Intracranial pressure monitoring in severe traumatic brain injury: results from the American College of Surgeons Trauma Quality Improvement Program. J Neurotrauma. 2013;30(20):1737–46.
12. Farahvar A, Gerber LM, Chiu YL, Carney N, Härtl R, Ghajar J. Increased mortality in patients with severe traumatic brain injury treated without intracranial pressure monitoring. J Neurosurg. 2012;117(4):729–34.
13. Gerber LM, Chiu YL, Carney N, Härtl R, Ghajar J. Marked reduction in mortality in patients with severe traumatic brain injury. J Neurosurg. 2013;119(6):1583–90.
14. Talving P, Karamanos E, Teixeira PG, Skiada D, Lam L, Belzberg H, et al. Intracranial pressure monitoring in severe head injury: compliance with brain trauma foundation guidelines and effect on outcomes: a prospective study. J Neurosurg. 2013;119(5):1248–54.
15. Chesnut RM, Temkin N, Carney N, Dikmen S, Rondina C, Videtta W, et al. A trial of intracranial-pressure monitoring in traumatic brain injury. N Engl J Med. 2012;367(26):2471–81.
16. Rosner MJ, Daughton S. Cerebral perfusion pressure management in head injury. J Trauma. 1990;30(8):933–40; discussion 940–931.
17. Robertson CS, Valadka AB, Hannay HJ, Contant CF, Gopinath SP, Cormio M, et al. Prevention of secondary ischemic insults after severe head injury. Crit Care Med. 1999;27(10):2086–95.
18. Contant CF, Valadka AB, Gopinath SP, Hannay HJ, Robertson CS. Adult respiratory distress syndrome: a complication of induced hypertension after severe head injury. J Neurosurg. 2001;95(4):560–8.
19. Brain Trauma Foundation, American Association of Neurological Surgeons, Congress of Neurological Surgeons, Joint Section on Neurotrauma and Critical Care, AANS/CNS, Bratton SL, et al. Guidelines for the management of severe traumatic brain injury. IX. Cerebral perfusion thresholds. J Neurotrauma. 2007;24(Suppl 1):S59–64.
20. Huang SJ, Hong WC, Han YY, Chen YS, Wen CS, Tsai YS, et al. Clinical outcome of severe head injury using three different ICP and CPP protocol-driven therapies. J Clin Neurosci. 2006;13(8):818–22.
21. Johnson U, Nilsson P, Ronne-Engstrom E, Howells T, Enblad P. Favorable outcome in traumatic brain injury patients with impaired cerebral pressure autoregulation when treated at low cerebral perfusion pressure levels. Neurosurgery. 2011;68(3):714–21; discussion 721–712.
22. Bullock R, Sakas D, Patterson J, Wyper D, Hadley D, Maxwell W, et al. Early post-traumatic cerebral blood flow mapping: correlation with structural damage after focal injury. Acta Neurochir Suppl (Wien). 1992;55:14–7.
23. Robertson C. Desaturation episodes after severe head injury: influence on outcome. Acta Neurochir Suppl (Wien). 1993;59:98–101.
24. Robertson CS, Gopinath SP, Goodman JC, Contant CF, Valadka AB, Narayan RK. SjvO$_2$ monitoring in head-injured patients. J Neurotrauma. 1995;12(5):891–6.
25. Cruz J. The first decade of continuous monitoring of jugular bulb oxyhemoglobin saturation: management strategies and clinical outcome. Crit Care Med. 1998;26(2):344–51.
26. Le Roux PD, Newell DW, Lam AM, Grady MS, Winn HR. Cerebral arteriovenous oxygen difference: a predictor of cerebral infarction and outcome in patients with severe head injury. J Neurosurg. 1997;87(1):1–8.
27. Kiening KL, Unterberg AW, Bardt TF, Schneider GH, Lanksch WR. Monitoring of cerebral oxygenation in patients with severe head injuries: brain tissue PO$_2$ versus jugular vein oxygen saturation. J Neurosurg. 1996;85(5):751–7.
28. Gupta AK, Hutchinson PJ, Al-Rawi P, Gupta S, Swart M, Kirkpatrick PJ, et al. Measuring brain

tissue oxygenation compared with jugular venous oxygen saturation for monitoring cerebral oxygenation after traumatic brain injury. Anesth Analg. 1999;88(3):549–53.

29. Longhi L, Pagan F, Valeriani V, Magnoni S, Zanier ER, Conte V, et al. Monitoring brain tissue oxygen tension in brain-injured patients reveals hypoxic episodes in normal-appearing and in peri-focal tissue. Intensive Care Med. 2007;33(12):2136–42.

30. Ponce LL, Pillai S, Cruz J, Li X, Julia H, Gopinath S, et al. Position of probe determines prognostic information of brain tissue PO$_2$ in severe traumatic brain injury. Neurosurgery. 2012;70(6):1492–502; discussion 1502–1493.

31. Sarrafzadeh AS, Kiening KL, Bardt TF, Schneider GH, Unterberg AW, Lanksch WR. Cerebral oxygenation in contusioned vs. nonlesioned brain tissue: monitoring of PtiO$_2$ with Licox and Paratrend. Acta Neurochir Suppl. 1998;71:186–9.

32. Martini RP, Deem S, Yanez ND, Chesnut RM, Weiss NS, Daniel S, et al. Management guided by brain tissue oxygen monitoring and outcome following severe traumatic brain injury. J Neurosurg. 2009;111(4):644–9.

33. Lee HC, Chuang HC, Cho DY, Cheng KF, Lin PH, Chen CC. Applying cerebral hypothermia and brain oxygen monitoring in treating severe traumatic brain injury. World Neurosurg. 2010;74(6):654–60.

34. Green JA, Pellegrini DC, Vanderkolk WE, Figueroa BE, Eriksson EA. Goal directed brain tissue oxygen monitoring versus conventional management in traumatic brain injury: an analysis of in hospital recovery. Neurocrit Care. 2013;18(1):20–5.

35. McCarthy MC, Moncrief H, Sands JM, Markert RJ, Hall LC, Wenker IC, et al. Neurologic outcomes with cerebral oxygen monitoring in traumatic brain injury. Surgery. 2009;146(4):585–91.

36. Meixensberger J, Vath A, Jaeger M, Kunze E, Dings J, Roosen K. Monitoring of brain tissue oxygenation following severe subarachnoid hemorrhage. Neurol Res. 2003;25(5):445–50.

37. Narotam PK, Morrison JF, Nathoo N. Brain tissue oxygen monitoring in traumatic brain injury and major trauma: outcome analysis of a brain tissue oxygen-directed therapy clinical article. J Neurosurg. 2009;111(4):672–82.

38. Spiotta AM, Stiefel MF, Gracias VH, Garuffe AM, Kofke WA, Maloney-Wilensky E, et al. Brain tissue oxygen-directed management and outcome in patients with severe traumatic brain injury. J Neurosurg. 2010;113(3):571–80.

39. Nangunoori R, Maloney-Wilensky E, Stiefel M, Park S, Andrew Kofke W, Levine JM, et al. Brain tissue oxygen-based therapy and outcome after severe traumatic brain injury: a systematic literature review. Neurocrit Care. 2012;17(1):131–8.

40. Oddo M, Milby A, Chen I, Frangos S, MacMurtrie E, Maloney-Wilensky E, et al. Hemoglobin concentration and cerebral metabolism in patients with aneurysmal subarachnoid hemorrhage. Stroke. 2009;40(4):1275–81.

41. Cormio M, Valadka AB, Robertson CS. Elevated jugular venous oxygen saturation after severe head injury. J Neurosurg. 1999;90(1):9–15.

42. Chang JJ, Youn TS, Benson D, Mattick H, Andrade N, Harper CR, et al. Physiologic and functional outcome correlates of brain tissue hypoxia in traumatic brain injury. Crit Care Med. 2009;37(1):283–90.

43. van den Brink WA, van Santbrink H, Steyerberg EW, Avezaat CJ, Suazo JA, Hogesteeger C, et al. Brain oxygen tension in severe head injury. Neurosurgery. 2000;46(4):868–76; discussion 876–868.

44. Eriksson EA, Barletta JF, Figueroa BE, Bonnell BW, Sloffer CA, Vanderkolk WE, et al. The first 72 hours of brain tissue oxygenation predicts patient survival with traumatic brain injury. J Trauma Acute Care Surg. 2012;72(5):1345–9.

45. Stocchetti N, Canavesi K, Magnoni S, Valeriani V, Conte V, Rossi S, et al. Arterio-jugular difference of oxygen content and outcome after head injury. Anesth Analg. 2004;99(1):230–4.

46. Goodnough LT. Risks of blood transfusion. Crit Care Med. 2003;31(12):S678–86.

47. Soderberg-Naucler C, Fish KN, Nelson JA. Reactivation of latent human cytomegalovirus by allogeneic stimulation of blood cells from healthy donors. Cell. 1997;91(1):119–26.

48. Bowden RA, Sayers M, Flournoy N, Newton B, Banaji M, Thomas ED, et al. Cytomegalovirus immune globulin and seronegative blood products to prevent primary cytomegalovirus-infection after marrow transplantation. N Engl J Med. 1986;314(16):1006–10.

49. Phelan HA, Gonzalez RP, Patel HD, Caudill JB, Traylor RK, Yancey LR, et al. Prestorage leukoreduction ameliorates the effects of aging on banked blood. J Trauma. 2010;69(2):330–5.

50. Shander A, Popovsky MA. Understanding the consequences of transfusion-related acute lung injury. Chest. 2005;128(5):598s–604s.

51. Johnston AJ, Gupta AK. Advanced monitoring in the neurology intensive care unit: microdialysis. Curr Opin Crit Care. 2002;8(2):121–7.

52. Reinstrup P, Stahl N, Mellergard P, Uski T, Ungerstedt U, Nordstrom CH. Intracerebral microdialysis in clinical practice: baseline values for chemical markers during wakefulness, anesthesia, and neurosurgery. Neurosurgery. 2000;47(3):701–9; discussion 709–710.

53. Schulz MK, Wang LP, Tange M, Bjerre P. Cerebral microdialysis monitoring: determination of normal and ischemic cerebral metabolisms in patients with aneurysmal subarachnoid hemorrhage. J Neurosurg. 2000;93(5):808–14.

54. Chamoun R, Suki D, Gopinath SP, Goodman JC, Robertson C. Role of extracellular glutamate measured by cerebral microdialysis in severe traumatic brain injury. J Neurosurg. 2010;113(3):564–70.

55. Hlatky R, Valadka AB, Goodman JC, Robertson CS. Evolution of brain tissue injury after evacuation of acute traumatic subdural hematomas. Neurosurgery. 2004;55(6):1318–1323; discussion 1324.

56. Sarrafzadeh A, Haux D, Kuchler I, Lanksch WR, Unterberg AW. Poor-grade aneurysmal subarachnoid hemorrhage: relationship of cerebral metabolism to outcome. J Neurosurg. 2004;100(3):400–6.

57. Timofeev I, Carpenter KL, Nortje J, Al-Rawi PG, O'Connell MT, Czosnyka M, et al. Cerebral extracellular chemistry and outcome following traumatic brain injury: a microdialysis study of 223 patients. Brain. 2011;134(Pt 2):484–94.

58. Adamides AA, Rosenfeldt FL, Winter CD, Pratt NM, Tippett NJ, Lewis PM, et al. Brain tissue lactate elevations predict episodes of intracranial hypertension in patients with traumatic brain injury. J Am Coll Surg. 2009;209(4):531–9.

59. Skjoth-Rasmussen J, Schulz M, Kristensen SR, Bjerre P. Delayed neurological deficits detected by an ischemic pattern in the extracellular cerebral metabolites in patients with aneurysmal subarachnoid hemorrhage. J Neurosurg. 2004;100(1):8–15.

60. Kull LL, Emerson RG. Continuous EEG monitoring in the intensive care unit: technical and staffing considerations. J Clin Neurophysiol. 2005;22(2):107–18.

61. Vespa PM, Nuwer MR, Nenov V, Ronne-Engstrom E, Hovda DA, Bergsneider M, et al. Increased incidence and impact of nonconvulsive and convulsive seizures after traumatic brain injury as detected by continuous electroencephalographic monitoring. J Neurosurg. 1999;91(5):750–60.

62. Ronne-Engstrom E, Winkler T. Continuous EEG monitoring in patients with traumatic brain injury reveals a high incidence of epileptiform activity. Acta Neurol Scand. 2006;114(1):47–53.

63. Vespa PM, Boscardin WJ, Hovda DA, McArthur DL, Nuwer MR, Martin NA, et al. Early and persistent impaired percent alpha variability on continuous electroencephalography monitoring as predictive of poor outcome after traumatic brain injury. J Neurosurg. 2002;97(1):84–92.

64. Steudel WI, Kruger J. Using the spectral analysis of the EEG for prognosis of severe brain injuries in the first post-traumatic week. Acta Neurochir Suppl (Wien). 1979;28(1):40–2.

65. Beridze M, Khaburzania M, Shakarishvili R, Kazaishvili D. Dominated EEG patterns and their prognostic value in coma caused by traumatic brain injury. Georgian Med News. 2010;186:28–33.

66. Gutling E, Gonser A, Imhof HG, Landis T. EEG reactivity in the prognosis of severe head injury. Neurology. 1995;45(5):915–8.

67. Rothstein TL, Thomas EM, Sumi SM. Predicting outcome in hypoxic-ischemic coma. A prospective clinical and electrophysiologic study. Electroencephalogr Clin Neurophysiol. 1991;79(2):101–7.

68. Rossetti AO, Oddo M, Logroscino G, Kaplan PW. Prognostication after cardiac arrest and hypothermia: a prospective study. Ann Neurol. 2010;67(3):301–7.

69. Fugate JE, Wijdicks EF, Mandrekar J, Claassen DO, Manno EM, White RD, et al. Predictors of neurologic outcome in hypothermia after cardiac arrest. Ann Neurol. 2010;68(6):907–14.

70. Young GB. Continuous EEG monitoring in the ICU. Acta Neurol Scand. 2006;114(1):67–8.

71. Vespa P, Tubi M, Claassen J, Buitrago-Blanco M, McArthur D, Velazquez AG, et al. Metabolic crisis occurs with seizures and periodic discharges after brain trauma. Ann Neurol. 2016;79(4):579–90.

72. Cruccu G, Aminoff MJ, Curio G, Guerit JM, Kakigi R, Mauguiere F, et al. Recommendations for the clinical use of somatosensory-evoked potentials. Clin Neurophysiol. 2008;119(8):1705–19.

73. Zandbergen EG, Hijdra A, Koelman JH, Hart AA, Vos PE, Verbeek MM, et al. Prediction of poor outcome within the first 3 days of postanoxic coma. Neurology. 2006;66(1):62–8.

74. Carter BG, Butt W. Review of the use of somatosensory evoked potentials in the prediction of outcome after severe brain injury. Crit Care Med. 2001;29(1):178–86.

75. Wijdicks EF. Brain death worldwide: accepted fact but no global consensus in diagnostic criteria. Neurology. 2002;58(1):20–5.

76. Buchner H, Ferbert A, Hacke W. Serial recording of median nerve stimulated subcortical somatosensory evoked potentials (SEPs) in developing brain death. Electroencephalogr Clin Neurophysiol. 1988;69(1):14–23.

77. Sonoo M, Tsai-Shozawa Y, Aoki M, Nakatani T, Hatanaka Y, Mochizuki A, et al. N18 in median somatosensory evoked potentials: a new indicator of medullary function useful for the diagnosis of brain death. J Neurol Neurosurg Psychiatry. 1999;67(3):374–8.

78. Goldie WD, Chiappa KH, Young RR, Brooks EB. Brainstem auditory and short-latency somatosensory responses in brain death. Neurology. 1981;31(3):248–56.

79. Machado C, Valdes P, Garcia-Tigera J, Virues T, Biscay R, Miranda J, et al. Brain-stem auditory evoked potentials and brain death. Electroencephalogr Clin Neurophysiol. 1991;80(5):392–8.

80. Facco E, Munari M, Gallo F, Volpin SM, Behr AU, Baratto F, et al. Role of short latency evoked potentials in the diagnosis of brain death. Clin Neurophysiol. 2002;113(11):1855–66.

Choice of Intracranial Pressure Monitoring Modality: Parenchymal Monitor vs. Parenchymal Monitor with Brain Tissue Oxygen Monitor vs. External Ventricular Drain

Christian B. Ricks and David O. Okonkwo

Introduction

A primary focus of intensive care unit (ICU) management of severe traumatic brain injury (TBI) is avoidance of secondary injury in the hours to days following injury. Intracranial pressure (ICP) has been the cornerstone of neuromonitoring in TBI. The Monro-Kellie hypothesis states that the interior volume of the cranium is fixed, and its constituents (blood, cerebrospinal fluid [CSF], brain parenchyma) maintain an equilibrium. As brain volume expands from trauma, intracranial pressures rise, and cerebral ischemia and/or brain herniation syndromes may ensue. Since the pioneering work of Lundberg et al. in the 1960s, the measurement of ICP has become an essential monitoring tool in TBI patients [1]. ICP elevation is observed in approximately 50% of severe TBI patients with an abnormal computed tomography (CT) scan [2]. Many studies have correlated elevated intracranial pressures to systemic and cerebral derangements, hypoxia, hypotension, fevers, reduced cerebral perfusion pressure (CPP), and overall poor outcomes [3, 4]. The maintenance of ICP below 20 mmHg and CPP above 55 mmHg is strongly correlated to improved mortality rates [5], though this has evolved to include an assessment of autoregulation in determining the ideal CPP for an individual patient.

The Fourth Edition of the Brain Trauma Foundation (BTF) Guidelines for the Management of Severe Traumatic Brain Injury [6] note:

1. Management of severe TBI patients using information from ICP monitoring is recommended to reduce in-hospital and 2-week post-injury mortality (Level IIB recommendation).
2. Management of severe TBI patients using guideline-based recommendations for CPP monitoring is recommended to decrease 2-week mortality (Level IIB recommendation).
3. Treating ICP above 22 mmHg is recommended because values above this level are associated with increased mortality (Level IIB recommendation).
4. The recommended target cerebral perfusion pressure (CPP) value for survival and favorable outcomes is between 60 and 70 mmHg. Whether 60 or 70 mmHg is the minimum optimal CPP threshold is unclear and may depend upon the patient's autoregulatory status (Level IIB recommendation).

C. B. Ricks, MD, MS · D. O. Okonkwo, MD, PhD (✉)
Department of Neurological Surgery, University of Pittsburgh, Pittsburgh, PA, USA
e-mail: rickscb@upmc.edu; okonkwodo@upmc.edu

© Springer International Publishing AG, part of Springer Nature 2018
S. D. Timmons (ed.), *Controversies in Severe Traumatic Brain Injury Management*,
https://doi.org/10.1007/978-3-319-89477-5_4

Role of Intracraial Pressure Monitoring in Management of Severe Traumatic Brain Injury

Goal-directed therapy in patients with moderate or severe TBI includes managing ICP and systemic blood pressure to maintain cerebral perfusion pressure, cerebral blood flow (CBF), and thus oxygen delivery to at-risk tissue to prevent brain ischemia and secondary injury [7]. While the dangers of untreated elevated ICP and its correlation with lower CPP and increased disability and mortality seem well established, the methods of monitoring and treatment are still the subject of much debate and contradictory evidence. In a randomized controlled study, Benchmark Evidence from South American Trials: Treatment of Intracranial Pressure (BEST:TRIP), Chestnut et al. showed equivalence between a protocol to manage ICP with the use of an intraparenchymal monitor (IPM) and a protocol involving clinical and radiographic assessment of ICP [8]. Cremer et al. in a retrospective cohort study also analyzed ICP-monitored versus clinically assessed cohorts sent to two different Dutch hospitals and found no differences in Glasgow Outcome Scale (GOS) scores at 12 months after injury [9]. There was, however, increased use of sedatives, vasopressors, mannitol, and barbiturates and a longer use of mechanical ventilation in those with managed with ICP monitors. Shafi et al. retrospectively analyzed the National Trauma Data Bank between 1994 and 2001 for those with Glasgow Coma Scale (GCS) $\leq$ 8 treated with ICP monitoring ($n = 708$) and without ($n = 938$) [10]. After controlling for severity, craniotomy, and other comorbidities, ICP monitoring was associated with a 45% reduction in survival. Of note, many of these studies have been criticized for being single-study centers, using retrospectively gathered data, exclusion of patients who died in the first 24 h, and baseline differences between groups known to affect outcomes.

Several studies have shown the benefit of ICP monitoring and by extension aggressive ICP treatment using objective data. Farahvar et al. looked at 2134 patients admitted to New York State trauma centers who were entered into a prospec-tive database administered by the Brain Trauma Foundation (BTF). A total of 1446 were treated with ICP-lowering therapies, with 1202 having an ICP monitor inserted. They found that even after adjusting for all other factors confounding mortality, the insertion of an ICP monitor was associated with a lower 2-week mortality [11]. Stein et al. reviewed case series of severe closed TBI patients after 1970 analyzing 6-month mortality and favorable outcomes [12]. Retrospective analysis of 127 case series involving more than 125,000 patients showed a consistent reduction in mortality by 12%, and 6% improved favorable outcomes in ICP-monitored patients. This suggests some patients who were saved had persistent poor outcomes. Meta-analysis by Yuan et al. [13] identified 14 studies that compared ICP monitoring with no ICP monitoring for the treatment of severe TBI; the 7 studies published after 2012 did demonstrate a lower mortality in patients with ICP monitors placed. Another recent meta-analysis showed that ICP monitoring reduced the risk of electrolyte disturbances and renal failure and improved prognosis [14]. The largest study to date, conducted by the American College of Surgeons Trauma Quality Improvement Program (ACS TQIP), retrospectively analyzed 10,628 adults with severe TBI from 2009 to 2011. Some 1874 patients (17.6%) had ICP monitors placed, with a mortality of 32%. After adjusting for confounders, the adjusted odds ratio for mortality was 0.44 (95% confidence interval between 0.31 and 0.63) compared to those patients managed without ICP monitoring [15].

The literature, as a whole, remains without clear consensus on the extent to which ICP monitoring should be employed in severe TBI patients. As mentioned previously, the BEST:TRIP trial was a randomized, prospective clinical trial comparing two ICP treatment protocols, one involving an ICP monitor and one with serial clinical assessment and radiographic studies. There was no difference in outcomes noted. Following publication of the BEST:TRIP trial, many centers began to question the use of ICP monitors. A consensus group was organized by the BEST:TRIP investigators, wherein international thought leaders in the field attempted to provide context [16]. The consensus was that, for those currently using ICP monitors, the results of the BEST:TRIP trial should not change clinical practice and ICP monitoring should continue to be a mainstay of severe TBI management, particularly in higher-income countries.

The literature does not offer clear guidelines regarding what type of monitors to use, treatment objectives, and pressure management algorithms. This ambiguity has impacted those managing these patients, with one survey showing that only 20% of Canadian neurosurgeons are highly confident that the routine use of ICP monitoring improves patient outcomes [17]. Though there is wide variability in ICP monitoring practices across centers, hospitals with higher rates of ICP monitoring have lower rates of TBI related mortality [18].

Options for Neuromonitoring

In the following sections, we summarize the evidence and advantages of various intracranial pressure monitoring systems, including external ventricular drain (EVD), intraparenchymal monitor, or the addition of a brain tissue oxygen (PbO2) monitor:

Intraparenchymal Monitor

While the dangers of untreated elevated ICP and its correlation with lower CPP and increased disability and mortality seem well established, the methods of monitoring and treatment are still the subject of much debate and contradictory evidence.

Intraparenchymal monitoring is a method of inserting a fiber-optic pressure or miniaturized strain gauge monitor at the tip of a fine metallic wire several centimeters into the brain parenchyma. This allows for continuous transduction of pressures to a bedside monitor. Compared to EVDs, intraparenchymal monitors are easier to place, less likely to become infected or require repositioning, and do not need to be adjusted with changes in patient positioning. Intraparenchymal

monitors are also reported to have lower rates of hemorrhage (0.6% vs. 1.6%), lower rates of malfunction (11.9% vs. 19.7%), and lower infection rates (0% vs. 2.6%) [19]. Replacement of a malfunctioning intraparenchymal monitor is relatively straightforward. The relative safety has led some to suggest that placement can be done without neurosurgeon involvement and have shown comparable outcomes when placed by neurointensivists [20].

However, once an intraparenchymal monitor is "zeroed" and inserted, no additional recalibrations can be performed, and no external means of validating the transduced pressure is available. An additional concern is that most are not compatible with magnetic resonance imaging (MRI) given the risk of excessive heating or movement within the brain [21]. The biggest difference between the two methods relies on the ability of an EVD to therapeutically drain CSF, which is a powerful tool for lowering ICP. In some centers where the intraparenchymal monitor is the standard ICP monitoring technique, insertion of an EVD may be required to manage refractory elevated ICP, and patients are sometimes managed with both devices.

External Ventricular Drain

The external ventricular drain can be both a monitor and a therapeutic intervention. An EVD connected to an external gauge is the most accurate and economic measurement of intracranial pressure and can be validated manually, unlike parenchymal monitors. In addition, an EVD has inherent therapeutic function and is able to drain CSF as an additional powerful tool to lower ICP and thus maintain CPP, CBF, and brain tissue oxygenation. The therapeutic benefit of drainage is increased when intraventricular hemorrhage (IVH) is present. The placement of an EVD can be more challenging than an intraparenchymal monitor, especially in patients with effaced or shifted ventricles or diffuse brain swelling; EVDs also require repositioning in up to 12% of patients [22]. There are higher complication rates including catheter-related hemorrhages and infection [23], although the latter can be reduced with antibiotic impregnated catheters [24]. Radiographic hemorrhage rates may be as high as 21.6% with insertion and 22.5% with removal of EVDs [25]. EVDs can also become obstructed with blood or debris, with attendant need for replacement.

The impact of management with an EVD on mortality is still debated, with some studies showing survival benefit and other increased mortality. Griesdale et al. retrospectively examined the relationship between EVD and mortality by evaluating 171 patients admitted with severe TBI at a single university-affiliated hospital. They found that EVD use was associated with higher mortality for patients with an initial GCS $\geq$ 6, while use in more severely comatose patients demonstrated a statistically insignificant trend for lower mortality. Liu et al. performed a prospective randomized analysis of 122 patients who were treated with either an EVD or ICP monitor and otherwise managed identically except for the drainage of CSF when ICP reached above 20 [26]. This group found that those managed with placement of EVD had a statistically lower rate of refractory intracranial hypertension (21.0% compared to 51.7%), lower rates of surgical decompression (40.3% compared to 58.3%), higher 1-month survival rates (90.3% compared to 76.4%), and improved 6-month Glasgow Outcome Scales (3.79 compared with 3.07). Importantly, the length of hospitalization or duration of ICU stay did not change in this study. This contradicts the retrospective analysis of Kasotakis et al., who after reviewing 253 patients managed with IPM and 124 with EVD found longer duration of ICP monitoring and ICU length of stay with EVD [19]. This difference is explained by the weaning of the EVD gradually over several days before clamping and removal by the Kasotakis group—a common clinical practice in other disorders. The Liu group, however, removed the EVD without weaning once ICP had been controlled for 24 h and thus did not extend the duration of ICP monitoring or ICU stay. Complications were higher with EVD use in both studies, notably, higher catheter-related hemorrhages and infections, which are predictable

based on the larger diameter of the EVD tubing, the deep site of insertion, and external drainage posing contamination risk.

External ventricular drainage management can include continuous or intermittent drainage. In the "open" position cerebrospinal fluid can drain continually, in theory maintaining a more constant intracranial pressure. In the "closed" position, the intracranial pressure can be continuously monitored but must be intermittently opened for drainage. A third option is for the addition of IPM to allow for continuous drainage via EVD and ICP monitoring via IPM. In one retrospective cohort study by Nwachuku et al., open EVD was compared to a closed, intermittently drained EVD [27]. When matched for age, sex, and severity of injury, patients with the closed EVD had higher mean ICP (15.8 mmHg) than the open EVD (10.14 mmHg), even after adjusting for initial GCS and whether the patient had a craniectomy. Shore et al. showed that, compared to continuous drainage, intermittent drainage was associated with increased markers of neuronal injury, lower volumes of CSF drained, and increased mean ICPs in a pediatric severe TBI cohort study [28].

Taken together the 4th Edition Brain Trauma Foundation Guidelines recommend [6]:

1. An EVD system zeroed at the midbrain with continuous drainage of CSF may be considered to lower ICP burden more effectively than intermittent use (Level III recommendation).
2. The use of CSF drainage to lower ICP in patients with an initial Glasgow Coma Scale <6 during the first 12 h after injury may be considered (Level III recommendation).

Brain Tissue Oxygenation Monitor

Treating elevated ICP is designed to maintain CPP and thus prevent secondary cerebral ischemia. However, several studies have demonstrated that cerebral ischemia may occur in spite of optimized ICP and CPP [29, 30]. Thus perfusion-related ischemia is only one cause of cellular hypoxia in the TBI patient [31]. This is further validated by studies showing elevated lactate/pyruvate ratios and thus anaerobic metabolism, which is independent of CPP [32]. Parallel to the body of evidence showing poor outcomes in patients with elevated ICP, exist many studies linking duration, number, and intensity of cerebral hypoxia episodes to poor outcomes [33, 34]. (See also chapter "Oxygen Management and Prevention of Cerebral Ischemia".) This work was first demonstrated using jugular bulb saturations [35]. Normal brain oxygen values are between 20 and 40 mmHg, while episodes of $pB_tO_2 < 15$ mmHg are associated with worse outcomes [36]. The insertion of a brain parenchyma oxygen saturation monitor allows for the continuous measurement of local partial pressure brain tissue oxygen (pB_tO_2) levels. This can be done through the same bolt and burr hole as an ICP monitor and is typically combined with a brain temperature monitor. Given the evidence for treatment of elevated ICP, these monitors are usually inserted in addition to an ICP monitoring device (intraparenchymal monitor or EVD). Simply increasing CPP in a TBI patient, however, is frequently inadequate to ensure oxygenation due to the altered autoregulation capacity. In these patients a comprehensive approach to optimizing brain oxygen levels involves maintaining CPP, adjusting the fraction of inspired O_2 (FiO_2), maintaining fluid status, altering demand (reducing fevers, seizures, etc.), increasing hemoglobin level, or, if needed, surgical decompression.

Steiffel et al. showed in a prospective study using a historical control that the addition of a pB_tO_2 monitor and treatment to maintain oxygenation greater than 25 mmHg, compared to an ICP monitor alone, was associated with decreased mortality (25% vs. 44%) [37] and in a subsequent analysis by Spiotta et al. improved short-term outcomes [38]. Narotam et al. published similar results, comparing prospectively gathered data with historical controls, and showed that treating both ICP (goal <20 mmHg) and pB_tO_2 (goal >20 mmHg) led to improved mortality (25.9% vs. 41.5%) and 6-month Glasgow Outcome Scales [39]. Unfortunately comparisons to historical values have many potential confounding factors. Green et al. tried to avoid this criticism by a retrospective review of two different attending neurosurgeon practices over the same time period [40]. This produced two matched cohorts, with and without pB_tO_2 monitors, using goal-directed therapies to maintain ICP > 20 mmHg and CPP > 60 mmHg, as well as $pB_tO_2 > 20$ mmHg in that cohort. They did not find a benefit in survival or functional status improvement at discharge. Martini et al. had similar findings, adding only that pB_tO_2 monitoring increased the duration of hospitalization [41]. These contradictory results undermine the importance of a randomized control trial, which has recently been completed (brain tissue oxygen monitoring in traumatic brain injury (BOOST 2)), although not yet published.

The additional data provided by pB_tO_2 is important to place the ICP and CPP values into context. Patients with moderately elevated ICP (20–30 mmHg) or reduced CPP may not require aggressive management with a normal pB_tO_2. This distinction is important when considering the known risks of ICP-lowering and CPP-elevating therapies [42, 43]. The use of pB_tO_2 monitors may thus be able to individualize ICP and CPP thresholds instead of dogmatically adhering to recommendations to keep ICP < 20 mmHg and CPP > 55 mmHg. This is appealing given the heterogenous nature of TBI and the underlying differences or comorbidities of the patients it affects.

pB_tO_2 monitoring is not without its risks and shortcomings. Devices can be improperly inserted, become damaged, or infected. In addition, information may only reflect a small area of brain tissue or reflect O_2 diffusion more effectively than brain ischemia [44]. Many questions exist regarding the proper thresholds for pB_tO_2 treatment and the most effective treatment strategies.

Advances in Neuromonitoring Technology

The choice among available neuromonitoring technologies is a false choice. Multiple monitors may be inserted, and a single patient can have an EVD, intraparenchymal monitor, pB_tO_2 monitor, and brain temperature probe all inserted simultaneously through multiple lumen bolts. One product (Raumedic; Helmbrechts, Germany) has simplified this approach with a single catheter with multiple functions to simultaneously measures intracranial pressure, intracranial temperature, and oxygen partial pressure via ventricular catheters containing a microchip that allows ICP or temperature measurements in addition to standard EVD functionality. Other combined fiber-optic ICP and EVD devices are also on the market. The technological advances in these areas ensure that the future of neuromonitoring will not require deciding between what type of information to receive but what to do with the variety of information obtained.

Conclusions

Intracranial pressure monitoring has been a mainstay of management of severe traumatic brain injury for four decades. The guidelines for severe TBI management again emphasize the indication for use of ICP monitoring in the care of severe TBI patients [6]. There is no clear advantage to the use of an intraparenchymal monitor versus an external ventricular drain. Rather, individual patient characteristics may suggest the use of one, the other, or both. Goal-directed therapy for ICP, CPP, brain tissue oxygenation, and cerebral blood flow will continue to mature with the advances in technology available to clinicians.

References

1. Lundberg N. Continuous recording and control of ventricular fluid pressure in neurosurgical practice. Acta Psychiatr Scand Suppl. 1960;36(149):1–193.
2. Narayan RK, Kishore PR, Becker DP, Ward JD, Enas GG, Greenberg RP, et al. Intracranial pressure: to monitor or not to monitor? A review of our experience with severe head injury. J Neurosurg. 1982;56(5):650–9.
3. Juul N, Morris GF, Marshall SB, Marshall LF. Intracranial hypertension and cerebral perfusion pressure: influence on neurological deterioration and outcome in severe head injury. The executive committee of the international selfotel trial. J Neurosurg. 2000;92(1):1–6.
4. Murray GD, Butcher I, McHugh GS, Lu J, Mushkudiani NA, Maas AI, et al. Multivariable prognostic analysis in traumatic brain injury: results from the impact study. J Neurotrauma. 2007;24(2):329–37.
5. Balestreri M, Czosnyka M, Hutchinson P, Steiner LA, Hiler M, Smielewski P, et al. Impact of intracranial pressure and cerebral perfusion pressure on severe disability and mortality after head injury. Neurocrit Care. 2006;4(1):8–13.
6. Carney N, Totten AM, O'Reilly C, Ullman JS, Hawryluk GW, Bell MJ, Bratton SL, Chesnut R, Harris OA, Kissoon N, Rubiano AM, Shutter L, Tasker RC, Vavilala MS, Wilberger J, Wright DW, Ghajar J. Guidelines for the management of severe traumatic brain injury, fourth edition. Neurosurgery. 2017;80(1):6–15.
7. Mehta A, Kochanek PM, Tyler-Kabara E, Adelson PD, Wisniewski SR, Berger RP, et al. Relationship of intracranial pressure and cerebral perfusion pressure with outcome in young children after severe traumatic brain injury. Dev Neurosci. 2010;32(5–6):413–9.
8. Chesnut RM, Temkin N, Carney N, Dikmen S, Rondina C, Videtta W, et al. A trial of intracranial-pressure monitoring in traumatic brain injury. N Engl J Med. 2012;367(26):2471–81.
9. Cremer OL, van Dijk GW, van Wensen E, Brekelmans GJ, Moons KG, Leenen LP, et al. Effect of intracranial pressure monitoring and targeted intensive care on functional outcome after severe head injury. Crit Care Med. 2005;33(10):2207–13.
10. Shafi S, Diaz-Arrastia R, Madden C, Gentilello L. Intracranial pressure monitoring in brain-injured patients is associated with worsening of survival. J Trauma. 2008;64(2):335–40.
11. Farahvar A, Gerber LM, Chiu YL, Carney N, Hartl R, Ghajar J. Increased mortality in patients with severe traumatic brain injury treated without intracranial pressure monitoring. J Neurosurg. 2012;117(4):729–34.
12. Stein SC, Georgoff P, Meghan S, Mirza KL, El Falaky OM. Relationship of aggressive monitoring and treatment to improved outcomes in severe traumatic brain injury. J Neurosurg. 2010;112(5):1105–12.
13. Yuan Q, Wu X, Sun Y, Yu J, Li Z, Du Z, et al. Impact of intracranial pressure monitoring on mortality in patients with traumatic brain injury: a systematic review and meta-analysis. J Neurosurg. 2015;122(3):574–87.
14. Han J, Yang S, Zhang C, Zhao M, Li A. Impact of intracranial pressure monitoring on prognosis of patients with severe traumatic brain injury: a prisma systematic review and meta-analysis. Medicine (Baltimore). 2016;95(7):e2827.
15. Alali AS, Fowler RA, Mainprize TG, Scales DC, Kiss A, de Mestral C, et al. Intracranial pressure monitoring in severe traumatic brain injury: results from the American College of Surgeons Trauma Quality Improvement Program. J Neurotrauma. 2013;30(20):1737–46.
16. Chesnut RM, Bleck TP, Citerio G, Classen J, Cooper DJ, Coplin WM, et al. A consensus-based interpreta-

tion of the benchmark evidence from south American trials: treatment of intracranial pressure trial. J Neurotrauma [Research Support, Non-US Gov't]. 2015;32(22):1722–4.

17. Sahjpaul R, Girotti M. Intracranial pressure monitoring in severe traumatic brain injury—results of a Canadian survey. Can J Neurol Sci. 2000;27(2): 143–7.

18. Lingsma HF, Roozenbeek B, Perel P, Roberts I, Maas AI, Steyerberg EW. Between-centre differences and treatment effects in randomized controlled trials: a case study in traumatic brain injury. Trials. 2011;12:201.

19. Kasotakis G, Michailidou M, Bramos A, Chang Y, Velmahos G, Alam H, et al. Intraparenchymal vs extracranial ventricular drain intracranial pressure monitors in traumatic brain injury: less is more? J Am Coll Surg. 2012;214(6):950–7.

20. Sadaka F, Kasal J, Lakshmanan R, Palagiri A. Placement of intracranial pressure monitors by neurointensivists: case series and a systematic review. Brain Inj. 2013;27(5):600–4.

21. Newcombe VF, Hawkes RC, Harding SG, Willcox R, Brock S, Hutchinson PJ, et al. Potential heating caused by intraparenchymal intracranial pressure transducers in a 3-tesla magnetic resonance imaging system using a body radiofrequency resonator: assessment of the codman microsensor transducer. J Neurosurg. 2008;109(1):159–64.

22. Saladino A, White JB, Wijdicks EF, Lanzino G. Malplacement of ventricular catheters by neurosurgeons: a single institution experience. Neurocrit Care. 2009;10(2):248–52.

23. Guyot LL, Dowling C, Diaz FG, Michael DB. Cerebral monitoring devices: analysis of complications. Acta Neurochir Suppl. 1998;71:47–9.

24. Zabramski JM, Whiting D, Darouiche RO, Horner TG, Olson J, Robertson C, et al. Efficacy of antimicrobial-impregnated external ventricular drain catheters: a prospective, randomized, controlled trial. J Neurosurg. 2003;98(4):725–30.

25. Miller C, Tummala RP. Risk factors for hemorrhage associated with external ventricular drain placement and removal. J Neurosurg. 2017;126(1): 289–97.

26. Liu H, Wang W, Cheng F, Yuan Q, Yang J, Hu J, et al. External ventricular drains versus intraparenchymal intracranial pressure monitors in traumatic brain injury: a prospective observational study. World Neurosurg. 2015;83(5):794–800.

27. Nwachuku EL, Puccio AM, Fetzick A, Scruggs B, Chang YF, Shutter LA, et al. Intermittent versus continuous cerebrospinal fluid drainage management in adult severe traumatic brain injury: assessment of intracranial pressure burden. Neurocrit Care. 2014;20(1):49–53.

28. Shore PM, Thomas NJ, Clark RS, Adelson PD, Wisniewski SR, Janesko KL, et al. Continuous versus intermittent cerebrospinal fluid drainage after severe traumatic brain injury in children: effect on biochemical markers. J Neurotrauma. 2004;21(9): 1113–22.

29. Gopinath SP, Robertson CS, Contant CF, Hayes C, Feldman Z, Narayan RK, et al. Jugular venous desaturation and outcome after head injury. J Neurol Neurosurg Psychiatry. 1994;57(6):717–23.

30. Le Roux PD, Newell DW, Lam AM, Grady MS, Winn HR. Cerebral arteriovenous oxygen difference: a predictor of cerebral infarction and outcome in patients with severe head injury. J Neurosurg. 1997;87(1):1–8.

31. Menon DK, Coles JP, Gupta AK, Fryer TD, Smielewski P, Chatfield DA, et al. Diffusion limited oxygen delivery following head injury. Crit Care Med. 2004;32(6):1384–90.

32. Vespa PM, O'Phelan K, McArthur D, Miller C, Eliseo M, Hirt D, et al. Pericontusional brain tissue exhibits persistent elevation of lactate/pyruvate ratio independent of cerebral perfusion pressure. Crit Care Med. 2007;35(4):1153–60.

33. Bardt TF, Unterberg AW, Hartl R, Kiening KL, Schneider GH, Lanksch WR. Monitoring of brain tissue po2 in traumatic brain injury: effect of cerebral hypoxia on outcome. Acta Neurochir Suppl. 1998;71:153–6.

34. Kiening KL, Hartl R, Unterberg AW, Schneider GH, Bardt T, Lanksch WR. Brain tissue po2-monitoring in comatose patients: implications for therapy. Neurol Res. 1997;19(3):233–40.

35. Cruz J. The first decade of continuous monitoring of jugular bulb oxyhemoglobinsaturation: management strategies and clinical outcome. Crit Care Med. 1998;26(2):344–51.

36. Valadka AB, Gopinath SP, Contant CF, Uzura M, Robertson CS. Relationship of brain tissue po2 to outcome after severe head injury. Crit Care Med. 1998;26(9):1576–81.

37. Stiefel MF, Spiotta A, Gracias VH, Garuffe AM, Guillamondegui O, Maloney-Wilensky E, et al. Reduced mortality rate in patients with severe traumatic brain injury treated with brain tissue oxygen monitoring. J Neurosurg. 2005;103(5):805–11.

38. Spiotta AM, Stiefel MF, Gracias VH, Garuffe AM, Kofke WA, Maloney-Wilensky E, et al. Brain tissue oxygen-directed management and outcome in patients with severe traumatic brain injury. J Neurosurg. 2010;113(3):571–80.

39. Narotam PK, Morrison JF, Nathoo N. Brain tissue oxygen monitoring in traumatic brain injury and major trauma: outcome analysis of a brain tissue oxygen-directed therapy. J Neurosurg. 2009;111(4):672–82.

40. Green JA, Pellegrini DC, Vanderkolk WE, Figueroa BE, Eriksson EA. Goal directed brain tissue oxygen monitoring versus conventional management in traumatic brain injury: an analysis of in hospital recovery. Neurocrit Care. 2013;18(1):20–5.

41. Martini RP, Deem S, Yanez ND, Chesnut RM, Weiss NS, Daniel S, et al. Management guided by brain tissue oxygen monitoring and outcome following severe traumatic brain injury. J Neurosurg. 2009;111(4):644–9.

42. Contant CF, Valadka AB, Gopinath SP, Hannay HJ, Robertson CS. Adult respiratory distress syndrome: a complication of induced hypertension after severe head injury. J Neurosurg. 2001;95(4): 560–8.

43. Cruz J. Adverse effects of pentobarbital on cerebral venous oxygenation of comatose patients with acute traumatic brain swelling: relationship to outcome. J Neurosurg. 1996;85(5):758–61.

44. Rosenthal G, Hemphill JC 3rd, Sorani M, Martin C, Morabito D, Obrist WD, et al. Brain tissue oxygen tension is more indicative of oxygen diffusion than oxygen delivery and metabolism in patients with traumatic brain injury. Crit Care Med. 2008;36(6):1917–24.

Oxygen Management and Prevention of Cerebral Ischemia

Ashley Ralston and M. Ross Bullock

Introduction

Management of traumatic brain injury (TBI) patients encompasses a multifaceted, interdisciplinary approach, including several controversial areas, some with limited support from "level I evidence-based" data. Despite advancements in medical care, mortality in severe TBI ranges from 25 to 40%, though recent papers have suggested a decrease in mortality by approximately 10–12% with intracranial pressure (ICP) monitoring and aggressive medical management [1, 2]. These findings have not been substantiated with randomized controlled trials and are still controversial.

A significant concern for practitioners managing these patients is the prevention of secondary injury. Proposed mechanisms of secondary injury include mitochondrial damage, free oxygen radical generation, and ischemia. There are several intracranial and extracranial causes of secondary injury. Decreased perfusion, contributing to global and focal brain ischemia, is caused not only by increased intracranial pressure but also by uncontrolled hypertension resulting in loss of autoregulation or arterial hypotension commonly seen in polytrauma. Direct injury to neuronal cells leads to release of neuropeptides (e.g., inflammasomes, neurokinin, and substance P), which ultimately stimulate systemic inflammatory cytokines (tumor necrosis factor alpha [TNFα] and interleukin-1beta [IL-1β]) [3]. Overall, the neuroinflammatory and systemic inflammatory pathways increase blood-brain barrier (BBB) permeability and may increase cerebral edema or hyperemia, thus increasing ICP hours and days later.

Mitochondrial damage causes dysregulation of cellular homeostasis and cell death pathways [4]. Mitochondrial dysregulation also affects calcium transport, decreasing the mitochondrial membrane potential. This leads to increased oxidative phosphorylation and inhibits cellular respiration. In normal tissue, anaerobic glycolysis produces 2 moles of adenosine triphosphate (ATP), whereas mitochondria can produce 34 ATP with aerobic metabolism. Mitochondrial dysfunction due to oxidative stress also increases the formation of radical oxygen species (ROS) and radical nitrogen species (RNS). The oxidative stress disrupts normal ATP formation and transport channels, leading to the formation of pores exposing the mitochondrial matrix to the cytosol and initiating apoptosis [4].

Despite the small percentage of body weight, the brain encompasses only 2%; cerebral

A. Ralston, MD · M. R. Bullock, MD, PhD (✉)
Department of Neurosurgery, University of
Miami-Miller School of Medicine, Miami, FL, USA
e-mail: ashley.ralston@jhsmiami.org;
RBullock@med.miami.edu

© Springer International Publishing AG, part of Springer Nature 2018
S. D. Timmons (ed.), *Controversies in Severe Traumatic Brain Injury Management*,
https://doi.org/10.1007/978-3-319-89477-5_5

metabolism requires 20% of cardiac output and oxygen consumption. Hypoperfusion, in combination with oxidative stress, and consequent local cytotoxic edema can lead to secondary and delayed brain tissue hypoxia, which may occur despite adequate cerebral perfusion pressure (CPP) and control of ICP.

Decreased cerebral oxygenation may also result from systemic factors, such as decreased cerebral blood flow (e.g., due to shock), decreased delivery (anemia or hemoglobin dysfunction), or decreased diffusion within the brain (e.g., perivascular edema and endothelial swelling) [5]. Increasing the oxygen tension gradient may facilitate diffusion across edematous pericapillary brain tissue [6]. Hyperbaric oxygen treatment has been suggested for TBI patients, as it appears to decrease local inflammation and edema and may increase the oxygen diffusion gradient, with positive effects upon brain metabolism at the mitochondrial level and, more recently, promising clinical outcomes as a result.

In this chapter, the current practices, controversies, active research, and future projects concerning oxygen management of traumatic brain injury patients are discussed.

Current Practice

Prevention of hypoxia is a widely accepted practice in all forms of critical care; however, the optimal partial pressure of oxygen in the blood (PaO_2) has not been fully determined, and brain tissue oxygen (pB_tO_2) monitoring has not been adopted as a standard of care, although one recent trial suggested it to be beneficial (BOOST, see later) [7].

Prolonged cerebral hypoxia, including pB_tO_2 less than 15 mmHg, has an increased likelihood of poor outcomes [8]. An initial pB_tO_2 measurement of less than 10 mmHg for more than 30 min was correlated with an increased risk of death or poor outcomes. Hyperoxia has also been associated with complications (see later) and is not currently recommended.

Airway management of comatose traumatic brain injury patients, and ventilated patients in general, is centered on oxygenation and ventilation; however, carbon dioxide (CO_2) management and ventilation are also extremely important in TBI patients. Briefly, there have been a variety of recommendations for optimal CO_2. Prior work recommended hyperventilation to induce hypocarbia and thus reduce intracranial pressure. However, more recent studies demonstrated that CO_2 levels below about 25 mmHg can significantly decrease cerebral blood flow leading to cerebral ischemia. Therefore, the Guidelines for Management of Severe TBI recommend against a $PaCO_2$ below 25 mmHg [9]. However, temporarily hyperventilating patients to a $PaCO_2$ of 30–35 mmHg for shorter periods remains an accepted practice for acute refractory elevations in ICP [9].

In general, ventilator strategies in TBI patients—high tidal volume (V_T) and low positive end-expiratory pressure (PEEP) to keep ICP low—contradict lung-protective strategies (low V_T and higher PEEP) [10]. Concern for an increase in ICP related to increasing PEEP has not been validated and may usually be offset by positioning the patient head up at 25–40° to promote venous drainage from the head. However, high tidal volumes may increase the risk of lung injury, and recommendations include tidal volumes from 6 to 10 mL/kg, in order to decrease overdistension of alveoli [11]. Current fractional inspired oxygen concentration (FiO_2) recommendations are to start at 100% and titrate down as quickly as possible to maintain peripheral saturations above 95% or PaO_2 above 80 mmHg.

Complications of Prolonged Hyperoxia

An important consideration of any treatment includes the side effects or risks associated with it. Prolonged hyperoxia ($PaO_2 > 200$ mmHg or hyperbaric oxygen) has been associated with complications in multiple systems, mainly central nervous system (CNS) and pulmonary. A rat study found extensive pulmonary inflammation with hyperoxia at 1.5 atmosphere absolute (ATA), with a disruption of the alveolar-capillary barrier leading to respiratory failure and death [12]. There have been reports of injury to the lens of the eye, described as retrolental fibroplasia, especially in neonates. A small study examined the effects of different oxygen concentrations and pressures on bovine lenses in culture. Lenses exposed to higher concentrations, under higher pressures (hyperbaric), for longer periods of time demonstrated decreased lenticular transparency in a centripetal orientation [13]. Hyperoxia has also been shown to cause cerebral peripheral vasoconstriction, which may decrease cerebral perfusion pressure (CPP), nullifying the beneficial effects of improved oxygen delivery.

Recently, a multicenter retrospective review evaluated the effect of arterial hyperoxia on mortality in ventilated TBI patients managed in a general (non-neurologic/neurosurgical) ICU setting from 2003 to 2008. Some 403 were normoxic (PaO_2 60–300 mmHg), 256 were hyperoxic ($PaO_2 > 300$ mmHg), and 553 were hypoxic ($PaO_2 < 60$ mmHg). Fatality rates were higher in the hypoxia group (41%), followed by the hyperoxia group (32%), with best outcomes seen in the normoxia group (23%). (See also chapter "Management to Optimal Parameters: Euboxia?".) After a multivariate analysis, Rincon et al. concluded that arterial hyperoxia is independently associated with higher in-hospital case fatality [14]. There are many criticisms to this study, including the absence of neurocritical care and the lack of cerebral pB_tO_2 monitoring or $CMRO_2$ evaluation and lack of control for lung injury or severity of TBI. The range for normoxia in this study was very wide and begins at a relatively low value ($PaO2$ 60–300 mmHg). A study evaluating neurologic outcomes in cardiac arrest patients with return of spontaneous circulation found the optimal range to be from 70 to 240 mmHg, which correlated with improved outcomes in this specific population [15].

Hyperbaric oxygen (HBO) has also been associated with barotrauma to multiple organs. These include injuries to the middle and inner ear, as well as ocular effects listed previously. Patients with sensory deficits (e.g., in coma or sedated) may be at increased risk for rupture of the tympanic membrane, as visualized on otoscopy in almost 4% of patients. Oxygen toxicity at hyperbaric levels may also result in lung and central nervous system (CNS) complications, including an increased risk of seizures, which can be problematic in a TBI patient already at risk for seizures [16].

Invasive Oxygen Delivery Monitoring

Since evidence exists to suggest an optimal PaO_2 range, several techniques have been developed and are clinically available for monitoring cerebral oxygenation, mostly indirectly. Global evaluation can be performed with jugular bulb hemoglobin oxygen saturation (SjO_2), and focal evaluation of pB_tO_2 has been performed with several types of intracranial monitors. Both of these techniques provide an indirect or direct measure of brain tissue oxygen delivery to the brain.

Prior work demonstrated ventilation with 100% FiO_2 also decreased brain lactate levels, suggesting an improvement in cerebral oxidative metabolism, with lactate consumption [17]. However, the oxygen-carrying capacity of red blood cells is very high at full saturation, which is achieved at ambient oxygen tension (~3 mL per 100 mL of blood), and may be only minimally improved with higher inspired oxygen concentrations of over ~40%. For this reason, the minimal increase in oxygen transport achieved by hyperoxia remains controversial as a method to improve oxygen delivery or utilization (Fig. 1). For example, Magnoni et al. found a slight decrease in lactate levels, with no significant change in the lactate-to-pyruvate (LP) ratio, leading to an overall picture of decreased cerebral glucose metabolism but not improved oxidative function [18].

One small prospective, randomized trial compared outcomes when directing care based on pB_tO_2 versus ICP monitoring. The pB_tO_2 goal was >20 mmHg for adequate brain oxygenation, as a pB_tO_2 less than 15 mmHg and, more significantly, less than 10 mmHg, has been shown to contribute to worse outcomes [19]. With this in mind, a PaO_2 between 100 and 300 mmHg maintained the pB_tO_2 from 15 to 35 mmHg for

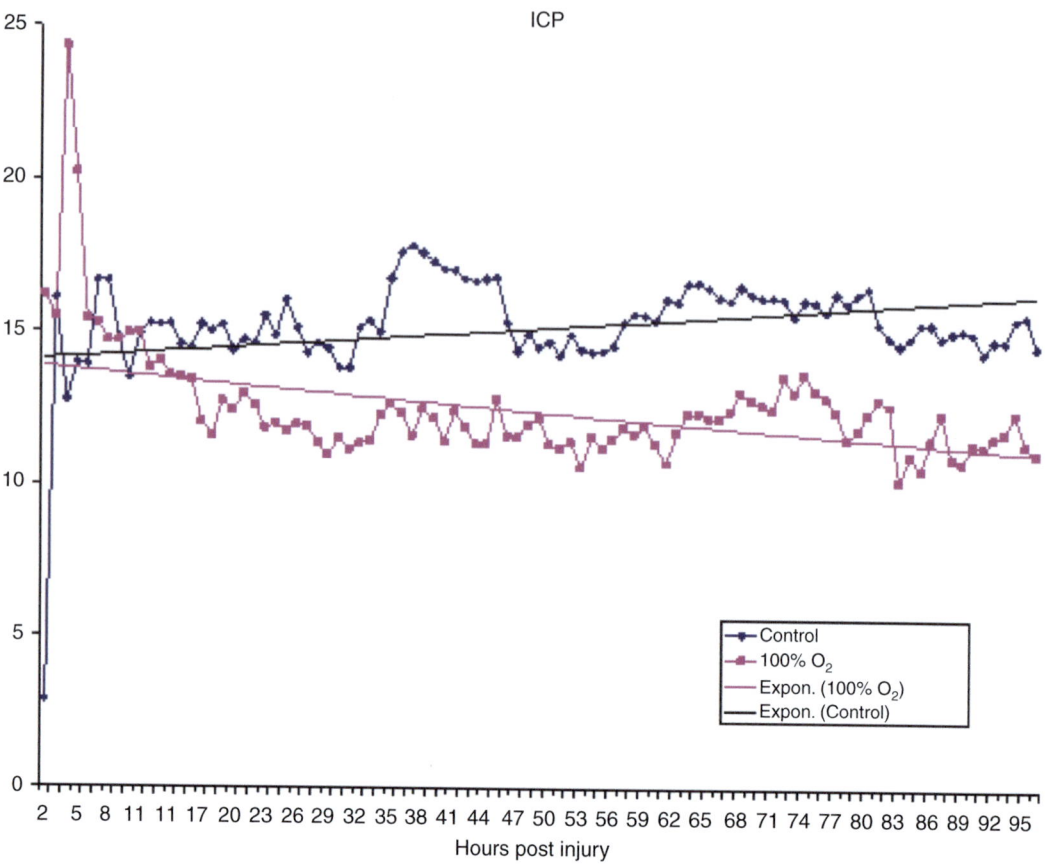

Fig. 1 Comparison of intracranial pressure in 26 patients with normoxia (control) compared with 25 patients with hyperoxia (100% FiO$_2$)

most patients. Though a small study (only 23 patients with pB$_t$O$_2$ monitoring and 27 with ICP monitoring), there was a significant decrease in mortality at 6 months in the pB$_t$O$_2$-directed group. There was also a trend toward increased favorable outcomes, though this was not statistically significant, possibly related to the low power from a small sample size. Importantly, there was no increase in pulmonary complications in the pB$_t$O$_2$-driven treatment group (one patient with pB$_t$O$_2$-driven treatment and three patients with ICP-driven treatment experienced pulmonary complications). Despite the small nature of this study, it has demonstrated safety, and potential benefit, to monitoring pB$_t$O$_2$ and increasing the PaO$_2$ in moderate to severe TBI patients [7].

Further comparison between ICP monitoring alone and ICP monitoring in conjunction with pB$_t$O$_2$ monitoring was completed during the BOOST-II trial (currently under review for publication). A tiered medical management protocol was standardized between the two groups, while the control group had management based on ICP monitoring alone, and the treatment group included ICP and pB$_t$O$_2$ monitor-based management. Though not statistically significant, likely due to small sample size, mortality was lower, and more favorable outcomes were seen in the combined ICP- and pB$_t$O$_2$-based treatment group.

Jugular Bulb Oximetry

Despite numerous publications on this subject, in the 1980s and 1990s by Robertson and others, the general consensus of the field is now that global changes in cerebral oxygenation, as inferred from jugular bulb hemoglobin oxygen saturation ($S_{jv}O_2$) do not correlate with pB_tO_2 in normal-appearing or perilesional tissue. No significant systemic events (hypotension, hypoxemia, anemia, or hypocapnia) were associated with periods of focal brain hypoxia, as measured by intracerebral $PbtO_2$ sensors. pB_tO_2 was lower in perilesional/peri-contusional tissue than normal tissue and was unexpectedly low despite a normal $S_{jv}O_2$, indicating a benefit of focal monitoring over global oxygenation monitoring at the jugular bulb [20]. Longhi et al. conclude that emphasis should be placed on evaluation of the brain microcirculation, instead of macrocirculation, specifically focusing on local alterations in oxygen diffusion that may be related to local vasoconstriction, edema, and microthrombi formation [20].

Microdialysis

Microdialysis (MD) catheters are relatively small (<1 mm diameter), minimally invasive, and safe. When used with systems such as the ISCUS or CMA 100 analyzer (M Dialysis AB, Stockholm, Sweden) and a microinfusion pump, they can indirectly measure the effects of oxidative stress, ischemia, and neurochemical/mitochondrial dysfunction on the nervous system, by quantifying the metabolites of mitochondrial metabolism, namely, lactate, pyruvate, glucose, and glutamate (marker of excitotoxicity) [21]. The lactate-pyruvate (LP) ratio is a marker of anaerobic metabolism, as pyruvate is metabolized to lactate in the event of hypoxia or mitochondrial damage [21]. This leads to an increased lactate level and a variable pyruvate level. Two types of elevated LP ratios are recognized: type I, related to hypoxia, is an elevated lactate level with a very low pyruvate level; and type II, related to mitochondrial dysfunction, is an elevated lactate with a normal or increased pyruvate level [22, 23].

A recent paper by Magnoni et al. examined the concordance of microdialysis and diffusion tensor imaging (DTI) by magnetic resonance imaging (MRI) [24]. MD catheters were placed

into normal-appearing frontal white matter, and samples were collected for at least 72 h. Eleven patients underwent DTI between 2 and 9 weeks post injury and were compared with age- and sex-matched controls. Tau protein levels (a marker of brain injury) were significantly elevated on insertion and decreased slowly over time. A significant inverse correlation was found between MD levels of tau and the anisotropy reductions compared with controls. No significant correlation was found with other MD measurements, including lactate, pyruvate, LP ratio, glucose, or glutamate. They postulate that both increased levels of tau and decreased anisotropy reflect traumatic axonal injury, but conclusions from this study are degraded by the long interval between the early post-acute microdialysis and the late MRI studies. Further studies have yet to be completed to determine the clinical significance of these findings [24].

Combining Invasive Monitoring and Noninvasive Imaging Techniques

Advances in positron emission tomography (PET) imaging capabilities have increased their applications in TBI, and at least three centers worldwide have PET installations located in or very near the neurocritical care unit. Nearby location of imaging equipment to the ICU allows studies in acute and subacute TBI patients, leading researchers to investigate the validity of direct, noninvasive, regional measures of brain metabolism. For example, the cerebral metabolic rate for oxygen ($CMRO_2$) can be measured using oxygen-15 positron emission tomography (^{15}O-PET) and hydrogen-1 magnetic resonance spectroscopy (1H-MRS) to evaluate metabolism in controls and in injured and peri-contusional brain after removal of acute subdural hematoma. In the same patient, regional cerebral blood flow and glucose utilization can be mapped regionally [25]. These evolving imaging modalities thus allow in-depth, noninvasive investigation into traumatic brain injury, demonstrating the metabolic effects of diffuse axonal injury, contusions, and subdural hematoma. In general, severe TBI reduces brain oxygen consumption by around 40%. In some patients this occurs with simultaneous increase in glucose utilization, especially under acute subdural hematomas. Post-TBI hyperglycolysis has led to treatment strategies using lactate and ketones as "alternate brain fuels" to allow more effective alternate pathways into the Krebs cycle for aerobic metabolism [26, 27].

Perilesional neurons, including those under subdural hematomas, have increased vulnerability to mitochondrial impairment, as demonstrated by lesser increase in pB_tO_2 when compared with normal areas demonstrating unimpaired regional cerebral blood flow [28]. A reduction in N-acetylaspartate (NAA) peaks, as shown by MRS or microdialysis, indicates dysfunction or loss of normal neural tissue and has been noted peripheral to contusions [29, 30]. Insufficient oxygen delivery with maximum oxygen extraction results in ischemia, characterized by a large oxygen extraction fraction (OEF), and low $CMRO_2$ (as demonstrated by PET) [31, 32].

In a group of 35 TBI patients undergoing MRI, ^{15}O-PET images were also obtained on 4 patients. PET measurements demonstrated a decrease in cerebral blood flow (CBF), cerebral blood volume (CBV), and OEF surrounding the contusions. Comparing these findings with apparent diffusion coefficient (ADC) MRI sequences, the reductions were present outside the peri-contusional edema and included areas with reduced ADC coefficients representing presumed cytotoxic edema. These findings suggest the potential salvageable nature of the perilesional tissue [33]. This argues in favor of strategies such as hyperoxia (see later).

Nortje et al. conducted a prospective trial investigating the effects of hyperoxia on cerebral MD, pB_tO_2, and ^{15}O-PET in 11 patients with severe TBI [34]. Hyperoxia did increase the mean pB_tO_2 (from 28 to 57 mmHg), but this did not directly translate into a change in MD lactate or pyruvate levels. Microdialysis measurements of lactate and pyruvate did not significantly change. The LP ratio was minimally decreased, which was statistically significant, but likely not clinically relevant. Initial ^{15}O-PET images were obtained at baseline FiO_2 (0.35–0.5), followed by

an increase in FiO_2 (0.6–0.8) for a median time of 50 min before repeating the ^{15}O-PET. Several parameters were evaluated for focal and global regions of interest (ROI), including CBV, CBF, $CMRO_2$, and OEF. $CMRO_2$ was significantly increased in the focal ROI in patients after undergoing hyperoxia, which may indicate a metabolic benefit in at-risk tissue. The volume of the "at-risk" tissue was significantly decreased, by 10–50 mL in some patients, with hyperoxia. The time period of hyperoxia, as well as the change in FiO_2, was relatively short and not constant between patients. This was a small study, and therefore it is difficult to generalize the results, especially in regard to neurologic outcomes [34].

Another small study investigating the effects of hyperoxia on brain oxygen metabolism included five patients undergoing PET with baseline oxygenation and after an hour of 100% FiO_2. Measurements of CBF, CBV, OEF, and $CMRO_2$ were performed and were not significantly different after hyperoxia, despite an increase in the PaO_2 from 117 to 371 [5].

In summary, although hyperoxia has been demonstrated to increase pB_tO_2, this does not equate to an increase in cerebral oxygen utilization, as revealed by recent PET studies. pB_tO_2 changes can be observed shortly after changes in FiO_2, while changes in metabolites (as measured by MD) or $CMRO_2$ may lag behind [6]. This may suggest an effect on mitochondrial metabolism, such as protein induction, that requires many minutes or hours to become established, rather than an enzyme activity rate increase. However, detailed determination of the molecular basis of these post-TBI changes has not been performed in animal models or TBI humans to our knowledge.

Recent and Future Laboratory and Clinical Trials: Hyperbaric Hyperoxia

Several studies have been completed examining cognitive function after TBI in rat models. One such rat study, using a fluid percussion TBI model, documented a decrease in cerebral edema on MRI. HBO therapy was applied for 1 h every day for 2 weeks. There was significantly higher water content, or cerebral edema, in both TBI and TBI treated with HBO therapy groups compared with the control rats. The TBI rats treated with HBO therapy had a statistically significant reduction in the edema at 24 and 48 h after injury when compared with the untreated TBI group. They also demonstrated a functional improvement in water maze testing [35]. This argues in favor of a putative effect of hyperoxia on metabolism, which in turn may assist in clearance of cytotoxic intracellular edema in the treated group.

To support this hypothesis, another study comparing normobaric normoxia (30% FiO_2), normobaric hyperoxia (100% FiO_2), and hyperbaric hyperoxia treatments for 4 h after fluid percussion injury revealed higher levels of adenosine triphosphate (ATP) in both the normobaric hyperoxia and hyperbaric hyperoxia groups. There was a significant improvement in water maze testing, as well as decreased hippocampal neuronal loss, in the hyperbaric hyperoxia group when compared with the normobaric normoxia or normobaric hyperoxia groups [36].

Recently, an examination of inflammatory markers and neurological outcomes was performed on rats undergoing modified Feeney's free-fall brain injury model. HBO significantly inhibited the TLR4/NFkB signaling pathway with reduced expression of TNFα (alpha), IL-6, and IL-1β (beta). Also examined were histological slices of brain tissue that demonstrated decreased neuronal apoptosis in the HBO group. Neurological tests were performed at 12 and 24 h, with improved testing in the HBO group [37]. Overall, the rat studies suggest decreased cerebral edema and neuronal loss with an improvement in neurologic outcomes in rats undergoing hyperbaric oxygen treatment after TBI.

Limited investigation in five normal patients using single-photon emission computed tomography (SPECT) with 99^{m}Tc-d,l-hexamethylpropylene-amine oxime (HMPAO) investigated changes in regional cerebral blood flow. The marker was injected after 40 min of exposure to normoxia or HBO—100% FiO_2 at 2.5 atmospheres absolute (ATA)—and regional blood flow was assessed. A preferential increase in CBF was seen in the left hemisphere, specifically, in the superior frontal, ventral premotor, parietal, and middle temporal cortices. Together, these areas comprise the dorsal attention system (DAS) [38]. A second attention system, the default mode network (DMN), including areas of the prefrontal, posterior cingulate, and middle temporal cortices, had a detectable increase in rCBF. Recent TBI work has suggested that the DMN may be vulnerable in brain injury, with decreased volumes after TBI, and may also be reflective of level of consciousness. Also noted was a regional hypoperfusion in the nondominant hemisphere, including the cingulate, hippocampal, temporal, and insular cortices as well as the basal ganglia, which may be related to selectively increased CBF to the dominant hemisphere.

Rockswold et al. conducted several prospective, randomized phase I and II trials comparing hyperbaric hyperoxia (HBO) with normobaric hyperoxia (NBO) or standard treatment in severe TBI patients. In the first trial, patients with severe TBI (mean GCS 5.7) were randomized within 24 h to either HBO with 60 min of HBO at 1.5 ATA (26 patients), NBO with 3 h of 100% FiO_2 at 1.0ATA (21 patients), or standard care (variable FiO_2, 22 patients). HBO and NBO treatments were performed for 3 days, at 24-h intervals. Of note, to decrease the known risk of inner ear damage from the HBO treatment, all patients in the HBO treatment group underwent bilateral myringotomies [39]. Intracranial pressure, pB_tO_2, and MD values for lactate, pyruvate, glucose, and glycerol were monitored and recorded. CBF was significantly elevated in the HBO group and was not significantly changed in the NBO or standard treatment groups. When evaluating $CMRO_2$ response, there was no significant change overall; however, when broken down to evaluate patients who began with a low or normal CBF, the $CMRO_2$ did significantly increase in both the HBO and NBO groups, but not the standard treatment group. Both the NBO and HBO groups demonstrated a decrease in cerebrospinal fluid (CSF) lactate, but only the HBO group revealed a decrease in MD lactate levels and LP ratio. Patients in the HBO group experienced a decrease in ICP, which was maintained until the next treatment.

In the phase II trial, HBO and NBO treatments were combined and compared with standard treatment. Twenty patients underwent combined HBO/NBO treatment, consisting of 60 min of HBO at 1.5 ATA followed by 3 h of 100% FiO_2 at 1.0 ATA, and 22 patients were treated with standard care. Similar findings to the preliminary study included a reduction in ICP in the HBO/NBO group compared with standard treatment, as well as decreased lactate and LP ratios. Mortality was significantly lower in the HBO/NBO group (16%) as compared with standard care (42%). Using the Glasgow Outcome Scale (GOS) at 6 months, more patients in the HBO/NBO group had a favorable outcome (74%) when compared with standard care (38%) [40].

The hyperbaric oxygen brain injury treatment (HOBIT) trial is poised to evaluate the optimal treatment model, comparing standard treatment with varied combinations of HBO with or without NBO. Hyperbaric treatment options will include different atmospheric pressures (from 1.5 to 2.5 ATA), at different frequencies (once or twice daily), with or without concurrent normobaric hyperoxia for 5 days.

Conclusions

In conclusion, many of the data regarding brain tissue oxygen monitoring and directed management are still controversial, yet a collage of evidence from various techniques in TBI humans and animal models suggests the strong possibility of biological effect, and possible benefit, from hyperoxia. Recent studies with newer techniques such as MD, PET, and MRS highlight the potential benefits and relative safety of hyperbaric oxygen treatment for severely injured TBI patients. Hopefully the HOBIT trial, if funded, with its modern multicenter design, will clarify the value of hyperoxia.

It is extremely clear, however, that hypoxia and reduced oxygen delivery to the injured brain, even when brief and transient, result in worsened outcomes and increased death of neurons after

TBI [41]. Modern neurocritical care for severe TBI is thus based upon delivery of adequate oxygenation to the injured brain, more than any other single fundamental principle.

References

1. Gerber LM, Chiu YL, Carney N, Hartl R, Ghajar J. Marked reduction in mortality in patients with severe traumatic brain injury. J Neurosurg. 2013;119(6):1583–90.
2. Lawrence T, Helmy A, Bouamra O, Woodford M, Lecky F, Hutchinson PJ. Traumatic brain injury in England and Wales: prospective audit of epidemiology, complications and standardised mortality. BMJ Open. 2016;6(11):e012197.
3. Corrigan F, Mander KA, Leonard AV, Vink R. Neurogenic inflammation after traumatic brain injury and its potentiation of classical inflammation. J Neuroinflammation. 2016;13(1):264.
4. Yonutas HM, Vekaria HJ, Sullivan PG. Mitochondrial specific therapeutic targets following brain injury. Brain Res. 2016;1640(Pt A):77–93.
5. Diringer MN, Aiyagari V, Zazulia AR, Videen TO, Powers WJ. Effect of hyperoxia on cerebral metabolic rate for oxygen measured using positron emission tomography in patients with acute severe head injury. J Neurosurg. 2007;106(4):526–9.
6. Diringer MN. Hyperoxia: good or bad for the injured brain? Curr Opin Crit Care. 2008;14(2):167–71.
7. Lin CM, Lin MC, Huang SJ, Chang CK, Chao DP, Lui TN, et al. A prospective randomized study of brain tissue oxygen pressure-guided management in moderate and severe traumatic brain injury patients. Biomed Res Int. 2015;2015:529580.
8. Valadka AB, Gopinath SP, Contant CF, Uzura M, Robertson CS. Relationship of brain tissue po2 to outcome after severe head injury. Crit Care Med. 1998;26(9):1576–81.
9. Carney N, Totten AM, O'Reilly C, Ullman JS, Hawryluk GW, Bell MJ, et al. Guidelines for the management of severe traumatic brain injury, fourth edition. Neurosurgery. 2016;80(1):6–15.
10. Haddad SH, Arabi YM. Critical care management of severe traumatic brain injury in adults. Scand J Trauma Resusc Emerg Med. 2012;20:12.
11. Jallo J, Loftus CM. Neurotrauma and critical care of the brain. New York: Thieme; 2009.
12. Demchenko IT, Welty-Wolf KE, Allen BW, Piantadosi CA. Similar but not the same: normobaric and hyperbaric pulmonary oxygen toxicity, the role of nitric oxide. Am J Physiol Lung Cell Mol Physiol. 2007;293(1):L229–38.

13. Schaal S, Beiran I, Rubinstein I, Miller B, Dovrat A. Lenticular oxygen toxicity. Invest Ophthalmol Vis Sci. 2003;44(8):3476–84.

14. Rincon F, Kang J, Vibbert M, Urtecho J, Athar MK, Jallo J. Significance of arterial hyperoxia and relationship with case fatality in traumatic brain injury: a multicentre cohort study. J Neurol Neurosurg Psychiatry. 2014;85(7):799–805.

15. Wang CH, Huang CH, Chang WT, Tsai MS, Lu TC, Yu PH, et al. Association between early arterial blood gas tensions and neurological outcome in adult patients following in-hospital cardiac arrest. Resuscitation. 2015;89:1–7.

16. Plafki C, Peters P, Almeling M, Welslau W, Busch R. Complications and side effects of hyperbaric oxygen therapy. Aviat Space Environ Med. 2000;71(2):119–24.

17. Menzel M, Doppenberg EM, Zauner A, Soukup J, Reinert MM, Bullock R. Increased inspired oxygen concentration as a factor in improved brain tissue oxygenation and tissue lactate levels after severe human head injury. J Neurosurg. 1999;91(1): 1–10.

18. Magnoni S, Ghisoni L, Locatelli M, Caimi M, Colombo A, Valeriani V, et al. Lack of improvement in cerebral metabolism after hyperoxia in severe head injury: a microdialysis study. J Neurosurg. 2003;98(5):952–8.

19. Figaji AA, Fieggen AG, Argent AC, Leroux PD, Peter JC. Does adherence to treatment targets in children with severe traumatic brain injury avoid brain hypoxia? A brain tissue oxygenation study. Neurosurgery. 2008;63(1):83–91; discussion 91–82.

20. Longhi L, Pagan F, Valeriani V, Magnoni S, Zanier ER, Conte V, et al. Monitoring brain tissue oxygen tension in brain-injured patients reveals hypoxic episodes in normal-appearing and in peri-focal tissue. Intensive Care Med. 2007;33(12):2136–42.

21. Hlatky R, Valadka AB, Goodman JC, Contant CF, Robertson CS. Patterns of energy substrates during ischemia measured in the brain by microdialysis. J Neurotrauma. 2004;21(7):894–906.

22. Stahl N, Mellergard P, Hallstrom A, Ungerstedt U, Nordstrom CH. Intracerebral microdialysis and bedside biochemical analysis in patients with fatal traumatic brain lesions. Acta Anaesthesiol Scand. 2001;45(8):977–85.

23. Nordstrom CH, Nielsen TH, Schalen W, Reinstrup P, Ungerstedt U. Biochemical indications of cerebral ischaemia and mitochondrial dysfunction in severe brain trauma analysed with regard to type of lesion. Acta Neurochir. 2016;158(7):1231–40.

24. Magnoni S, Mac Donald CL, Esparza TJ, Conte V, Sorrell J, Macri M, et al. Quantitative assessments of traumatic axonal injury in human brain: concordance of microdialysis and advanced MRI. Brain. 2015;138(Pt 8):2263–77.

25. Vespa P, Bergsneider M, Hattori N, Wu HM, Huang SC, Martin NA, et al. Metabolic crisis without brain ischemia is common after traumatic brain injury: a combined microdialysis and positron emission tomography study. J Cereb Blood Flow Metab. 2005;25(6):763–74.

26. Bergsneider M, Hovda DA, Shalmon E, Kelly DF, Vespa PM, Martin NA, et al. Cerebral hyperglycolysis following severe traumatic brain injury in humans: a positron emission tomography study. J Neurosurg. 1997;86(2):241–51.

27. Glenn TC, Kelly DF, Boscardin WJ, McArthur DL, Vespa P, Oertel M, et al. Energy dysfunction as a predictor of outcome after moderate or severe head injury: indices of oxygen, glucose, and lactate metabolism. J Cereb Blood Flow Metab. 2003;23(10):1239–50.

28. Tolias CM, Kumaria A, Bullock MR. Hyperoxia and traumatic brain injury. J Neurosurg. 2009;110(3):607–9; author reply 609–611.

29. Kubas B, Lebkowski W, Lebkowska U, Kulak W, Tarasow E, Walecki J. Proton MR spectroscopy in mild traumatic brain injury. Pol J Radiol. 2010;75(4):7–10.

30. Horska A, Barker PB. Imaging of brain tumors: MR spectroscopy and metabolic imaging. Neuroimaging Clin N Am. 2010;20(3):293–310.

31. Ghosh A, Highton D, Kolyva C, Tachtsidis I, Elwell CE, Smith M. Hyperoxia results in increased aerobic metabolism following acute brain injury. J Cereb Blood Flow Metab. 2016;37(8):2910–20.

32. Coles JP, Fryer TD, Smielewski P, Rice K, Clark JC, Pickard JD, et al. Defining ischemic burden after traumatic brain injury using 15O pet imaging of cerebral physiology. J Cereb Blood Flow Metab. 2004;24(2):191–201.

33. Newcombe VF, Williams GB, Outtrim JG, Chatfield D, Gulia Abate M, Geeraerts T, et al. Microstructural basis of contusion expansion in traumatic brain injury: insights from diffusion tensor imaging. J Cereb Blood Flow Metab. 2013;33(6):855–62.

34. Nortje J, Coles JP, Timofeev I, Fryer TD, Aigbirhio FI, Smielewski P, et al. Effect of hyperoxia on regional oxygenation and metabolism after severe traumatic brain injury: preliminary findings. Crit Care Med. 2008;36(1):273–81.

35. Liu S, Liu Y, Deng S, Guo A, Wang X, Shen G. Beneficial effects of hyperbaric oxygen on edema in rat hippocampus following traumatic brain injury. Exp Brain Res. 2015;233(12):3359–65.

36. Zhou Z, Daugherty WP, Sun D, Levasseur JE, Altememi N, Hamm RJ, et al. Protection of mitochondrial function and improvement in cognitive recovery in rats treated with hyperbaric oxygen following lateral fluid-percussion injury. J Neurosurg. 2007;106(4):687–94.

37. Meng XE, Zhang Y, Li N, Fan DF, Yang C, Li H, et al. Hyperbaric oxygen alleviates secondary brain injury after trauma through inhibition of Tlr4/nf-kappab signaling pathway. Med Sci Monit. 2016;22:284–8.

38. Micarelli A, Jacobsson H, Larsson SA, Jonsson C, Pagani M. Neurobiological insight into hyperbaric hyperoxia. Acta Physiol (Oxf). 2013;209(1):69–76.

39. Rockswold SB, Rockswold GL, Zaun DA, Zhang X, Cerra CE, Bergman TA, et al. A prospective, randomized clinical trial to compare the effect of hyperbaric to normobaric hyperoxia on cerebral metabolism, intracranial pressure, and oxygen toxicity in severe traumatic brain injury. J Neurosurg. 2010;112(5):1080–94.

40. Rockswold SB, Rockswold GL, Zaun DA, Liu J. A prospective, randomized phase ii clinical trial to evaluate the effect of combined hyperbaric and normobaric hyperoxia on cerebral metabolism, intracranial pressure, oxygen toxicity, and clinical outcome in severe traumatic brain injury. J Neurosurg. 2013;118(6):1317–28.

41. Graham DI, Ford I, Adams JH, Doyle D, Teasdale GM, Lawrence AE, et al. Ischaemic brain damage is still common in fatal non-missile head injury. J Neurol Neurosurg Psychiatry. 1989;52(3):346–50.

What Is the Optimal Sedative Regimen in Severe Traumatic Brain Injury Patients?

Bradley A. Boucher

Sedative Indications in Patients with Severe Traumatic Brain Injury

Sedatives are commonly used in the acute management of patients with severe TBI. General indications for use of sedatives in critically ill patients include control of anxiety, pain, agitation, and ventilation management. The latter indication is particularly important in TBI patients to prevent hypoxia and hypercapnia, which may worsen the brain injury secondarily. Specific indications in severe TBI patients include management of intracranial pressure (ICP), seizures, and temperature control and reduction of cerebral metabolic demand [1]. Optimization of cerebral metabolic rate ($CMRO_2$) and cerebral blood flow (CBF) is also a priority [2].

The ideal sedative in TBI patients would be effective in producing high-quality, consistent sedation, have a rapid onset and offset of action with no accumulation of active metabolites, and have no systemic side effects [3]. Moreover, the ideal sedative would reduce $CMRO_2$, CBF, and ICP and reduce seizure activity [3]. Unfortunately, no agent meets all of these demands. Furthermore, a comprehensive review of the randomized clinical trials evaluating sedative use in severe TBI patients was conducted

in 2011 [4]. This systematic review concluded that no single sedative agent has been demonstrated to have clear superiority over another in TBI. This conclusion is complicated, however, by the paucity of randomized, controlled, comparative trials in critically ill patients in general [4]. In addition, sedatives are often used in combination making the study of a single agent difficult in TBI patients. As such, selection of agents is primarily based on extrapolation of the differential effects on cerebral and systemic hemodynamics, pharmacodynamic and pharmacokinetic properties, and side effects in other critically ill patient subsets. Avoidance of hypotension, which is a common side effect with many of these agents, is particularly important based on its strong association with poor outcomes in TBI patients [5]. Balancing beneficial effects versus attenuating neurologic dysfunction and development of complications remains some of the biggest challenges in the use of these central nervous system (CNS)-acting agents in TBI patients [1].

Pharmacodynamic, Pharmacokinetic Poperties and Side Effect Profile of Sedatives Commonly Used in TBI Patients

Propofol

Propofol is a highly lipophilic, γ(gamma)-aminobutyric acid (GABA) receptor agonist formu-

B. A. Boucher, PharmD, FCCP, FNAP, MCCM, BCPS
Department of Clinical Pharmacy and Translational Science, College of Pharmacy,
University of Tennessee Health Science Center,
Memphis, TN, USA
e-mail: bboucher@uthsc.edu

© Springer International Publishing AG, part of Springer Nature 2018
S. D. Timmons (ed.), *Controversies in Severe Traumatic Brain Injury Management*,
https://doi.org/10.1007/978-3-319-89477-5_6

lated as an oil-in-water emulsion [6]. It is also available as a phosphorylated prodrug known as fos-propofol that does not have a lipid vehicle [6]. GABA$_A$ receptors are located on neurons throughout the CNS modulating chloride channel opening [6]. In addition to its dose-dependent sedative, hypnotic, and amnestic properties, propofol has also been demonstrated to have anticonvulsant properties including control of status epilepticus [7]. Pharmacologic properties include decreased ICP, decreased cerebral metabolic rate oxygen (CMRO$_2$), and decreased cerebral electrical activity. Propofol may also have neuroprotective effects by limiting oxidative stress [2]. Since its approval in 1986, propofol has historically become one of the most popular sedatives used in severe TBI patients, largely because of its ability to readily cross the blood-brain barrier, resulting in a very rapid onset and short offset. This pharmacokinetic profile is ideal in severe TBI patients to allow for an accurate neurological assessment shortly after its discontinuation. Elimination is largely independent of both renal and hepatic functions, i.e., liver conjugation to inactive glucuronide and sulfate metabolites that are eliminated by the kidneys [6, 8]. Side effects include decreases in mean arterial pressure (MAP) and cerebral perfusion pressure (CPP), which may be detrimental in severe TBI patients, especially in patients with loss of autoregulation of CBF. Other side effects are increases in serum triglycerides and caloric intake (1.1 kcal/mL) because of its lipid vehicle [8]. A potentially life-threatening event with administration of propofol is known as the propofol infusion syndrome (PRIS) with signs including bradycardia, acidosis, lactatemia, elevated creatinine phosphokinase, and myocardial failure [9]. Furthermore, PRIS may be common in TBI patients [10]. Among numerous risk factors are doses exceeding 4–5 mg/kg/h, prolonged infusions, and concomitant use of therapeutic hypothermia [9, 11, 12].

While early animal studies suggested a neuroprotective role for propofol after TBI, and it has clearly become the mainstay of sedation in TBI, concerns from subsequent animal studies have surfaced concerning the potential neurotoxicity of propofol following TBI. Two recent TBI rodent studies have demonstrated worse outcomes—i.e., apoptotic cell and neuronal cell death and 28-day mortality—in animals receiving propofol compared with unsedated controls [13, 14]. The proposed mechanism for the worsened outcomes relates to expression of the p75 neurotropin receptor and upregulation of the precursor of brain-derived neurotrophic factor, thereby impairing neurogenesis [13]. Noteworthy is that in one animal study, propofol was administered as a single 10 mg/kg intravenous (IV) dose 24 h after TBI [13], while a high-dose infusion (36 and 72 mg/kg/h) was used in the other animal study without a control group [14]. Impairment of neutrophil and macrophage function may be yet another potential adverse consequence of propofol [15]. Propofol's lipid vehicle may be responsible for its immunosuppressant effects [8].

In a prospective clinical investigation in moderate TBI patients requiring mechanical ventilation, propofol was significantly associated with adrenal insufficiency compared to patients receiving mechanical ventilation alone [16]. Lastly, a recent editorial issued an "urgent" call for randomized clinical trials of propofol to alternative sedatives following discovery of a potential statistical error in a landmark study questioning its beneficial effects in moderate to severe TBI patients receiving propofol and morphine compared to a group of patients receiving morphine alone [17]. The latter study has been widely cited and contributed to the Level II recommendation for propofol in controlling ICP in TBI patients within the most recent TBI management guidelines [18, 19]. While these reports will likely not alter propofol use as a first-line sedative therapy in TBI patients in the short term, a paradigm shift may eventually occur to using sedatives with more favorable side effect profiles as new medications become available and existing ones undergo further study.

Benzodiazepines

For decades, benzodiazepines have been a mainstay of therapy for sedation in critically ill patients because of their potent anxiolytic, hypnotic, and anticonvulsant effects. As a sedative class, benzodiazepines tend to lower CBF, cerebral metabolic rate of oxygen ($CRMO_2$), and ICP in addition to raising the seizure threshold [2]. The pharmacologic effects of benzodiazepines occur via dose-dependent augmentation of GABA at the $GABA_A$ receptors as well as stimulation of κ(kappa) receptors in the CNS [2]. While sharing pharmacologic properties, the benzodiazepines commonly used in TBI patients—i.e., midazolam and lorazepam—vary significantly in their physiochemical prop-

erties (see Tables 1 and 2) [2, 3, 6, 20]. These differences result in substantially different pharmacokinetic properties including onset and offset. For example, midazolam has a much shorter effective half-life and more rapid onset and offset than lorazepam and diazepam due to the high lipid solubility at physiologic pH of the parent compound [2, 6]. Because of its rapid onset, midazolam may be administered as an IV bolus but is more commonly administered as a

Table 1 Summary of pharmacology and safety of sedatives used in TBI patients[a] [2, 3, 6]

Sedative	Receptor pharmacology	CBF^b	$CMRO_2{}^b$	ICP^b	MAP^b	Other effects	Side effects
Propofol	$GABA_A$ agonist	↓	↓	↓	↓	Raise seizure threshold Neuroprotection (?) Neurotoxicity (?) Neutrophil, macrophage impairment (?) Adrenal suppression No significant drug interactions	Respiratory suppression PRIS Lipid vehicle: ↑ TGs, calories
Midazolam	$GABA_A$, κ(kappa) agonist	↓	↓	↓	↓	Raise seizure threshold	Respiratory/cough suppression Tolerance/ withdrawal Delirium
Lorazepam	$GABA_A$, κ(kappa) agonist	↓	↓	↓	↓	Raise seizure threshold	Respiratory/cough suppression Tolerance/ withdrawal Delirium Propylene glycol toxicity (↓ renal function, long-term infusions)
Morphine	μ(mu)$_1$, μ(mu)$_2$, κ(kappa) ε(epsilon), Δ(Delta) agonist	↔	↔	↓ ↑	$(↓)^c$	Analgesia	Respiratory/cough suppression ↓ GI motility Histamine release
Fentanyl	μ(mu)$_1$, μ(mu)$_2$, κ(kappa) ε(epsilon), Δ(Delta) agonist	↔	↔	↓ ↑	$(↓)^c$	Analgesia	Respiratory/cough suppression ↓ GI motility
Sufentanil	μ(mu)$_1$, μ(mu)$_2$, κ(kappa) ε(epsilon), Δ(Delta) agonist	↔	↔	↓ ↑	$(↓)^c$	Analgesia	Respiratory/cough suppression ↓ GI motility

(continued)

Table 1 (continued)

Sedative	Receptor pharmacology	CBF[b]	CMRO$_2$[b]	ICP[b]	MAP[b]	Other effects	Side effects
Remifentanil	μ(mu)$_1$, μ(mu)$_2$, κ(kappa) ε(epsilon), Δ(Delta) agonist	↔	↔	↓ ↑	(↓)[c]	Unique non-hepatic metabolism	Respiratory/cough suppression ↓ GI motility
Dexmedetomidine	Central α(alpha)$_2$ agonist	↓	↔	↓	↓	Minimal respiratory depression Opiate-sparing effects Loading doses associated with hypotension, bradycardia Neuroprotective (?) Neurotoxicity (?)	
Pentobarbital	GABA$_A$ agonist AMPA antagonist	↓	↓	↓	↓	Raise seizure threshold Immunosuppression	GI hypermotility Hepatic enzyme induction
Ketamine	NMDA antagonist	↑	↑	↑	↑↔[d]	Lower seizure threshold Neuroprotective (?)	Hallucinations, delirium, Emergence phenomenon ↑ salivation, ↑ lacrimation, ↑ myocardial O$_2$ demand
Etomidate	GABA$_A$ agonist	↓	↓	↓	↓	Lower seizure threshold	Adrenal suppression Propylene glycol toxicity (↓ renal function, long-term infusions)

[a]*GABA* γ(gamma)-aminobutyric acid, *AMPA* α(alpha)-amino-3-hydroxy-5-methyl-4-isoxazolepropionic acid, *NMDA* N-methyl-D-aspartate, *PRIS* propofol infusion syndrome, *TGs* triglycerides
[b]*CBF* cerebral blood flow, *CMRO$_2$* cerebral metabolic rate, *ICP* intracranial pressure, *MAP* mean arterial pressure. CBF and CMRO$_2$ ceiling effect for opioids and benzodiazepines
[c]Rapid infusions, large opioid doses may reduce MAP, CPP
[d]High ketamine doses may reduce MAP

continuous infusion. Consequently, due to accumulation of active metabolites, midazolam's effects may be significantly prolonged when given in high dosage for protracted infusion periods. The benzodiazepines differ in their metabolism by the liver, with diazepam and midazolam undergoing cytochrome P450 (CYP) enzyme system with lorazepam being conjugated to a glucuronide metabolite. As such, the latter may be less susceptible to drug interactions with other drugs metabolized by the CYP enzymes [6]. Both diazepam and midazolam have active metabolites that are primarily eliminated by the kidneys as is the inactive lorazepam glucuronide metabolite. Lorazepam has a unique potential problem related to accumulation of its formulation vehicle, propylene glycol, which is used as a diluent. Propylene glycol toxicity primarily manifests as a metabolic acidosis with an elevated osmolar gap and renal dysfunction. This typically occurs in patients receiving high-dose lorazepam infu-

Table 2 Selected pharmacokinetics of sedatives used in TBI patients[a] [2, 3, 6, 20]

Sedative	Bolus dose onset (minutes)	Dosage	Elimination $t_{1/2}$	Active metabolites	Effect of end-stage liver disease
Propofol	1–2	5–50 µg/kg/min (0.3–3 mg/kg/h)	3–12 h (short term) 50 h (long term)	–	None
Midazolam	2–5	0.02–0.1 mg/kg/h	3–11 h	+	Major
Lorazepam	15–20	0.01–0.1 mg/kg/h	8–15 h	–	Major
Morphine	5–10	2–4 mg q1–2 h	3–4 h	+	Major
Fentanyl	1–2	0.7–10 µg/kg/h	2–4 h	–	Major
Sufentanil	5	4 µg/kg (induction)	2.2 h	–	Major
Remifentanil	1–3	0.5–15 µg/kg/h	3–10 min	–	None
Dexmedetomidine	5–10	0.2–0.7 µg/kg/h	2 h	–	Major
Pentobarbital	20–60	30–40 mg/kg loading dose 1–2 mg/kg/h maintenance	11.7–19.6 h	–	Major
Ketamine	<1	2 mg/kg (induction) 50 µg/kg/min	2.6 h	+	No data
Etomidate	<1	0.2–0.4 mg/kg (induction)	4.8 h	–	Moderate

sions for extended periods, although may occur at lower dosages as well [6, 20].

While benzodiazepines generally have beneficial effects on ICP, they also have the potential to reduce mean arterial pressure (MAP) thereby lowering the CPP in TBI patients, especially when administered as bolus IV doses. In addition, benzodiazepines may induce respiratory depression that may compromise the ability to extubate TBI patients. While flumazenil can be used to reverse adverse effects of benzodiazepines, this agent should not be relied upon in TBI patients because of its potential to increase ICP and decrease CPP [3]. Tolerance and withdrawal symptoms upon abrupt discontinuation may also occur with prolonged infusion of benzodiazepines. While these side effects are important concerns in critically ill patients, the major controversy that exists with their use as sedatives relates to their association with delirium [21, 22]. Delirium (both hyperactive and hypoactive delirium) has received immense attention among critical care practitioners to the point of recognition as a "…major public health care problem…" [20] because of its associated increased mor-

bidity and mortality [23, 24]. Recognition of the association of benzodiazepines with delirium in critically ill patients resulted in a major reversal from benzodiazepines recommended as first-line therapy in the 2002 clinical practice guidelines published by the American College of Critical Care Medicine to use of analgesics followed by non-benzodiazepine sedatives in the 2013 clinical practice guidelines as first-line therapy [20, 25]. While the potential for delirium should be considered with the use of benzodiazepines in TBI patients by inference, discerning development of this complication independent of the underlying CNS in this subset of critically ill patients is extremely challenging since coma has been demonstrated as an independent risk factor for delirium development [21]. An additional challenge is that no delirium screening tools have been validated for TBI patients distinct from other critically ill patients [1]. Nonetheless, benzodiazepines play some role in the sedation of TBI patients presently lacking suitable alternatives, especially while patients are still in coma, but their use in TBI is limited, as for other critically ill patient subsets [26].

Opiate Narcotics

Opiates act a number of receptors including the $\mu(mu)_1$ (supraspinal analgesia), $\mu(mu)_2$ (ventilator depression, bradycardia), κ(kappa) (sedation, spinal analgesia), ϵ(epsilon) (dysphoria, hallucinations, respiratory stimulation), and Δ(Delta) (analgesia, behavioral effects, epileptogenic) [2, 8]. Stimulation of these receptors can result in desired pharmacologic effects but undesired adverse effects as well. Regardless, management of pain is essential in critically ill patients since inadequate analgesia may result in development of agitation [6]. Furthermore, while primarily used in critically ill patients for their analgesic properties, opiates also have significant sedative properties as well. This has resulted in the general recommendation for analgesic first sedation ("analgosedation") in mechanically ventilated intensive care unit (ICU) patients [20]. Opiate narcotics that are commonly used in TBI patients include morphine, fentanyl, sufentanil, and remifentanil (see Tables 1 and 2). All will provide analgesia at equipotent doses and the potential to decrease the use of non-opiate sedatives. However, the latter agents have advantages over morphine and hydromorphone based on their more rapid onset and offset. Prolonged sedation can occur with prolonged infusions, especially fentanyl [2]. Furthermore, all are metabolized to inactive metabolites, except morphine that is metabolized to an active metabolite, morphine-6-glucuronide, that can accumulate in patients with concurrent renal insufficiency. The opiate narcotic that has received the most attention in TBI patients in recent years is remifentanil based on its unique metabolism, i.e., hydrolysis by tissue and plasma esterases [2]. This property has the potential to diminish accumulation and sustain the rapid offset upon discontinuation of the remifentanil infusion facilitating neurological exam of the patient. Data include favorable comparisons to hypnotic-based regimens (i.e., propofol, midazolam) in a randomized clinical trial [27].

While suitable for monotherapy, in moderate to severe TBI patients, opiates are typically used in combination with the previously discussed sedative hypnotic agents (e.g., propofol, benzodiazepines, etc.). One major reason is the potential for hypotension secondary to a reduction in sympathetic tone in TBI patients receiving opiate narcotics, especially when given as high bolus doses and in patients with relative hypovolemia [2]. Hypotension may in turn have deleterious effect on ICP and CPP. Several comparative studies of opiate narcotics within class or other non-opiate sedatives have documented an increase in ICP in severe TBI patients [4]. In contrast, blunting of noxious stimuli by opiate analgesics may have a beneficial effect on preventing intracranial hypertension. One advantage of opiates over some of the other sedatives is the ability to reverse their activity with antagonists such as naloxone. While effective, use of reversal agents may have the deleterious effect of raising ICP in TBI patients. In summary, based upon the benefit-to-risk ratio, opiate narcotics will undoubtedly continue to have an adjunctive role in sedating TBI patients based on available studies to date.

Barbiturates

Among the oldest sedatives used in TBI patients are the barbiturates. In particular, pentobarbital has had a prominent role in managing patients with refractory elevations in ICP and status epilepticus, although it can be used in lower doses intermittently as a sedative. Pharmacologically, barbiturates work by stimulating GABA receptors and inhibiting α(alpha)-amino-3-hydroxy-5-methyl-4-isoxazolepropionic acid (AMPA) receptors [2]. Both effects produce dose-dependent sedation. Furthermore, pentobarbital may have a favorable effect on $CRMO_2$, thereby lowering ICP. Akin to propofol, pentobarbital is highly lipophilic, readily crosses the blood-brain barrier, and has a rapid onset of action. While pentobarbital has a rapid onset, it can accumulate with repeated doses or when given as an infusion. The result is the potential for a prolonged effective half-life, which may be unwelcome relative to performing a serial neurologic exam in TBI patients. This long duration of action is one major factor in pentobarbital being reserved for those TBI patients with refractory elevated ICP. The therapeutic goal for this indication is burst suppression on the electroencephalogram (EEG), which requires high pentobarbital loading doses (25–40 mg/kg) and maintenance doses beginning at 1–2 mg/kg/h thereafter [28]. In addition, monitoring of serum concentrations to attain concentrations of 20–40 mg/L is typically performed along with EEG monitoring. At these concentrations, pentobarbital may exhibit saturable metabolism prolonging its elimination even more. Consequently, upon discontinuation of the pentobarbital infusion, it may be several days before a neurological exam can be accurately performed, which is a major consideration before inducing a "pentobarbital coma" [2]. One of the other major side effects with pentobarbital that limits its utility in TBI is hypotension, with the potential to lower CPP and increase ICP to unacceptable values. A systematic review of the literature suggested that one of every four patients receiving barbiturate therapy will develop hypotension [29]. The hypotension is a consequence of direct myocardial and peripheral vasodilation [2]. Pentobarbital can also cause gastroparesis and hypokalemia that can lead to myocardial dysrhythmias, as wells as venous irritation mandating central IV administration. Extravasation can result in serious tissue damage. On emergence from coma, there may be a period of gastrointestinal (GI) hypermotility. Lastly, barbiturates are well-known inducers of hepatic enzymes that may affect the metabolism of other concomitant drugs. Despite these undesirable adverse effects, high-dose barbiturate administration has a Level II recommendation by the Brain Trauma Foundation to control elevated ICP refractory to maximum standard medical and surgical treatment in adults, because it is effective in doing so when other modalities have failed [18]. Initiation of barbiturate therapy withdrawal can occur when ICP has been controlled satisfactorily for 24–48 h. Barbiturates should be tapered over 24–72 h to prevent ICP spikes.

Ketamine

The pharmacologic effects of ketamine are a consequence of competitive antagonism of the glutamatergic N-methyl-D-aspartate (NMDA) receptor [6]. Blockade of the NMDA receptor also inhibits cellular influx of calcium, which coincidentally is generally considered to be a key pathophysiologic event in TBI patients. This mechanism of action is distinctly different than other sedatives commonly used in critically ill patients. Pharmacologic effects include amnesia, analgesia, and sedation. It may also have beneficial effects in patients with status epilepticus via blockage of the NMDA receptor. This effect is in contrast to other reports that ketamine may actually be epileptogenic [2]. Ketamine also induces a state of "dissociative anesthesia" in which non-comatose patients are conscious and maintain respiration and motor reflexes [6]. Other pharmacologic effects include increases in mean arterial pressure and heart rate as well as bronchodilation secondary to a stimulatory effect on the sympathetic nervous system. Furthermore, there are data suggesting that ketamine may have anti-inflammatory properties as well [6]. Ketamine is highly lipid soluble, which is responsible for a very rapid onset of action. It is metabolized in the liver via N-demethylation to the active metabolites norketamine and hydroxyl-norketamine that are subsequently renally eliminated [6]. The potential for accumulation of these active metabolites is thus a concern in patients with renal insufficiency.

Despite having several desirable pharmacologic effects relative to the CNS and cardiovascular system, ketamine use historically has been limited by its adverse drug reactions. Among the side effects are hallucinations, delirium, out-of-body experiences, and unpleasant flashbacks [6]. Other side effects include hypersalivation, lacrimation, and increased myocardial oxygen demand.

A major controversy related to the use of ketamine in TBI patients relates to its effect on ICP. Early reports suggested that ketamine was associated with an increase in ICP [1]. However, more recent data suggests that ketamine has a neutral effect on ICP and CPP [20]. For example, in a randomized study comparing TBI patients receiving sufentanil and midazolam versus ketamine and midazolam, no significant changes were observed in ICP or CPP between the two groups [30]. Further support for the use of ketamine emanates from a recent meta-analysis of 101 adult and 55 pediatric TBI patients that concluded that ketamine does not increase ICP in severe TBI patients and may actually lower ICP in selected cases [31]. These findings were corroborated by a second independent meta-analysis of five randomized studies of ketamine trials compared to opiates in 198 TBI patients. Thus, there is renewed interest in ketamine minimally as an induction agent, especially in hemodynamically unstable TBI patients versus alternative agents such as propofol or etomidate [32]. The potential for ketamine to be neuroprotective because of its antagonism of glutamate (widely accepted as an excitatory neurotoxin in TBI) patients is also intriguing [33]. Regardless, while evidence exists in animal studies of a neuroprotective effect with ketamine, improvement in outcome in humans following TBI is lacking [33]. As such, ketamine presently should be considered only as adjunctive to other sedatives in TBI patients. A more expanded role is possible in the future as further evidence emerges, but currently it is not in common usage.

Dexmedetomidine

Dexmedetomidine is a centrally acting, α(alpha)$_2$-adrenergic receptor agonist that has both sedating and anxiolytic, as well as analgesic/opiate-sparing properties [20]. While approved in the USA for only short-term use (<24 h) at a dose of 0.7 μg/kg/h, numerous studies have been performed with dexmedetomidine administered for longer durations and higher dosages (up to 1.5 μg/kg/h) without any significant adverse events [6]. Among its desirable therapeutic attributes is a relative lack of respiratory depression, which is relatively uncommon among the other sedative alternatives in critically ill patients [6]. This allows the dexmedetomidine infusion to be continued post-extubation. Critically ill patients are generally more arousable with the use of dexmedetomidine compared with other sedatives, although this is less well documented in TBI patients. Another favorable attribute of dexmedetomidine is its association with a lower prevalence of delirium compared to the benzodiazepines [20]. Metabolism of dexmedetomidine occurs in the liver by hydroxylation and N-glucuronidation to inactive metabolites [6]. Among the most concerning side effects with dexmedetomidine are its sympatholytic effects. This can lead to systemic hypotension and bradycardia [20]. Hypotension is particularly problematic when dexmedetomidine infusions are preceded by a loading dose [20]. As such, loading doses should be avoided in TBI patients receiving dexmedetomidine as a sedative. Dexmedetomidine can also cause xerostomia [6].

As the newest sedative available for general use in the critically ill patient, fewer randomized clinical trials are available for dexmedetomidine compared with other sedatives. This is particularly true for TBI patients. In a very small randomized, crossover, pilot study involving only eight patients (four TBI, three subarachnoid hemorrhage, one intracerebral hemorrhage), dexmedetomidine was equally effective in its sedating effects without any adverse physiologic systemic or cerebral effects [34]. Thereafter, a retrospective study of the hemodynamic effects of dexmedetomidine compared with propofol was conducted [35]. A total of 105 neurocritical care patients receiving dexmedetomidine were compared 1:1 with patients receiving propofol, matched based on propensity scoring of baseline characteristics. Most patients included in this two-center study were stroke patients with only approximately 5% TBI patients. No differences in the composite out of hypotension (mean arterial pressure <60 mmHg) and bradycardia (heart rate <50 beats/min) were observed between the two groups. More recently, a prospective observational single-center study of dexmedetomidine plus propofol ($N = 148$), dexmedetomidine only ($N = 222$), or propofol only ($N = 39$) was conducted in severe TBI patients [36]. The dexmedetomidine-only group significantly achieved the target sedation level compared with the other groups ($p = 0.001$). However, dexmedetomidine with or without propofol was also associated with a significantly higher incidence of hypotension ($p = 0.01$). The potential for dexmedetomidine as a neuroprotective agent is also being investigated with limited in vitro data supporting this hypothesis [37]. While dexmedetomidine holds promise as a potential first-line sedative in TBI patients, additional randomized clinical trials are needed before this practice can be advocated. This is particularly true in the absence of superiority trials with this unique sedative [38]. Additionally, effects on long-term outcome after TBI are totally unknown with this medication. Given its mechanism of action as an $\alpha(alpha)_2$-adrenergic receptor agonist, there are broad implications for cellular chemistry (specifically the effect of blocking alpha receptors on calcium transport and metabolism) and neuronal function (e.g., recovery from hypoxemia, firing, and plasticity); this is not an insignificant problem. (See also chapter "Oxygen Management and Prevention of Cerebral Ischemia".)

Etomidate

Etomidate is used primarily as an induction agent for rapid sequence intubation in patients with hemodynamic instability [2, 6]. Considering the importance of avoiding hypotension in TBI patients, etomidate therefore does have a potential role as a sedative in this patient subset akin to that of ketamine. Pharmacologically, etomidate is a $GABA_A$ receptor agonist with a rapid onset (1 min) and offset (10–15 min) of action secondary to its high lipid solubility [6]. Similar to the other sedatives used in critically ill patients, it is primarily metabolized by the liver [6]. Beneficial effects in TBI patients include maintenance of CPP with a decrease in ICP, CBF, and $CMRO_2$ [6]. Despite these potential advantages, etomidate has been associated with adrenal suppression through inhibition of 11-β(beta)-hydroxylase, which converts 11-deoxycortisol to cortisol [2]. This effect has been demonstrated with single dose as well as infusions [39]. Adrenocortical insufficiency thereafter has the potential to induce hypotension, which is one of the primary disadvantages to using etomidate in TBI patients [2]. Thus, while having a role as sedative in TBI patients, the risk-to-benefit ratio must be carefully weighed compared to alternative sedatives, e.g., ketamine. This includes not using etomidate as a continuous infusion [2].

Monitoring of Pain, Sedation, and Delirium in the Traumatic Brain Injury Patient

Inadequate analgesia is an important contributing factor to discomfort and agitation in critically ill patients. Thus, monitoring pain is an important mainstay in the management of critically ill patients. Since patients with moderate to severe TBI are unable to respond to questions regarding their level of comfort, use of the Behavioral Pain Scale (BPS) or the Critical-Care Pain Observation Tool (CPOT) has been advocated in these patients [40]. Other emerging tools that may have merit in severe TBI patients are the Nociception Coma Scale (NCS) [41] and the Nociception Coma Scale-Revised (NCS-R) [42].

Monitoring of sedation may be an even greater challenge than analgesia in TBI patients based on their underlying diminished levels of consciousness. Another important consideration is a body of evidence that uninterrupted sedation in critically ill patients is associated with worse outcomes [43]. Over time, this led to a paradigm shift in critical care medicine advocating daily interruption of sedation and maintenance of light levels of sedation when feasible [20, 44]. The practice of daily interruption has been challenged, however, based on more recent conflicting data [45]. Furthermore, these data apply to general critical care patients, and not TBI patients. In a study of 12 patients with severe TBI undergoing repeated awakening procedures, ICP increased from 13.4± 6 to 22.7 ± 12 mmHg (p <0.05) with a significant but modest increase in CPP from 75.6 ± 11 to 79.1 ± 21 mmHg (p <0.05) [46]. The risks of daily sedation interruption were corroborated in a study of 20 severe TBI patients including cessation in one-third of the daily interruption trials due to a significant increase in ICP [47]. However, these were very small studies without significantly adverse changes in physiological parameters, and the goals of ICU observation of severe

TBI patients often encompass frequent (hourly) neurological checks, which require at least temporary cessation of sedation to glean an accurate examination. This is one reason that propofol is in such wide usage in this patient population.

Numerous sedation-monitoring scales have been developed, although the Richmond Agitation-Sedation Scale (RASS) and Sedation-Agitation Scale (SAS) have been deemed to be the most valid and reliable tools for assessing quality and depth of sedation in critically ill patients [20]. Unfortunately, much of the clinical research related to sedation in critically ill patients has been derived in medical and surgical ICU patients, making evaluation of pain and sedation particularly problematic in TBI patients. Nonetheless, a recent consensus statement provides some degree of confidence relative to the utility of the RASS and SAS in TBI patients along with conventional neurologic assessment tools, e.g., Glasgow Coma Scale and Full Outline of Unresponsiveness (FOUR) score [40]. Further complicating evaluation of TBI patients is the use of neuromuscular blocking agents, which would essentially invalidate the motor elements of the RASS and SAS, as well as the presence of speech, motor, and sensory deficits. In these patients or patients in a deeply sedated state, the utility of electroencephalogram monitoring has been suggested including the bispectral index monitoring [1]. Nevertheless, validation of this latter technique in TBI patients and other critically ill patients is not particularly robust [6].

Delirium is yet another challenging issue to discern in TBI patients. Inherently, delirium—defined as a disturbance of consciousness and impaired cognitive functioning—will be layered upon an already disturbed underlying pathology in neurologically injured patients. The screening tool most often advocated for delirium in other unresponsive critically ill patients is known as the Intensive Care Delirium Screening Checklist (ICDSC) [48]. However, attributing delirium to sedative use, in particular the use of benzodiazepines, is often impossible to do in severe and some moderate TBI patients.

Considering the major obstacles facing clinical investigators related to evaluating pain, seda-tion, and delirium in neurologically critically ill patient monitoring, it is not surprising that there is a dearth of data available. Nonetheless, an ambitious prospective study was conducted in three centers to assess the feasibility and reliability of pain and sedation scales in 151 neuro-critical care patients [49]. Unfortunately, only 26 TBI patients were included in the study, with the majority of the patients having intracerebral or subarachnoid hemorrhages. Screening for delirium also occurred. Overall findings were that pain and sedation could be routinely evaluated in neurocritical care patients using tools designed for other critical care patient populations (e.g., BPS, RASS, etc.). Delirium could also be evaluated in the majority of the patients, although it required the patients to be sufficiently alert. This resulted in no evaluation for delirium in 6 of 24 patients who were deeply sedated throughout the study. Nonetheless, a longer length of stay was associated with an increased proportion of items recorded on the ICDSC, although this may be correlation without causation. This study provides important data supporting the routine use of pain, sedation, and monitoring evaluation in TBI patients when feasible during their ICU stay.

Pharmacokinetic Considerations in Traumatic Brain Injury Patients Receiving Sedatives

The potential for pharmacokinetic alterations in critically ill patients has been recognized for decades [50]. These alterations are particularly important in this patient subset secondary to their relative instability as well as being at risk for baseline or secondary organ dysfunction. The organs of greatest concern relative to drug disposition are the liver for agents undergoing hepatic metabolism and the kidneys for drugs undergoing renal elimination of the parent compound or metabolites. In general, the greatest concern relates to a reduction in drug clearance resulting in increased drug concentrations. This could be due to diminished hepatic or renal blood flow or decreases in intrinsic metabolism [51]. Nonetheless, increases in drug clearance have also been observed.

The first consideration for sedative drugs is to know the pharmacokinetic disposition of each individual agent (see Fig. 1). Additionally, for drugs undergoing metabolism, it is imperative to know if the metabolites are pharmacologically active. Table 2 summarizes the pharmacokinetic profiles for the sedatives used in TBI patients. All except propofol are metabolized by the liver with midazolam, morphine, and ketamine having active metabolites. Unlike estimation of renal function, estimating hepatic metabolism is challenging. If hepatic dysfunction is suspected, use of the Child-Pugh score is recommended to guide dosing to avoid excessive sedation and/or other concentration-dependent effects [52]. One additional advantage with sedative use relates to titration of dose to response following initial dosing. Relative to estimation of renal elimination of metabolites, the use of the Cockcroft-Gault equation is recommended [53]. In instances of rapidly changing renal function, an alternative to the use of this equation is the method by Jelliffe and Jelliffe [54]. In cases of severe acute kidney failure, renal replacement therapies may be employed to maintain homeostasis. Conventional hemodialysis will generally require a dosage reduction for water-soluble agents. Nevertheless, continuous renal replacement therapies (CRRT) are being used in many intensive care units. Depending on the CRRT conditions (e.g., membrane, flow rate, etc.), dosage reductions may not be warranted.

As a subset of critically ill patients, pharmacokinetic alterations have been also been studied in TBI patients as well as animal models of TBI [51]. Not only are these patients at risk of the same alterations documented in other critically ill patients, but they may have some unique changes. For example, alteration in the blood-brain barrier may occur in TBI patients that would enhance CNS drug distributions. The presence of the acute phase response is another consideration in TBI patients. Pro-inflammatory cytokines (e.g., interleukin-1-ß[beta] (IL-ß[beta]), interleukin-6 (IL-6), and tumor necrosis factor-α[alpha] (TNF α[alpha])) are released following TBI, resulting in inhibition of oxidative metabolism [50]. Effects on hepatic conjugative metabolism (e.g., glucuronidation, sulfation, and acetylation) have also been observed, although the effect is usually less profound than for oxidative reactions [50]. While inhibition of metabolism secondary to the acute phase response may be evident early following TBI, increases in metabolism have been observed for pentobarbital over several days, which also has been documented for the anticonvulsant phenytoin (see Fig. 2) [55]. A study of antipyrine, a cytochrome P450 substrate, in TBI patients suggests this phenomenon is dynamic and general in nature with a likely decrease in metabolism initially following the TBI with increasing metabolism over time [56, 57]. Drug interactions are yet another concern, especially since sedatives are often given concurrently

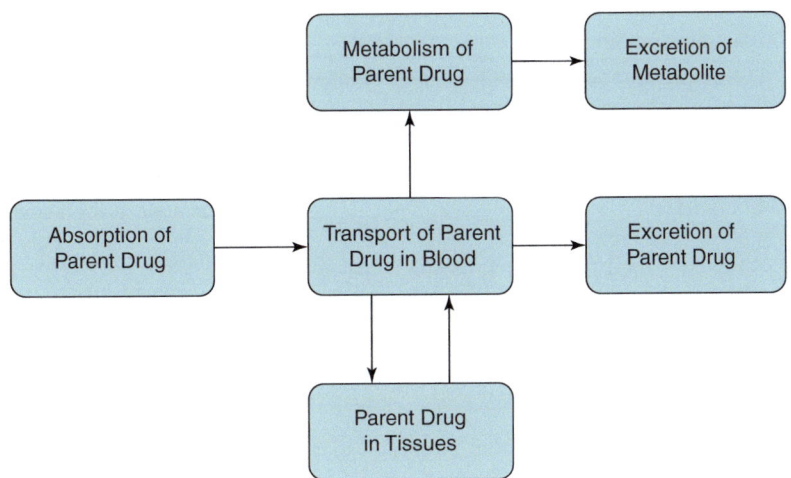

Fig. 1 Simplified pharmacokinetic model of the interactions between the four basic pharmacokinetic processes of drug absorption, distribution, metabolism, and excretion. Reprinted with permission from Boucher BA, Wood GC, Swanson JM. Pharmacokinetic changes in critical illness. Crit Care Clin. 2006 Apr;22(2):255–271

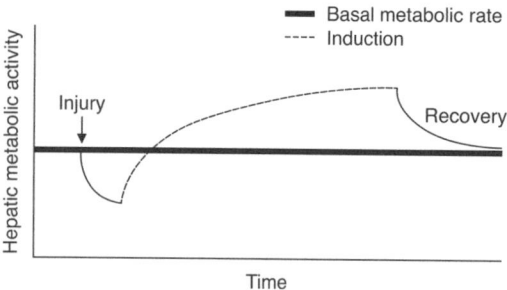

Fig. 2 Representation of possible changes in phenytoin metabolism over time following acute traumatic brain injury. Reprinted with permission from Boucher BA, Hanes SD. Pharmacokinetic alterations after severe head injury. Clinical relevance. Clin Pharmacokinet. 1998 Sep;35(3):209–221

[51]. While pharmacokinetic alterations may not be evident, there is the potential for additive or antagonistic CNS pharmacologic effects in the TBI patients. Lastly, the role of precision medicine is presently unclear for sedative use in TBI patients. Nonetheless, data are growing for selected agents—e.g., propofol, midazolam, remifentanil, etc.—that may explain some of the variability in dose and response in critically ill patients [58].

Conclusions

While sedation is a mainstay for TBI patients in the ICU, clinical trials in this patient are notoriously difficult to conduct. However, using sound pharmacological principles and having a thorough understanding of mechanisms of action and pharmakokinetcs can help clinicians select agents for various clinical scenarios.

References

1. Oddo M, Crippa IA, Mehta S, Menon D, Payen JF, Taccone FS, et al. Optimizing sedation in patients with acute brain injury. Crit Care. 2016;20(1):128.
2. Flower O, Hellings S. Sedation in traumatic brain injury. Emerg Med Int. 2012;2012:637171.
3. Urwin SC, Menon DK. Comparative tolerability of sedative agents in head-injured adults. Drug Saf. 2004;27(2):107–33.
4. Roberts DJ, Hall RI, Kramer AH, Robertson HL, Gallagher CN, Zygun DA. Sedation for critically ill adults with severe traumatic brain injury: a systematic review of randomized controlled trials. Crit Care Med. 2011;39(12):2743–51.
5. Chesnut RM, Marshall LF, Klauber MR, Blunt BA, Baldwin N, Eisenberg HM, et al. The role of secondary brain injury in determining outcome from severe head injury. J Trauma. 1993;34(2):216–22.
6. Roberts DJ, Haroon B, Hall RI. Sedation for critically ill or injured adults in the intensive care unit: a shifting paradigm. Drugs. 2012;72(14):1881–916.
7. Meierkord H, Boon P, Engelsen B, Gocke K, Shorvon S, Tinuper P, et al. EFNS guideline on the management of status epilepticus in adults. Eur J Neurol. 2010;17(3):348–55.
8. Devlin JW, Roberts RJ. Pharmacology of commonly used analgesics and sedatives in the ICU: benzodiazepines, propofol, and opioids. Crit Care Clin. 2009;25(3):431–49, vii.
9. Corbett SM, Montoya ID, Moore FA. Propofol-related infusion syndrome in intensive care patients. Pharmacotherapy. 2008;28(2):250–8.
10. Cremer OL, Moons KG, Bouman EA, Kruijswijk JE, de Smet AM, Kalkman CJ. Long-term propofol infusion and cardiac failure in adult head-injured patients. Lancet. 2001;357(9250):117–8.
11. Dengler B, Garvin R, Seifi A. Can therapeutic hypothermia trigger propofol-related infusion syndrome? J Crit Care. 2015;30(4):823–4.
12. Krajcova A, Waldauf P, Andel M, Duska F. Propofol infusion syndrome: a structured review of experimental studies and 153 published case reports. Crit Care. 2015;19:398.
13. Sebastiani A, Granold M, Ditter A, Sebastiani P, Golz C, Pottker B, et al. Posttraumatic propofol neurotoxicity is mediated via the pro-brain-derived neurotrophic factor-p75 neurotrophin receptor pathway in adult mice. Crit Care Med. 2016;44(2):e70–82.
14. Thal SC, Timaru-Kast R, Wilde F, Merk P, Johnson F, Frauenknecht K, et al. Propofol impairs neurogenesis and neurologic recovery and increases mortality rate in adult rats after traumatic brain injury. Crit Care Med. 2014;42(1):129–41.
15. Sanders RD, Hussell T, Maze M. Sedation & immunomodulation. Crit Care Clin. 2009;25(3):551–70, ix.
16. Li M, Zhang Y, Wu KS, Hu YH. Assessment of the effect of continuous sedation with mechanical ventilation on adrenal insufficiency in patients with traumatic brain injury. J Investig Med. 2016;64(3):752–8.
17. Roberts DJ, Faris PD, Zygun DA. Propofol for severe traumatic brain injury. J Neurosurg. 2014;120(1):289–90.
18. Brain Trauma Foundation, American Association of Neurological Surgeons, Congress of Neurological Surgeons, Joint Section on Neurotrauma and Critical Care, AANS/CNS, Bratton SL, et al. Guidelines for the management of severe traumatic brain

injury. XI. Anesthetics, analgesics, and sedatives. J Neurotrauma. 2007;24(Suppl 1):S71–6.

19. Kelly DF, Goodale DB, Williams J, Herr DL, Chappell ET, Rosner MJ, et al. Propofol in the treatment of moderate and severe head injury: a randomized, prospective double-blinded pilot trial. J Neurosurg. 1999;90(6):1042–52.

20. Barr J, Fraser GL, Puntillo K, Ely EW, Gelinas C, Dasta JF, et al. Clinical practice guidelines for the management of pain, agitation, and delirium in adult patients in the intensive care unit. Crit Care Med. 2013;41(1):263–306.

21. Ouimet S, Kavanagh BP, Gottfried SB, Skrobik Y. Incidence, risk factors and consequences of ICU delirium. Intensive Care Med. 2007;33(1):66–73.

22. Van Rompaey B, Elseviers MM, Schuurmans MJ, Shortridge-Baggett LM, Truijen S, Bossaert L. Risk factors for delirium in intensive care patients: a prospective cohort study. Crit Care. 2009; 13(3):R77.

23. Ely EW, Shintani A, Truman B, Speroff T, Gordon SM, Harrell FE Jr, et al. Delirium as a predictor of mortality in mechanically ventilated patients in the intensive care unit. JAMA. 2004;291(14):1753–62.

24. Shehabi Y, Riker RR, Bokesch PM, Wisemandle W, Shintani A, Ely EW, et al. Delirium duration and mortality in lightly sedated, mechanically ventilated intensive care patients. Crit Care Med. 2010;38(12):2311–8.

25. Jacobi J, Fraser GL, Coursin DB, Riker RR, Fontaine D, Wittbrodt ET, et al. Clinical practice guidelines for the sustained use of sedatives and analgesics in the critically ill adult. Crit Care Med. 2002;30(1): 119–41.

26. Mehta S, McCullagh I, Burry L. Current sedation practices: lessons learned from international surveys. Crit Care Clin. 2009;25(3):471–88, vii–viii.

27. Karabinis A, Mandragos K, Stergiopoulos S, Komnos A, Soukup J, Speelberg B, et al. Safety and efficacy of analgesia-based sedation with remifentanil versus standard hypnotic-based regimens in intensive care unit patients with brain injuries: a randomised, controlled trial [isrctn50308308]. Crit Care. 2004;8(4):R268–80.

28. Boucher BA, Wood GC. Acute management of the brain injury patient. In: DiPiro JT, Talbert RL, Yee GC, Matze GR, Wells BG, Posey LM, editors. Pharmacotherapy: a pathophysiologic approach. New York: McGraw-Hill; 2014. p. 895–909.

29. Marshall GT, James RF, Landman MP, O'Neill PJ, Cotton BA, Hansen EN, et al. Pentobarbital coma for refractory intra-cranial hypertension after severe traumatic brain injury: mortality predictions and one-year outcomes in 55 patients. J Trauma. 2010;69(2):275–83.

30. Wang X, Ding X, Tong Y, Zong J, Zhao X, Ren H, et al. Ketamine does not increase intracranial pressure compared with opioids: meta-analysis of randomized controlled trials. J Anesth. 2014;28(6):821–7.

31. Zeiler FA, Teitelbaum J, West M, Gillman LM. The ketamine effect on ICP in traumatic brain injury. Neurocrit Care. 2014;21(1):163–73.

32. Filanovsky Y, Miller P, Kao J. Myth: ketamine should not be used as an induction agent for intubation in patients with head injury. CJEM. 2010;12(2): 154–7.

33. Himmelseher S, Durieux ME. Revising a dogma: ketamine for patients with neurological injury? Anesth Analg. 2005;101(2):524–34, table of contents.

34. James ML, Olson DM, Graffagnino C. A pilot study of cerebral and haemodynamic physiological changes during sedation with dexmedetomidine or propofol in patients with acute brain injury. Anaesth Intensive Care. 2012;40(6):949–57.

35. Erdman MJ, Doepker BA, Gerlach AT, Phillips GS, Elijovich L, Jones GM. A comparison of severe hemodynamic disturbances between dexmedetomidine and propofol for sedation in neurocritical care patients. Crit Care Med. 2014;42(7):1696–702.

36. Pajoumand M, Kufera JA, Bonds BW, Devabhakthuni S, Boswell S, Hesselton K, et al. Dexmedetomidine as an adjunct for sedation in patients with traumatic brain injury. J Trauma Acute Care Surg. 2016;81(2): 345–51.

37. Schoeler M, Loetscher PD, Rossaint R, Fahlenkamp AV, Eberhardt G, Rex S, et al. Dexmedetomidine is neuroprotective in an in vitro model for traumatic brain injury. BMC Neurol. 2012;12:20.

38. Longrois D, Quintin L. Dexmedetomidine: superiority trials needed? Anaesth Crit Care Pain Med. 2016;35(3):237–8.

39. Malerba G, Romano-Girard F, Cravoisy A, Dousset B, Nace L, Levy B, et al. Risk factors of relative adrenocortical deficiency in intensive care patients needing mechanical ventilation. Intensive Care Med. 2005;31(3):388–92.

40. Riker RR, Fugate JE, Participants in the International Multi-disciplinary Consensus Conference on Multimodality Monitoring. Clinical monitoring scales in acute brain injury: assessment of coma, pain, agitation, and delirium. Neurocrit Care. 2014;21(Suppl 2):S27–37.

41. Schnakers C, Chatelle C, Vanhaudenhuyse A, Majerus S, Ledoux D, Boly M, et al. The nociception coma scale: a new tool to assess nociception in disorders of consciousness. Pain. 2010;148(2):215–9.

42. Chatelle C, Majerus S, Whyte J, Laureys S, Schnakers C. A sensitive scale to assess nociceptive pain in patients with disorders of consciousness. J Neurol Neurosurg Psychiatry. 2012;83(12):1233–7.

43. Kollef MH, Levy NT, Ahrens TS, Schaiff R, Prentice D, Sherman G. The use of continuous i.v. sedation is associated with prolongation of mechanical ventilation. Chest. 1998;114(2):541–8.

44. Kress JP, Pohlman AS, O'Connor MF, Hall JB. Daily interruption of sedative infusions in critically ill patients undergoing mechanical ventilation. N Engl J Med. 2000;342(20):1471–7.

45. Mehta S, Burry L, Cook D, Fergusson D, Steinberg M, Granton J, et al. Daily sedation interruption in mechanically ventilated critically ill patients cared for with a sedation protocol: a randomized controlled trial. JAMA. 2012;308(19):1985–92.

46. Skoglund K, Enblad P, Marklund N. Effects of the neurological wake-up test on intracranial pressure and cerebral perfusion pressure in brain-injured patients. Neurocrit Care. 2009;11(2):135–42.

47. Helbok R, Kurtz P, Schmidt MJ, Stuart MR, Fernandez L, Connolly SE, et al. Effects of the neurological wake-up test on clinical examination, intracranial pressure, brain metabolism and brain tissue oxygenation in severely brain-injured patients. Crit Care. 2012;16(6):R226.

48. Bergeron N, Dubois MJ, Dumont M, Dial S, Skrobik Y. Intensive care delirium screening checklist: evaluation of a new screening tool. Intensive Care Med. 2001;27(5):859–64.

49. Yu A, Teitelbaum J, Scott J, Gesin G, Russell B, Huynh T, et al. Evaluating pain, sedation, and delirium in the neurologically critically ill-feasibility and reliability of standardized tools: a multi-institutional study. Crit Care Med. 2013;41(8):2002–7.

50. Boucher BA, Wood GC, Swanson JM. Pharmacokinetic changes in critical illness. Crit Care Clin. 2006;22(2):255–71, vi.

51. Boucher BA, Hanes SD. Pharmacokinetic alterations after severe head injury. Clinical relevance. Clin Pharmacokinet. 1998;35(3):209–21.

52. Pugh RN, Murray-Lyon IM, Dawson JL, Pietroni MC, Williams R. Transection of the oesophagus for bleeding oesophageal varices. Br J Surg. 1973;60(8):646–9.

53. Cockcroft DW, Gault MH. Prediction of creatinine clearance from serum creatinine. Nephron. 1976;16(1):31–41.

54. Jelliffe RW, Jelliffe SM. A computer program for estimation of creatinine clearance from unstable creatinine concentration. Math Biosci. 1972;14:17–24.

55. Heinemeyer G, Roots I, Dennhardt R. Monitoring of pentobarbital plasma levels in critical care patients suffering from increased intracranial pressure. Ther Drug Monit. 1986;8(2):145–50.

56. Boucher BA, Kuhl DA, Fabian TC, Robertson JT. Effect of neurotrauma on hepatic drug clearance. Clin Pharmacol Ther. 1991;50(5 Pt 1):487–97.

57. McKindley DS, Boucher BA, Hess MM, Rodman JH, Feler C, Fabian TC. Effect of acute phase response on phenytoin metabolism in neurotrauma patients. J Clin Pharmacol. 1997;37(2):129–39.

58. Cohen M, Sadhasivam S, Vinks AA. Pharmacogenetics in perioperative medicine. Curr Opin Anaesthesiol. 2012;25(4):419–27.

Fluid and Electrolyte Management: Hyperosmolar Euvolemia and the Use of Hypertonic Saline for Intracranial Hypertension

Hussain Shallwani, Justice O. Agyei, John F. Morrison, and Kevin J. Gibbons

Introduction

The management of raised intracranial pressures (ICPs) involves a series of steps pursued in series or in parallel that can lower the ICP. Routine measures include positioning the head in a neutral position, controlling ventilation to prevent hypoxia and hypercapnia, maintaining an adequate bowel regimen to prevent increased intra-abdominal pressure, and administering adequate sedation and analgesia, and preventing fever and hypertension may be enough to lower ICP below 20 mmHg in certain cases [1]. Persistent intracranial hypertension, however, may require other measures. These consist of medical therapies such as heavier sedation and/or paralysis, hyperventilation to maintain $PaCO_2$ (partial pressure of arterial carbon dioxide) at 30–35 mmHg, hyperosmolar therapy, barbiturate coma, and hypothermia or procedural or surgical therapies such as cerebrospinal fluid (CSF) drainage and decompressive cranial surgery [1]. This chapter focuses on the use of hypertonic saline to lower the ICP in patients with traumatic brain injury (TBI).

Over the past 10 years, hypertonic saline has become a primary therapy in the neurocritical care unit. From a rarely used rescue therapy, it has now largely supplanted the use of mannitol in many units. The main advantages are more rapid and prolonged ICP control and the coeffect of improved intravascular volume and perfusion versus the hypovolemic state that can be induced by mannitol.

The effect of hypertonic saline on reducing the brain volume was described in the early 1900s [2]. The idea behind using hypertonic solution to reduce intracranial pressure is based on reduction in cerebral edema; this is achieved by increasing the osmolarity of the intravascular compartment and drawing free water across the blood-brain barrier into the vessels, thereby reducing the water content in the brain parenchyma [2]. The use of hypertonic saline for refractory intracranial hypertension was introduced when Worthley et al. described the use of 50 and 20 mL infusion of 5 mmol/mL hypertonic saline in two patients in whom mannitol and furosemide failed to achieve long-term ICP control [3]. Since then, the use of hypertonic saline as an agent to reduce ICP has been the focus of numerous studies, yet a number of questions still remain unanswered.

H. Shallwani, MD · J. O. Agyei, MD · J. F. Morrison, MD
K. J. Gibbons, MD (✉)
Department of Neurological Surgery, Jacobs School of Medicine and Biomedical Sciences, Buffalo, NY, USA
e-mail: HShallwani@UBNS.com; JAgyei@UBNS.com; JMorrison@UBNS.com; kgibbons@ubns.com

© Springer International Publishing AG, part of Springer Nature 2018
S. D. Timmons (ed.), *Controversies in Severe Traumatic Brain Injury Management*,
https://doi.org/10.1007/978-3-319-89477-5_7

Benefecial Effects of Hypertonic Saline in Patients with Traumatic Brain Injury

Brain Water Content

The main advantages of using hypertonic saline over other hyperosmolar therapies included absence of diuresis and maintenance of intravascular volume. Hypertonic saline is known to have a higher reflection coefficient (1.0) than mannitol (0.9) [4, 5]. Reflection coefficient is defined as the ability of blood-brain barrier (BBB) to keep the substance from moving across; a reflection coefficient of 1 denotes complete impermeability, whereas that of 0 denotes complete permeability. A higher reflection coefficient makes hypertonic saline a better intravascular osmotic agent than mannitol [4]. Loss of free water from the brain parenchyma leads to a reduced total brain water content and total brain volume after infusion of hypertonic saline [6–8]. However, studies have shown that this loss of free water may be different between injured and uninjured areas of the brain [8–12]. Moreover, there may actually be an increase in water and sodium content in injured areas of the brain after treatment with hypertonic saline [9, 11, 13] and a possibility of worsening peri-contusional edema and hypoxia [14]. This may be due to the disruption of blood-brain barrier at the site of injury. Of note, the integrity of BBB is a prerequisite for success of hyperosmolar therapy in reducing ICP, and loss is known to correlate with failure of response to hypertonic saline and subsequently poor outcome after TBI [15].

Vasoregulatory and Microcirculatory Effects

Another mechanism of secondary injury in patients with TBI is reduced cerebral perfusion and consequent low oxygen delivery. When animal studies showed that hypertonic saline could increase pial arteriole diameter [16], along with cerebral perfusion and oxygen delivery [10, 16], it was thought to be due to the fluid shift from

endothelial cells to the capillary lumen ("endothelial dehydration") [17], thereby decreasing the endothelial thickness and increasing the capillary diameter [10, 17, 18]. Smooth muscle relaxation is also thought to contribute to reductions in cerebrovascular resistance [14, 19]. In addition, oxygen delivery is facilitated by the dehydrated red blood cells' increased ease of flow through the capillaries, termed improved rheology [10, 17]. In essence, hypertonic saline is thought to counteract hypoperfusion after TBI by increasing capillary vessel diameter and plasma volume and therefore cerebral blood flow [17]. A considerable increase in cerebral perfusion pressure (CPP) has been observed when hypertonic saline is used for treatment of intracranial hypertension [4, 9, 20–30].

Permissive Hypernatremia (Osmotic Effects)

Some have argued that hypertonic saline is useful in lowering ICP as long as high serum osmolarity is maintained via sustained hypernatremia [23, 31, 32]. While some studies show that high serum sodium concentration correlates with low ICP [32–36], other studies have identified no significant change in serum sodium concentration when hypertonic saline was successful in treating intracranial hypertension [14, 22, 25, 26]. Sousa et al. showed that when 3% hypertonic saline failed to reduce ICP in a porcine model of intracranial hypertension, there was no significant change in serum sodium concentration either [37]. Similarly, when Jagannatha et al. identified increased urinary sodium loss after hypertonic saline was used for refractory intracranial hypertension, they proposed concomitant therapy to retain sodium as the key to maintain hyperosmolar state after infusion of hypertonic saline [38]. Generalizations based on these studies become difficult owing to inconsistent patient population, intervention, and data sampling [39]. Continuous infusion of hypertonic saline for prolonged hypernatremia is reported to successfully reduce the ICP in pediatric patients with TBI [23, 31]; however, it failed to decrease the need for additional treatment and did not improve mortality outcomes in adult patients with head injury [40] or other types of cerebral edema [33] (but see also [41, 42]). Still, the optimal natremic state for patients with intracranial hypertension and its role in reducing ICP remain controversial [14].

Hemodynamic Effects

In patients with head trauma (either isolated or associated with polytrauma), hypovolemia and hypotension are notable predictors of poor clinical outcomes [17, 43–47]. The difficulty in treating shock in multisystem trauma patients is made worse as severe head injury may affect the cardiac index and blood pressure and, therefore, interfere with recovery from hemorrhagic shock [13, 48]. A bolus of hypertonic saline expands the plasma volume [49], normalizes the cardiovascular functions [50–58], and can be used to reverse the hemorrhagic and hypovolemic shock [59–61]. In a multicenter trial comparing the efficacy of 7.5% hypertonic saline versus normal saline for initial resuscitation of trauma patients, the subgroup of patients with severe head injury was seen to have statistically significant improvement in survival when hypertonic saline was used for resuscitation [54, 62–64]. However, when a single dose of 7.5% hypertonic saline was compared to Ringer's lactate solution for prehospital resuscitation in another randomized control trial of 229 TBI patients, there was no difference in mortality or functional outcome between both groups [65]; notably, conclusions based on the latter trial cannot be generalized as the intervention was limited to a single prehospital dose of hypertonic saline. All in all, the risk of increasing ICP with isotonic fluids and causing hypovolemia due to diuresis with mannitol makes hypertonic saline a good choice for fluid resuscitation in patients with head trauma, especially with its additional advantage of improved cerebral oxygenation and blood flow [13]; a low volume is sufficient to improve hemodynamic parameters without the detrimental effects on ICP that can be seen with large volumes of isotonic fluids such as 0.9% saline [13, 66, 67].

Immunomodulatory Effects

Trauma, specifically traumatic brain injury, is followed by a cascade of events that leads to systemic inflammatory response syndrome, along with leukocyte migration to injured areas of the brain and peroxidase-protease-mediated cell death [17, 68]. Moreover, release of inflammatory mediators such as eicosanoids from activated leukocytes leads to vasospasm and interstitial edema [17, 69]. Hypertonic saline is thought to have some anti-inflammatory effects and therefore reduce post-traumatic complications secondary to inflammation. In vitro studies of human leukocytes and animal studies have shown hypertonicity to decrease neutrophil activation/adherence [70–74], stimulate lymphocyte proliferation [75], inhibit pro-inflammatory cytokines, and stimulate anti-inflammatory cytokine production [76–82]. When a single dose of 250 mL of 7.5% NaCl and 6% dextran-70 was used in patients with hemorrhagic shock, pro-inflammatory tumor necrosis factor (TNF)-alpha production was seen to decrease, while anti-inflammatory IL-1ra and IL-10 were increased [82]. It is thought that hypertonic saline may also play a role in brain cell immune modulation, which may lead to anti-inflammatory effects and potentially better outcome for patients with TBI [17].

Neurochemical Effects

One of the mechanisms of secondary injury in patients with TBI is increasing extracellular levels of the amino acid glutamate in the brain [83, 84]. This can occur after extensive neuronal depolarization due to reduced cerebral perfusion pressure or seizures [17, 83]. When normal Na+/K+ active exchange pump becomes dysfunctional, low extracellular Na+ leads to reversal of the Na+/glutamate secondary cotransporter, and, as a result, glutamate levels in the extracellular space rise [17, 85]. The "excitotoxic surge" in TBI patients has also been shown to correlate with increased ICP levels in those patients and their functional outcome at 6 months [84]. Hypertonic saline increases the extracellular Na+

levels and is thought to restore the extracellular sodium concentration and the normal direction of Na+/glutamate cotransporter and thereby prevent the damage caused by high levels of extracellular glutamate [17].

Hypertonic Saline: Experimental Studies in Animals

There have been many animal studies showing efficacy of hypertonic saline in experimental models of TBI. In most of these studies, trauma conditions are emulated with animal models of cryogenic injury and hemorrhagic shock, and various factors directly correlated with cerebral edema are measured. Hypertonic saline has been shown to decrease cerebral water content and ICP in many animal studies [9, 12, 13, 86–88]. Its effects on ICP were also seen when it was used for resuscitation in the treatment of TBI [66, 67, 89–93].

In a sheep model of cryogenic injury and hemorrhagic shock treated with hypertonic saline versus lactated Ringer's, animals given with hypertonic saline achieved a decrease in initial ICP [90]. The authors also noted that after the initial resuscitation, these animals required less maintenance fluid to maintain their mean arterial pressure [90]. Other studies have focused on the efficacy of hypertonic saline as both a resuscitation fluid and maintenance fluid. In a randomized study between 7.5% hypertonic saline versus lactated Ringer's as resuscitation fluid, Walsh et al. found that initial hypertonic saline bolus prevented the ICP rise that is seen with isotonic fluid resuscitation; animals treated with hypertonic saline as both resuscitation and maintenance fluids achieved higher cerebral blood flow (CBF) and lower cortical water content and, most importantly, maintained near-normal ICP when compared to animals that received lactated Ringer's [91]. In a similar study, Shackford et al. also noted improved mean arterial pressure (MAP), higher CBF, and lower ICP values in animals treated with hypertonic saline as both resuscitation and maintenance fluids [92].

Further experimental models were used to test hypertonic saline in models of intracranial hypertension and to compare them with existing hyperosmolar agents such as mannitol [37, 94–96]. Berger et al. compared the use of 7.2% hypertonic saline/10% Dextran-60 versus 20% mannitol in an experimental model of rabbits with head injury and hemorrhagic hypovolemia [9]. The authors observed that although mannitol was more potent in lowering ICP for a longer duration after the first dose, no difference in longevity of their effects was noted after a second infusion [9]. Secondly, due to its effect on blood pressure, rabbits treated with hypertonic saline had a higher cerebral perfusion pressure than those treated with mannitol [9]. In contrast, Qureshi et al. showed a significant difference in ICP reduction in both groups that were treated with hypertonic saline as opposed to those treated with mannitol. Furthermore, rebound effect was noted when hypertonic saline was used in dog models of hemorrhagic shock and intracranial hypertension [97]. Prough et al. noted that animals that received hypertonic saline had significantly lower ICP and higher CBF at 30 min; however, the effect was short-lasting and not sustained at 60, 90, or 120 min [97].

The experimental studies in animal models of TBI have provided invaluable insight in the topic of hyperosmolar therapy for intracranial hypertension. The success of hypertonic saline in reducing ICP in animal models of brain injury led to subsequent work in clinical setting, initially for cases of refractory intracranial hypertension, and later as an adjunct to other therapies that make up the current standard of care.

Hypertonic Saline: Clinical Setting

Since Worthley et al. [3] described the use of hypertonic saline for refractory intracranial hypertension, several studies followed that showed the efficacy of this treatment when all else has failed [4, 23–25, 28, 41, 98–104]. These studies are significantly different in their selection of patient population, choice of concentration of hypertonic saline, addition of dextrose/ hydroxyethyl starch, and choice of administration (bolus vs. continuous infusion). Nevertheless, the results of consistently reduced ICP seen with hypertonic saline encouraged further research in this area. The use of hypertonic saline has since become a widespread treatment option for patients with raised ICP.

Hypertonic saline is available in a wide range of concentrations from 1% to 30%. Most commonly used concentrations in the United States are 3% and 23.4% [105]. There is a lack of data as to which concentration is the most efficacious in reducing ICP in patients with TBI. Studies have used varying concentrations including 1.6%, 3%, 7.5%, 10%, 14.6%, or 23.4%, with varying results. The conclusions from animal studies have influenced clinical practice. Qureshi et al. showed that a greater reduction in ICP was achieved within 15 min with 23.4% hypertonic saline infusion in dogs as compared to 3% hypertonic saline solution; however, the effect of 3% hypertonic saline was more sustained [95]. Similarly, Lewandowski-Belfer et al. showed no significant difference in efficacy of 23.4% hypertonic saline versus 14.6% hypertonic saline in treating patients with refractory intracranial hypertension [35]. The optimal concentration that can effectively reduce ICP in patients without any potential adverse effects continues to be a topic of debate. It is advisable to titer the concentration of hypertonic saline depending on the desired effect on ICP, serum osmolality, and sodium concentration. High concentrations are usually used as a bolus in acute setting, while low concentrations can be safely used for continuous infusions.

The administration of hypertonic saline as a bolus infusion or a continuous infusion is also unclear. Typically, bolus doses of hypertonic saline are intended to reduce ICP in an acute setting. Continuous infusion of hypertonic saline is used in situations where a stable level of serum sodium and serum osmolality is required in order to lower the ICP to desired level [23, 36]. Studies have shown that continuous infusion is also safe and effective in lowering ICP [19, 23, 31, 36, 106] and may also reduce the number of other interventions to lower ICP [19]. However, the risk of potential adverse effects with continuous infusion of hypertonic saline must be given

special attention, and patients should be closely monitored accordingly.

A double-blinded crossover study involving pediatric patients with TBI compared the effect of 3% saline and 0.9% saline on ICP. They observed a statistically significant reduction in ICP 2 h after bolus infusion of 3% saline, but not with 0.9% saline [36]. Subsequently, a randomized prospective trial involving pediatric patients with head injury showed that patients receiving continuous infusion of 1.7% hypertonic saline as maintenance fluids were more likely to have lower ICP, require fewer interventions to control ICP, and have a shorter length of intensive care unit (ICU) stay as compared to controls receiving lactated Ringer's solution [32]. The trial did not, however, show any survival benefit with use of hypertonic saline [32]. After further studies showed similar benefits of ICP reduction with continuous infusion of hypertonic saline [23, 31], guidelines for management of pediatric cases of TBI recommended the use of 3% hypertonic saline as a continuous infusion on a sliding scale with the range between 0.1 and 1.0 mL/ kg of body weight per hour, maintaining a serum osmolarity of up to 360 mOsm/L [107, 108]. Some authors continue to argue that the results of these small studies and trials may be missing or understating the risk of adverse effects associated with continuous infusion of hypertonic saline [109]; an increase in creatinine has been reported with increasing concentration of serum sodium [31, 109], along with other adverse effects such as acute renal failure, thrombocytopenia, neutropenia, anemia, and acute respiratory distress syndrome [110]; the risk of serious adverse events should not be ignored in these patients. Bolus doses of 23.4% hypertonic saline have been used to treat refractory intracranial hypertension in children with TBI [103]. More recently, Piper et al. described their experience with bolus infusion of 23.4% hypertonic saline in pediatric cases of TBI, fueling another debate of bolus vs. continuous infusion of hypertonic saline in this patient population.

Compared to other osmotic agents such as mannitol, there has been growing evidence that hypertonic saline may be a superior agent for the treatment of intracranial hypertension. Studies have compared these agents based on their time of onset of effect, magnitude and duration of effect, rebound effect, need for other therapies to reduce ICP, efficacy in recurrent and refractory intracranial hypertension, failure rates, and outcomes [105]. Harutjunyan et al. reported that the onset of effect of hypertonic saline on ICP was faster than that of mannitol [20]; but comparable times have been reported in the literature otherwise [25, 105, 111, 112]. Similarly, initial studies had contradicting results on the magnitude of effect of hypertonic saline as compared to mannitol [20, 38, 41, 42, 101, 113–118]. A recent meta-analysis of randomized controlled trials comparing mannitol versus hypertonic saline for treatment of intracranial hypertension after TBI showed that the magnitude of effect, albeit the same in the first 30 min after infusion, is significantly greater at the 1-h and 2-h periods when hypertonic saline is used for treatment of intracranial hypertension [119]. The authors also reported that hypertonic saline caused a greater overall reduction in ICP as compared to mannitol [119]. Moreover, studies have shown that hypertonic saline achieves a sustained reduction in ICP for a longer period than that seen with mannitol [41, 101, 113, 114, 120], although, equal duration of action has also been reported [27, 38, 42]. A systematic review by Burgess et al. reported a lower rate of ICP treatment failure when hypertonic saline was used instead of mannitol in patients with TBI [121]. Similarly, the number of other therapies needed to control ICP is reportedly lower with the use of hypertonic saline for intracranial hypertension as compared to mannitol [42, 98]. Mangat et al. reported a lower daily and cumulative ICP burden, along with a shorter duration of ICU stay, when hypertonic saline was used for treatment of intracranial hypertension [27], although length of hospital stay and rate of 2-week mortality were not different [27]. In contrast, Vialet et al. observed that hypertonic saline may have some mortality benefit in patients with intracranial hypertension after TBI [41].

Although a meta-analysis of 36 retrospective and prospective studies and trials concluded that hypertonic saline may be more effective than mannitol and have a lower rate of treatment failure [122], it is difficult to draw conclusions based on existing literature due to lack of consistency in the treatment protocol of all the studies and insufficient quality of the randomized controlled trials. Due to the lack of quality of data on use of hypertonic saline, the current guidelines from Brain Trauma Foundation have recommended the use of mannitol as the mainstay for the treatment of intracranial hypertension when hyperosmolar therapy is indicated [123]. Further studies on hypertonic saline with better design and good data quality may help better understand this treatment option for intracranial hypertension. Also, the use of one agent certainly does not preclude the use of the other in a given patient. While research studies have sometimes compared mannitol versus hypertonic saline, either agent may be appropriate at different times in the course of treatment for a single injury, depending upon the physiological scenario, and they are commonly used in conjunction with one another in clinical practice.

Our experience with hypertonic saline use has been primarily for herniation syndromes secondary to ischemic and hemorrhagic stroke, subarachnoid hemorrhage, and to a lesser degree, isolated traumatic brain injury. In certain other instances including sinus venous thrombosis, acute spontaneous hemorrhage, or hemorrhagic conversion of stroke whereby the degree of edema is significant and associated with neurologic change, hypertonic saline is oftentimes used to decrease ICP and cerebral edema. However, it must be noted that the use of this therapy may have different physiological consequences for different clinical problems.

We use continuous infusions of 2% saline and 3% saline typically with a serum sodium goal of 150–160 mEq/L. Utilizing hypertonics to obtain and maintain a hypernatremic state has become fairly routine, based on clinical state, ICP measurement, or imaging demonstrating mass effect or edema. Both 2% saline and 3% saline are used as first-line agents, with 2% saline being initially used if central venous access is unavailable. Once central venous access becomes available, patients are transitioned to 3% saline. Use of 23.4% saline may be reserved for the acute intervention when herniation is occurring or a rapid decline in neurological exam is noted. In situations, such as this, surgery is often warranted, and 23.4% saline is used while the operating room is prepared. In patients who are receiving continuous infusions of 2% or 3% saline and who fail to consistently meet the desired serum sodium goal, 23.4% bolus infusions are sometimes used to help achieve the targeted serum sodium goal. Monitoring of serum sodium levels occurs every 6 h for the first 24 h with serial serum sodium levels. If there is an appropriate rise in sodium levels, the frequency of monitoring is de-escalated to every 12 h for the remainder of time the patient remains on the therapy. Infusion is discontinued or infusion rate is decreased based upon achievement and maintenance of the targeted goal or when there is a rise greater than 12 mEq/L over a 24-h period.

Potential Adverse Effects

Central Pontine Myelinolysis

Central pontine myelinolysis (CPM) is a known complication of rapid correction of chronic hyponatremia. It is hypothesized that rapid rise in sodium levels secondary to hypertonic saline infusion may have the same effect causing pontine demyelination. Similarly, rapid changes in serum sodium levels have been associated with subdural and intracerebral hemorrhages in children [124] as a result of sheering of bridging veins from contracture of the brain [125]. However, there has not been any report of CPM on magnetic resonance imaging (MRI) or postmortem or any other neurological complication when hypertonic saline was used to treat intracranial hypertension, even with sodium levels as high as 183 mEq/L [23, 31]. CPM is not known to occur with rapid infusions of hypertonic saline in patients who are initially normonatremic, and studies have shown that prolonged hypernatremia in a controlled fashion was well tolerated by pediatric patients with TBI [23, 31]. Because of the risks of CPM when hyponatremia is corrected too rapidly (i.e., more than 10–20 mEq/L per day [126–128]), hyponatremia should be excluded

before administering hypertonic saline [123, 129] as part of a hypernatremic hyperosmolar euvolemic therapy regimen.

Rebound Intracranial Hypertension

Much like the rebound phenomenon seen with mannitol, there have been reports of rebound intracranial hypertension after hypertonic saline was used to reduce ICP. However, many of these reports involve non-traumatic intracranial hypertension or experimental models [95, 97, 130]. In a comparison of the effect of 3% saline versus 23.4% saline in a canine model of intracranial hypertension, a gradual rise in ICP was seen in the group that received 23.4% saline, but a sustained effect was noted in the group which received 3% saline [95]. In contrast, Qureshi et al. reported that in patients with head trauma, the beneficial effect of 3% saline was short-lasting [33]. Tolerance to hypertonic saline is thought to develop after 3 days of continuous hypertonic state as the cerebral osmolytes such as amino acids (glutamate, glutamine, γ[gamma]-aminobutyric acid, N-acetylaspartate, alanine, aspartate, taurine), polyhydric alcohols (myoinositol), and methyl amines (creatine and glycerophosphorylcholine) move into the intracellular space resulting in loss of the osmotic gradient [128, 131–134]. Moreover, in patients with significant damage to BBB, prolonged continuous infusion of hypertonic saline may pose a considerable risk of rebound intracranial hypertension [135]. Some authors have suggested limiting the use of continuous infusion of hypertonic saline solution to 24 h [130, 135], while others have recommended weaning it—slowing over another 24–48 h to prevent rebound effect secondary to hyponatremia [135]. Given that peak cerebral edema after traumatic brain injury occurs at around 72 h, cessation prior to this may result in rebound problems with intracranial hypertension, and safe use beyond this period is common in clinical practice. Other studies on patients with TBI have described hypertonic saline to have longer-lasting effect on ICP than mannitol [17, 27, 41, 94, 101, 113, 114, 120], and no rebound was seen with administration of multiple bolus doses [24, 25, 28, 30, 35, 99, 104], suggesting that administration method using boluses rather than continuous drips may be more beneficial in certain clinical scenarios.

Acute Renal Failure

Huang et al. showed that when hypertonic saline was used for resuscitation of patient with burns, the risk of developing renal failure increased by four times as compared to those patients receiving Ringer's lactate [136]. Large fluid losses in patients with burns make them a very different patient population as compared to patients with TBI; nevertheless, the risk of renal failure with hypertonic saline is noteworthy. When continuous infusion of hypertonic saline was used to achieve permissive hypernatremia in order to treat intracranial hypertension, two pediatric patients developed acute renal failure [23]; notably, the authors reported that both cases of renal failure followed sepsis and multi-organ failure [23]. Therefore, the effect of hypertonic saline on the risk of developing renal failure could not be established. When Peterson et al. described the use of continuous hypertonic saline infusion in pediatric cases of traumatic brain injury, they did not observe any cases of renal failure, even with the highest concentration of over 180 mEq/L [31]; however, they did report a positive correlation between serum sodium and creatinine concentrations [31]. In experimental models testing the use of hypertonic saline, renal insufficiency has not been observed until up to five times the therapeutic dose in humans [68]. However, a recent retrospective study showed an increased number of acute renal failure in patients whose serum sodium level exceeded 170 mEq/L [110]. Regular monitoring of renal function is strongly advised when using hypertonic saline in patients with TBI and, most importantly, maintenance of adequate intravascular volume.

Electrolyte Abnormalities

Studies have shown that hypokalemia or hyperchloremic acidosis may occur in patients receiving hypertonic saline without K+ or acetate replacement [4, 128]. It is, therefore, recommended that patients receiving hypertonic saline should be closely monitored for other electrolyte abnormalities and treated with replacement therapies appropriately. It is important to continue to monitor serum Na+ carefully for an appropriate length of time after discontinuation of therapy (on the order of days and depending upon the duration of use of hyperosmolar euvolemic therapy) as rebound hyponatremia may occur, with its attendant neurological risks.

Impairment of Platelet Function and Coagulation

In vitro experiments on canine blood have shown that mannitol and 3% hypertonic saline both have a significant effect on platelet function and whole blood coagulation in a dose-dependent fashion [137]. While both agents made the blood more hypocoagulable, mannitol had a significantly greater effect on platelet aggregation, clot formation time, clot strength, and fibrin formation than hypertonic saline [137]. Similarly, Reed et al. showed decreased platelet aggregation and increased prothrombin time/partial thromboplastin time (PT/PTT) when hypertonic saline was used for fluid resuscitation [138]. One hypothesis to explain this effect is expansion of plasma volume and dilution of coagulation factors [128, 139]. However, more studies are needed to elucidate this further.

Pulmonary Edema/Cardiac Failure (Fluid Overload)

As hypertonic saline causes the movement of free water out of the cells, there is a theoretical risk of fluid overload, especially given the fact that NaCl can freely cross the capillary bed in systemic tissues and move into the extracellular space. There have been reports of pulmonary edema in patients with poor cardiovascular reserve [33]. It is appropriate that the guidelines from the Brain Trauma Foundation warn of the risk of inducing or aggravating cardiac failure and/or pulmonary edema in patients with underlying cardiac or pulmonary conditions [33, 129]. Consideration must be given to diuretic use should fluid overload inadvertently occur, in order to maintain euvolemia.

Phlebitis

Thrombosis of peripheral veins can occur if concentrated solutions are administered through peripheral venous catheter. It is recommended that solutions of greater than 2% saline be infused through a central venous catheter to prevent the risk of phlebitis [105, 125, 135].

Conclusions

The use of hypertonic saline has become a routine therapy in the treatment of critically ill neurosurgical patients. Rapid and prolonged control of elevated ICP can be achieved with its use and is attributed to a number of different mechanisms. Hypertonic saline may be used for resuscitation, emergent ICP control, and sustained ICP and cerebral perfusion management. The desired effect can be obtained without the risk of systemic hypovolemia and decreased cerebral perfusion, which are potential concerns with mannitol if it is not used correctly. The risks of hypertonic saline therapy are well described, but achievement of the goals of therapy and avoidance of overtreatment are easily measured by serum sodium concentration, osmolarity, and creatinine. Further, risk is mitigated by maintenance of appropriate intravascular volume status to optimize renal perfusion.

References

1. Rangel-Castilla L, Gopinath S, Robertson CS. Management of intracranial hypertension. Neurol Clin. 2008;26(2):521–41, x.
2. Weed LH, McKibben PS. Experimental alteration of brain bulk. Am J Physiol. 1919;48(4):531–58.
3. Worthley LI, Cooper DJ, Jones N. Treatment of resistant intracranial hypertension with hypertonic saline. Report of two cases. J Neurosurg. 1988;68(3):478–81.
4. Suarez JI, Qureshi AI, Bhardwaj A, Williams MA, Schnitzer MS, Mirski M, et al. Treatment of refractory intracranial hypertension with 23.4% saline. Crit Care Med. 1998;26(6):1118–22.
5. Zornow MH. Hypertonic saline as a safe and efficacious treatment of intracranial hypertension. J Neurosurg Anesthesiol. 1996;8(2):175–7.
6. Toung TJ, Nyquist P, Mirski MA. Effect of hypertonic saline concentration on cerebral and visceral organ water in an uninjured rodent model. Crit Care Med. 2008;36(1):256–61.
7. Todd MM, Tommasino C, Moore S. Cerebral effects of isovolemic hemodilution with a hypertonic saline solution. J Neurosurg. 1985;63(6):944–8.
8. Saltarini M, Massarutti D, Baldassarre M, Nardi G, De Colle C, Fabris G. Determination of cerebral water content by magnetic resonance imaging after small volume infusion of 18% hypertonic saline solution in a patient with refractory intracranial hypertension. Eur J Emerg Med. 2002;9(3):262–5.
9. Berger S, Schurer L, Hartl R, Deisbock T, Dautermann C, Murr R, et al. 7.2% NaCl/10% dextran 60 versus 20% mannitol for treatment of intracranial hypertension. Acta Neurochir Suppl (Wien). 1994;60:494–8.
10. Shackford SR, Zhuang J, Schmoker J. Intravenous fluid tonicity: effect on intracranial pressure, cerebral blood flow, and cerebral oxygen delivery in focal brain injury. J Neurosurg. 1992;76(1):91–8.
11. Lescot T, Degos V, Zouaoui A, Preteux F, Coriat P, Puybasset L. Opposed effects of hypertonic saline on contusions and noncontused brain tissue in patients with severe traumatic brain injury. Crit Care Med. 2006;34(12):3029–33.
12. Wisner DH, Schuster L, Quinn C. Hypertonic saline resuscitation of head injury: effects on cerebral water content. J Trauma. 1990;30(1):75–8.
13. Berger S, Schurer L, Hartl R, Messmer K, Baethmann A. Reduction of post-traumatic intracranial hypertension by hypertonic/hyperoncotic saline/dextran and hypertonic mannitol. Neurosurgery. 1995;37(1):98–107; discussion 107–8.
14. Dias C, Silva MJ, Pereira E, Silva S, Cerejo A, Smielewski P, et al. Post-traumatic multimodal brain monitoring: response to hypertonic saline. J Neurotrauma. 2014;31(22):1872–80.
15. Saw MM, Chamberlain J, Barr M, Morgan MP, Burnett JR, Ho KM. Differential disruption of blood-brain barrier in severe traumatic brain injury. Neurocrit Care. 2014;20(2):209–16.
16. Shackford SR, Schmoker JD, Zhuang J. The effect of hypertonic resuscitation on pial arteriolar tone after brain injury and shock. J Trauma. 1994;37(6):899–908.
17. Boone MD, Oren-Grinberg A, Robinson TM, Chen CC, Kasper EM. Mannitol or hypertonic saline in the setting of traumatic brain injury: what have we learned? Surg Neurol Int. 2015;6:177.
18. Mazzoni MC, Borgstrom P, Intaglietta M, Arfors KE. Capillary narrowing in hemorrhagic shock is rectified by hyperosmotic saline-dextran reinfusion. Circ Shock. 1990;31(4):407–18.

19. Roquilly A, Mahe PJ, Latte DD, Loutrel O, Champin P, Di Falco C, et al. Continuous controlled-infusion of hypertonic saline solution in traumatic brain-injured patients: a 9-year retrospective study. Crit Care. 2011;15(5):R260.

20. Harutjunyan L, Holz C, Rieger A, Menzel M, Grond S, Soukup J. Efficiency of 7.2% hypertonic saline hydroxyethyl starch 200/0.5 versus mannitol 15% in the treatment of increased intracranial pressure in neurosurgical patients—a randomized clinical trial [ISRCTN62699180]. Crit Care. 2005;9(5):R530–40.

21. Bentsen G, Breivik H, Lundar T, Stubhaug A. Hypertonic saline (7.2%) in 6% hydroxyethyl starch reduces intracranial pressure and improves hemodynamics in a placebo-controlled study involving stable patients with subarachnoid hemorrhage. Crit Care Med. 2006;34(12):2912–7.

22. Hartl R, Ghajar J, Hochleuthner H, Mauritz W. Hypertonic/hyperoncotic saline reliably reduces ICP in severely head-injured patients with intracranial hypertension. Acta Neurochir Suppl. 1997;70: 126–9.

23. Khanna S, Davis D, Peterson B, Fisher B, Tung H, O'Quigley J, et al. Use of hypertonic saline in the treatment of severe refractory posttraumatic intracranial hypertension in pediatric traumatic brain injury. Crit Care Med. 2000;28(4):1144–51.

24. Horn P, Munch E, Vajkoczy P, Herrmann P, Quintel M, Schilling L, et al. Hypertonic saline solution for control of elevated intracranial pressure in patients with exhausted response to mannitol and barbiturates. Neurol Res. 1999;21(8):758–64.

25. Eskandari R, Filtz MR, Davis GE, Hoesch RE. Effective treatment of refractory intracranial hypertension after traumatic brain injury with repeated boluses of 14.6% hypertonic saline. J Neurosurg. 2013;119(2):338–46.

26. Huang SJ, Chang L, Han YY, Lee YC, Tu YK. Efficacy and safety of hypertonic saline solutions in the treatment of severe head injury. Surg Neurol. 2006;65(6):539–46; discussion 46.

27. Mangat HS, Chiu YL, Gerber LM, Alimi M, Ghajar J, Hartl R. Hypertonic saline reduces cumulative and daily intracranial pressure burdens after severe traumatic brain injury. J Neurosurg. 2015;122(1):202–10.

28. Major EH, O'Connor P, Mullan B. Single bolus 30% hypertonic saline for refractory intracranial hypertension. Ir J Med Sci. 2015;184(1):159–65.

29. Munar F, Ferrer AM, de Nadal M, Poca MA, Pedraza S, Sahuquillo J, et al. Cerebral hemodynamic effects of 7.2% hypertonic saline in patients with head injury and raised intracranial pressure. J Neurotrauma. 2000;17(1):41–51.

30. Shein SL, Ferguson NM, Kochanek PM, Bayir H, Clark RS, Fink EL, et al. Effectiveness of pharmacological therapies for intracranial hypertension in children with severe traumatic brain injury—results from an automated data collection system time-synched to drug administration. Pediatr Crit Care Med. 2016;17(3):236–45.

31. Peterson B, Khanna S, Fisher B, Marshall L. Prolonged hypernatremia controls elevated intracranial pressure in head-injured pediatric patients. Crit Care Med. 2000;28(4):1136–43.

32. Simma B, Burger R, Falk M, Sacher P, Fanconi S. A prospective, randomized, and controlled study of fluid management in children with severe head injury: lactated Ringer's solution versus hypertonic saline. Crit Care Med. 1998;26(7):1265–70.

33. Qureshi AI, Suarez JI, Bhardwaj A, Mirski M, Schnitzer MS, Hanley DF, et al. Use of hypertonic (3%) saline/acetate infusion in the treatment of cerebral edema: effect on intracranial pressure and lateral displacement of the brain. Crit Care Med. 1998;26(3):440–6.

34. Wells DL, Swanson JM, Wood GC, Magnotti LJ, Boucher BA, Croce MA, et al. The relationship between serum sodium and intracranial pressure when using hypertonic saline to target mild hypernatremia in patients with head trauma. Crit Care. 2012;16(5):R193.

35. Lewandowski-Belfer JJ, Patel AV, Darracott RM, Jackson DA, Nordeen JD, Freeman WD. Safety and efficacy of repeated doses of 14.6 or 23.4% hypertonic saline for refractory intracranial hypertension. Neurocrit Care. 2014;20(3):436–42.

36. Fisher B, Thomas D, Peterson B. Hypertonic saline lowers raised intracranial pressure in children after head trauma. J Neurosurg Anesthesiol. 1992;4(1):4–10.

37. Sousa LM Jr, de Andrade AF, Belon AR, Soares MS, Amorim RL, Otochi JP, et al. Evaluation of the maintained effect of 3% hypertonic saline solution in an animal model of intracranial hypertension. Med Sci Monit Basic Res. 2016;22:123–7.

38. Jagannatha AT, Kamath S, Devi I, Rao UG. 376 The salt versus sugar debate: urinary sodium losses following hypertonic saline administration curtails its superior osmolar effect in comparison to mannitol in severe traumatic brain injury. Neurosurgery. 2016;63(Suppl 1):212.

39. White H, Cook D, Venkatesh B. The use of hypertonic saline for treating intracranial hypertension after traumatic brain injury. Anesth Analg. 2006;102(6):1836–46.

40. Qureshi AI, Suarez JI, Castro A, Bhardwaj A. Use of hypertonic saline/acetate infusion in treatment of cerebral edema in patients with head trauma: experience at a single center. J Trauma. 1999;47(4):659–65.

41. Vialet R, Albanese J, Thomachot L, Antonini F, Bourgouin A, Alliez B, et al. Isovolume hypertonic solutes (sodium chloride or mannitol) in the treatment of refractory posttraumatic intracranial hypertension: 2 mL/kg 7.5% saline is more effective than 2 mL/kg 20% mannitol. Crit Care Med. 2003;31(6):1683–7.

42. Kerwin AJ, Schinco MA, Tepas JJ 3rd, Renfro WH, Vitarbo EA, Muehlberger M. The use of 23.4% hypertonic saline for the management of elevated intracranial pressure in patients with severe traumatic brain injury: a pilot study. J Trauma. 2009;67(2):277–82.

43. Kokoska ER, Smith GS, Pittman T, Weber TR. Early hypotension worsens neurological outcome in pediatric patients with moderately severe head trauma. J Pediatr Surg. 1998;33(2):333–8.

44. Miller JD, Sweet RC, Narayan R, Becker DP. Early insults to the injured brain. JAMA. 1978;240(5):439–42.

45. Marmarou A, Anderson RL, Ward JD, Choi SC, Young HF, Eisenberg HM, et al. Impact of ICP instability and hypotension on outcome in patients with severe head trauma. Spec Suppl. 1991;75(1s):S59–66.

46. Newfield P, Pitts L, Kaktis J, Hoff J. The influence of shock on mortality after head trauma. Crit Care Med. 1980;8(4):254.

47. Wald SL, Shackford SR, Fenwick J. The effect of secondary insults on mortality and long-term disability after severe head injury in a rural region without a trauma system. J Trauma. 1993;34(3):377–81; discussion 81–2.

48. Yuan XQ, Wade CE, Clifford CB. Suppression by traumatic brain injury of spontaneous hemodynamic recovery from hemorrhagic shock in rats. J Neurosurg. 1991;75(3):408–14.

49. Dubick MA, Davis JM, Myers T, Wade CE, Kramer GC. Dose response effects of hypertonic saline and dextran on cardiovascular responses and plasma volume expansion in sheep. Shock. 1995;3(2):137–44.

50. Holcroft JW, Vassar MJ, Turner JE, Derlet RW, Kramer GC. 3% NaCl and 7.5% NaCl/dextran 70 in the resuscitation of severely injured patients. Ann Surg. 1987;206(3):279–88.

51. Kramer GC, Perron PR, Lindsey DC, Ho HS, Gunther RA, Boyle WA, et al. Small-volume resuscitation with hypertonic saline dextran solution. Surgery. 1986;100(2):239–47.

52. Maningas PA, DeGuzman LR, Tillman FJ, Hinson CS, Priegnitz KJ, Volk KA, et al. Small-volume infusion of 7.5% NaCl in 6% dextran 70 for the treatment of severe hemorrhagic shock in swine. Ann Emerg Med. 1986;15(10):1131–7.

53. Smith GJ, Kramer GC, Perron P, Nakayama S, Gunther RA, Holcroft JW. A comparison of several hypertonic solutions for resuscitation of bled sheep. J Surg Res. 1985;39(6):517–28.

54. Vassar MJ, Perry CA, Gannaway WL, Holcroft JW. 7.5% sodium chloride/dextran for resuscitation of trauma patients undergoing helicopter transport. Arch Surg. 1991;126(9):1065–72.

55. Tollofsrud S, Tonnessen T, Skraastad O, Noddeland H. Hypertonic saline and dextran in normovolaemic and hypovolaemic healthy volunteers increases interstitial and intravascular fluid volumes. Acta Anaesthesiol Scand. 1998;42(2):145–53.

56. Schertel ER, Valentine AK, Rademakers AM, Muir WW. Influence of 7% NaCl on the mechanical properties of the systemic circulation in the hypovolemic dog. Circ Shock. 1990;31(2):203–14.

57. Cudd TA, Purinton S, Patel NC, Wood CE. Cardiovascular, adrenocorticotropin, and cortisol responses to hypertonic saline in euvolemic sheep are altered by prostaglandin synthase inhibition. Shock. 1998;10(1):32–6.

58. Allen DA, Schertel ER, Schmall LM, Muir WW. Lung innervation and the hemodynamic response to 7% sodium chloride in hypovolemic dogs. Circ Shock. 1992;38(3):189–94.

59. Messmer K, Kreimeier U. Microcirculatory therapy in shock. Resuscitation. 1989;18(Suppl):S51–61.

60. Kreimeier U, Messmer K. Small volume resuscitation. In: Kox W, Gamble J, editors. Fluid resuscitation, Baillière's clinical anesthesiology. 2. London: Baillière Tindall; 1988. p. 545–77.

61. Riou B, Carli P. [Hypertonic sodium chloride and hemorrhagic shock]. Ann Fr Anesth Reanim. 1990;9(6):536–46.

62. Vassar MJ, Fischer RP, O'Brien PE, Bachulis BL, Chambers JA, Hoyt DB, et al. A multicenter trial for resuscitation of injured patients with 7.5% sodium chloride. The effect of added dextran 70. The Multicenter Group for the study of hypertonic saline in trauma patients. Arch Surg. 1993;128(9):1003–11; discussion 11–3.

63. Wade CE, Grady JJ, Kramer GC, Younes RN, Gehlsen K, Holcroft JW. Individual patient cohort analysis of the efficacy of hypertonic saline/dextran in patients with traumatic brain injury and hypotension. J Trauma. 1997;42(5 Suppl):S61–5.

64. Vassar MJ, Perry CA, Holcroft JW. Prehospital resuscitation of hypotensive trauma patients with 7.5% NaCl versus 7.5% NaCl with added dextran: a controlled trial. J Trauma. 1993;34(5):622–32; discussion 32–3.

65. Cooper DJ, Myles PS, McDermott FT, Murray LJ, Laidlaw J, Cooper G, et al. Prehospital hypertonic saline resuscitation of patients with hypotension and severe traumatic brain injury: a randomized controlled trial. JAMA. 2004;291(11):1350–7

66. Prough DS, Johnson JC, Poole GV Jr, Stullken EH, Johnston WE Jr, Royster R. Effects on intracranial pressure of resuscitation from hemorrhagic shock with hypertonic saline versus lactated Ringer's solution. Crit Care Med. 1985;13(5):407–11.

67. Prough DS, Whitley JM, Taylor CL, Deal DD, DeWitt DS. Regional cerebral blood flow following resuscitation from hemorrhagic shock with hypertonic saline. Influence of a subdural mass. Anesthesiology. 1991;75(2):319–27.

68. Doyle JA, Davis DP, Hoyt DB. The use of hypertonic saline in the treatment of traumatic brain injury. J Trauma. 2001;50(2):367–83.

69. Hariri RJ, Ghajar JB, Pomerantz KB, Hajjar DP, Giannuzzi RF, Tomich E, et al. Human glial cell production of lipoxygenase-generated eicosanoids: a potential role in the pathophysiology of vascular changes following traumatic brain injury. J Trauma. 1989;29(9):1203–10.

70. Rizoli SB, Kapus A, Fan J, Li YH, Marshall JC, Rotstein OD. Immunomodulatory effects of hypertonic resuscitation on the development of lung inflammation following hemorrhagic shock. J Immunol. 1998;161(11):6288–96.

71. Rizoli SB, Kapus A, Parodo J, Rotstein OD. Hypertonicity prevents lipopolysaccharide-stimulated CD11b/CD18 expression in human neutrophils in vitro: role for p38 inhibition. J Trauma. 1999;46(5):794–8; discussion 8–9.

72. Angle N, Hoyt DB, Coimbra R, Liu F, Herdon-Remelius C, Loomis W, et al. Hypertonic saline resuscitation diminishes lung injury by suppressing neutrophil activation after hemorrhagic shock. Shock. 1998;9(3):164–70.

73. Rizoli SB, Kapus A, Parodo J, Fan J, Rotstein OD. Hypertonic immunomodulation is reversible and accompanied by changes in CD11b expression. J Surg Res. 1999;83(2):130–5.

74. Rizoli SB, Rotstein OD, Parodo J, Phillips MJ, Kapus A. Hypertonic inhibition of exocytosis in neutrophils: central role for osmotic actin skeleton remodeling. Am J Physiol Cell Physiol. 2000;279(3):C619–33.

75. Loomis WH, Namiki S, Hoyt DB, Junger WG. Hypertonicity rescues T cells from suppression by trauma-induced anti-inflammatory mediators. Am J Physiol Cell Physiol. 2001;281(3):C840–8.

76. Junger WG, Coimbra R, Liu FC, Herdon-Remelius C, Junger W, Junger H, et al. Hypertonic saline resuscitation: a tool to modulate immune function in trauma patients? Shock. 1997;8(4):235–41.

77. Cuschieri J, Gourlay D, Garcia I, Jelacic S, Maier RV. Hypertonic preconditioning inhibits macrophage responsiveness to endotoxin. J Immunol. 2002;168(3):1389–96.

78. Gushchin V, Stegalkina S, Alam HB, Kirkpatrick JR, Rhee PM, Koustova E. Cytokine expression profiling in human leukocytes after exposure to hypertonic and isotonic fluids. J Trauma. 2002;52(5):867–71.

79. Oreopoulos GD, Bradwell S, Lu Z, Fan J, Khadaroo R, Marshall JC, et al. Synergistic induction of IL-10 by hypertonic saline solution and lipopolysaccharides in murine peritoneal macrophages. Surgery. 2001;130(2):157–65.

80. Oreopoulos GD, Wu H, Szaszi K, Fan J, Marshall JC, Khadaroo RG, et al. Hypertonic preconditioning prevents hepatocellular injury following ischemia/reperfusion in mice: a role for interleukin 10. Hepatology. 2004;40(1):211–20.

81. Powers KA, Woo J, Khadaroo RG, Papia G, Kapus A, Rotstein OD. Hypertonic resuscitation of hemorrhagic shock upregulates the anti-inflammatory response by alveolar macrophages. Surgery. 2003;134(2):312–8.

82. Rizoli SB, Rhind SG, Shek PN, Inaba K, Filips D, Tien H, et al. The immunomodulatory effects of hypertonic saline resuscitation in patients sustaining traumatic hemorrhagic shock: a randomized, controlled, double-blinded trial. Ann Surg. 2006;243(1):47–57.

83. Vespa P, Prins M, Ronne-Engstrom E, Caron M, Shalmon E, Hovda DA, et al. Increase in extracellular glutamate caused by reduced cerebral perfusion pressure and seizures after human traumatic brain injury: a microdialysis study. J Neurosurg. 1998;89(6):971–82.

84. Koura SS, Doppenberg EM, Marmarou A, Choi S, Young HF, Bullock R. Relationship between excitatory amino acid release and outcome after severe human head injury. Acta Neurochir Suppl. 1998;71:244–6.

85. Nicholls D, Attwell D. The release and uptake of excitatory amino acids. Trends Pharmacol Sci. 1990;11(11):462–8.

86. Zornow MH, Scheller MS, Shackford SR. Effect of a hypertonic lactated Ringer's solution on intracranial pressure and cerebral water content in a model of traumatic brain injury. J Trauma. 1989;29(4):484–8.

87. Sheikh AA, Matsuoka T, Wisner DH. Cerebral effects of resuscitation with hypertonic saline and a new low-sodium hypertonic fluid in hemorrhagic shock and head injury. Crit Care Med. 1996;24(7):1226–32.

88. Bacher A, Wei J, Grafe MR, Quast MJ, Zornow MH. Serial determinations of cerebral water content by magnetic resonance imaging after an infusion of hypertonic saline. Crit Care Med. 1998;26(1):108–14.

89. Schurer L, Dautermann C, Hartl R, Murr R, Berger S, Rohrich F, et al. Treatment of hemorrhagic hypotension with hypertonic/hyperoncotic solutions: effects on regional cerebral blood flow and brain surface oxygen tension. Eur Surg Res. 1992;24(1):1–12.

90. Anderson JT, Wisner DH, Sullivan PE, Matteucci M, Freshman S, Hildreth J, et al. Initial small-volume hypertonic resuscitation of shock and brain injury: short- and long-term effects. J Trauma. 1997;42(4):592–600; discussion 600–1.

91. Walsh JC, Zhuang J, Shackford SR. A comparison of hypertonic to isotonic fluid in the resuscitation of brain injury and hemorrhagic shock. J Surg Res. 1991;50(3):284–92.

92. Shackford SR. Effect of small-volume resuscitation on intracranial pressure and related cerebral variables. J Trauma. 1997;42(5 Suppl):S48–53.

93. Gunnar W, Jonasson O, Merlotti G, Stone J, Barrett J. Head injury and hemorrhagic shock: studies of the blood brain barrier and intracranial pressure after resuscitation with normal saline solution, 3% saline solution, and dextran-40. Surgery. 1988;103(4):398–407.

94. Mirski AM, Denchev ID, Schnitzer SM, Hanley FD. Comparison between hypertonic saline and mannitol in the reduction of elevated intracranial pressure in a rodent model of acute cerebral injury. J Neurosurg Anesthesiol. 2000;12(4):334–44.

95. Qureshi AI, Wilson DA, Traystman RJ. Treatment of elevated intracranial pressure in experimental intracerebral hemorrhage: comparison between mannitol and hypertonic saline. Neurosurgery. 1999;44(5):1055–63; discussion 63–4.

96. da Silva JC, de Lima Fde M, Valenca MM, de Azevedo Filho HR. Hypertonic saline more efficacious than mannitol in lethal intracranial hypertension model. Neurol Res. 2010;32(2):139–43.

97. Prough DS, Whitley JM, Taylor CL, Deal DD, DeWitt DS. Rebound intracranial hypertension in dogs after resuscitation with hypertonic solutions from hemorrhagic shock accompanied by an intracranial mass lesion. J Neurosurg Anesthesiol. 1999;11(2):102–11.

98. Einhaus SL, Croce MA, Watridge CB, Lowery R, Fabian TC. The use of hypertonic saline for the treatment of increased intracranial pressure. J Tenn Med Assoc. 1996;89(3):81–2.

99. Hartl R, Ghajar J, Hochleuthner H, Mauritz W. Treatment of refractory intracranial hypertension in severe traumatic brain injury with repetitive hypertonic/hyperoncotic infusions. Zentralbl Chir. 1997;122(3):181–5.

100. Schatzmann C, Heissler HE, Konig K, Klinge-Xhemajli P, Rickels E, Muhling M, et al. Treatment of elevated intracranial pressure by infusions of 10% saline in severely head injured patients. Acta Neurochir Suppl. 1998;71:31–3.

101. Oddo M, Levine JM, Frangos S, Carrera E, Maloney-Wilensky E, Pascual JL, et al. Effect of mannitol and hypertonic saline on cerebral oxygenation in patients with severe traumatic brain injury and refractory intracranial hypertension. J Neurol Neurosurg Psychiatry. 2009;80(8):916–20.

102. Rockswold GL, Solid CA, Paredes-Andrade E, Rockswold SB, Jancik JT, Quickel RR. Hypertonic saline and its effect on intracranial pressure, cerebral perfusion pressure, and brain tissue oxygen. Neurosurgery. 2009;65(6):1035–41; discussion 41–2.

103. Nakagawa K, Chang CW, Koenig MA, Yu M, Tokumaru S. Treatment of refractory intracranial hypertension with 23.4% saline in children with severe traumatic brain injury. J Clin Anesth. 2012;24(4):318–23.

104. Valentino AK, Nau KM, Miller DA, Hanel RA, Freeman W. Repeated dosing of 23.4% hypertonic saline for refractory intracranial hypertension. A case report. J Vasc Interv Neurol. 2008;1(4):113–7.

105. Mangat HS, Hartl R. Hypertonic saline for the management of raised intracranial pressure after severe traumatic brain injury. Ann N Y Acad Sci. 2015;1345:83–8.

106. Froelich M, Ni Q, Wess C, Ougorets I, Hartl R. Continuous hypertonic saline therapy and the occurrence of complications in neurocritically ill patients. Crit Care Med. 2009;37(4):1433–41.

107. Kochanek PM, Carney N, Adelson PD, Ashwal S, Bell MJ, Bratton S, et al. Guidelines for the acute medical management of severe traumatic brain injury in infants, children, and adolescents—second edition. Pediatr Crit Care Med. 2012;13(Suppl 1):S1–82.

108. Adelson PD, Bratton SL, Carney NA, Chesnut RM, du Coudray HE, Goldstein B, et al. Guidelines for the acute medical management of severe traumatic brain injury in infants, children, and adolescents. Chapter 11. Use of hyperosmolar therapy in the management of severe pediatric traumatic brain injury. Pediatr Crit Care Med. 2003;4(3 Suppl):S40–4.

109. Dominguez TE, Priestley MA, Huh JW. Caution should be exercised when maintaining a serum sodium level >160 meq/L. Crit Care Med. 2004;32(6):1438–9; author reply 9–40.

110. Gonda DD, Meltzer HS, Crawford JR, Hilfiker ML, Shellington DK, Peterson BM, et al. Complications associated with prolonged hypertonic saline therapy in children with elevated intracranial pressure. Pediatr Crit Care Med. 2013;14(6):610–20.

111. Lin KC, Chou CH, Chang WL, Ke DS, Kuo JR. The early response of mannitol infusion in traumatic brain injury. Acta Neurol Taiwanica. 2008;17(1):26–32.

112. Sorani MD, Morabito D, Rosenthal G, Giacomini KM, Manley GT. Characterizing the dose-response relationship between mannitol and intracranial pressure in traumatic brain injury patients using a high-frequency physiological data collection system. J Neurotrauma. 2008;25(4):291–8.

113. Battison C, Andrews PJ, Graham C, Petty T. Randomized, controlled trial on the effect of a 20% mannitol solution and a 7.5% saline/6% dextran solution on increased intracranial pressure after brain injury. Crit Care Med. 2005;33(1):196–202; discussion 57–8.

114. Ware ML, Nemani VM, Meeker M, Lee C, Morabito DJ, Manley GT. Effects of 23.4% sodium chloride solution in reducing intracranial pressure in patients with traumatic brain injury: a preliminary study. Neurosurgery. 2005;57(4):727–36; discussion 27–36.

115. Colton K, Yang S, Hu PF, Chen HH, Bonds B, Scalea TM, et al. Intracranial pressure response after pharmacologic treatment of intracranial hypertension. J Trauma Acute Care Surg. 2014;77(1):47–53; discussion.

116. Cottenceau V, Masson F, Mahamid E, Petit L, Shik V, Sztark F, et al. Comparison of effects of equiosmolar doses of mannitol and hypertonic saline on cerebral blood flow and metabolism in traumatic brain injury. J Neurotrauma. 2011;28(10):2003–12.

117. Sakellaridis N, Pavlou E, Karatzas S, Chroni D, Vlachos K, Chatzopoulos K, et al. Comparison of mannitol and hypertonic saline in the treatment of severe brain injuries. J Neurosurg. 2011;114(2):545–8.

118. Francony G, Fauvage B, Falcon D, Canet C, Dilou H, Lavagne P, et al. Equimolar doses of mannitol and hypertonic saline in the treatment of increased intracranial pressure. Crit Care Med. 2008;36(3):795–800.

119. Li M, Chen T, Chen SD, Cai J, Hu YH. Comparison of equimolar doses of mannitol and hypertonic saline for the treatment of elevated intracranial pressure after traumatic brain injury: a systematic review and meta-analysis. Medicine (Baltimore). 2015;94(17):e736.

120. Ichai C, Armando G, Orban JC, Berthier F, Rami L, Samat-Long C, et al. Sodium lactate versus mannitol in the treatment of intracranial hypertensive episodes in severe traumatic brain-injured patients. Intensive Care Med. 2009;35(3):471–9.

121. Burgess S, Abu-Laban RB, Slavik RS, Vu EN, Zed PJ. A systematic review of randomized controlled trials comparing hypertonic sodium solutions and

mannitol for traumatic brain injury: implications for Emergency Department Management. Ann Pharmacother. 2016;50(4):291–300.

122. Mortazavi MM, Romeo AK, Deep A, Griessenauer CJ, Shoja MM, Tubbs RS, et al. Hypertonic saline for treating raised intracranial pressure: literature review with meta-analysis. J Neurosurg. 2012;116(1):210–21.

123. Carney N, Totten AM, O'Reilly C, Ullman JS, Hawryluk GW, Bell MJ, et al. Guidelines for the management of severe traumatic brain injury, fourth edition. Neurosurgery. 2017;80(1):6–15.

124. Finberg L. Dangers to infants caused by changes in osmolal concentration. Pediatrics. 1967;40(6):1031–4.

125. Ziai WC, Toung TJ, Bhardwaj A. Hypertonic saline: first-line therapy for cerebral edema? J Neurol Sci. 2007;261(1–2):157–66.

126. Ayus JC, Krothapalli RK, Arieff AI. Changing concepts in treatment of severe symptomatic hyponatremia. Rapid correction and possible relation to central pontine myelinolysis. Am J Med. 1985;78(6 Pt 1):897–902.

127. Sterns RH, Riggs JE, Schochet SS Jr. Osmotic demyelination syndrome following correction of hyponatremia. N Engl J Med. 1986;314(24):1535–42.

128. Tyagi R, Donaldson K, Loftus CM, Jallo J. Hypertonic saline: a clinical review. Neurosurg Rev. 2007;30(4):277–89; discussion 89–90.

129. Brain Trauma Foundation, American Association of Neurological Surgeons, Congress of Neurological Surgeons, Joint Section on Neurotrauma and Critical Care AANS/CNS, Bratton SL, et al. Guidelines for the management of severe traumatic brain injury. II. Hyperosmolar therapy. J Neurotrauma. 2007;24(Suppl 1):S14–20.

130. Qureshi AI, Suarez JI, Bhardwaj A. Malignant cerebral edema in patients with hypertensive intracerebral hemorrhage associated with hypertonic saline infusion: a rebound phenomenon? J Neurosurg Anesthesiol. 1998;10(3):188–92.

131. Lien YH, Shapiro JI, Chan L. Study of brain electrolytes and organic osmolytes during correction of chronic hyponatremia. Implications for the pathogenesis of central pontine myelinolysis. J Clin Invest. 1991;88(1):303–9.

132. Trachtman H. Cell volume regulation: a review of cerebral adaptive mechanisms and implications for clinical treatment of osmolal disturbances: II. Pediatr Nephrol. 1992;6(1):104–12.

133. Trachtman H. Cell volume regulation: a review of cerebral adaptive mechanisms and implications for clinical treatment of osmolal disturbances. I. Pediatr Nephrol. 1991;5(6):743–50.

134. Trachtman H, Futterweit S, Tonidandel W, Gullans SR. The role of organic osmolytes in the cerebral cell volume regulatory response to acute and chronic renal failure. J Am Soc Nephrol. 1993;3(12):1913–9.

135. Ogden AT, Mayer SA, Connolly ES Jr. Hyperosmolar agents in neurosurgical practice: the evolving role of hypertonic saline. Neurosurgery. 2005;57(2):207–15; discussion 207–15.

136. Huang PP, Stucky FS, Dimick AR, Treat RC, Bessey PQ, Rue LW. Hypertonic sodium resuscitation is associated with renal failure and death. Ann Surg. 1995;221(5):543–54; discussion 54–7.

137. Adamik KN, Butty E, Howard J. In vitro effects of 3% hypertonic saline and 20% mannitol on canine whole blood coagulation and platelet function. BMC Vet Res. 2015;11:242.

138. Reed RL 2nd, Johnston TD, Chen Y, Fischer RP. Hypertonic saline alters plasma clotting times and platelet aggregation. J Trauma. 1991;31(1):8–14.

139. Hess JR, Dubick MA, Summary JJ, Bangal NR, Wade CE. The effects of 7.5% NaCl/6% dextran 70 on coagulation and platelet aggregation in humans. J Trauma. 1992;32(1):40–4.

Pituitary and Other Hormonal Derangements in Severe Traumatic Brain Injury

Courtney Pendleton and Jack Jallo

Introduction

Traumatic brain injury (TBI) remains a leading cause of death and disability in the United States, and it has been established that through various mechanisms, TBI may lead to dysfunction in various hormone axes in both the acute and chronic phases of injury [1–8]. However, acute and chronic hormone dysfunction is under-recognized in the TBI population. It is essential that clinicians treating patients with TBI understand the complex imbalances in pituitary function and hormone axes that occur, as early diagnosis and management may improve both the patients' clinical status and their ability to participate in the intensive post-injury rehabilitation programs necessary for most moderate to severe TBI injuries.

TBI is generally classified as mild, moderate, and severe. Although the majority of studies assess long-term hormone dysfunction in patients with moderate and severe TBI, those affected by mild TBI and repetitive TBI share disorders of hormone and pituitary function [9]. Notably, the repetitive mild to moderate TBI experienced by professional athletes appears to cause long-term hormone dysfunction in the limited reports available [10]. Military personnel are specifically at

C. Pendleton, MD · J. Jallo, MD, PhD, FACS (✉)
Department of Neurological Surgery, Thomas Jefferson University, Philadelphia, PA, USA
e-mail: Jack.Jallo@jefferson.edu

risk for blast-induced TBI (bTBI), caused largely by improvised explosive devices (IEDs), such as during the recent combat in Iraq and Afghanistan, which has been demonstrated to share similar hormone dysfunction and long-term sequelae as other forms of TBI [11, 12] despite the unique mechanism of injury.

The most common hormone dysfunction in TBI patients is growth hormone deficiency, but hypogonadotropic hypogonadism and hypopituitarism (primarily anterior pituitary hormones) have been described in the literature (Table 1) [8, 13].

Anatomy/Etiology

The mechanism of injury to the hypothalamic-pituitary system as a result of TBI remains incompletely understood. It is hypothesized that injury to the portal venous system surrounding the pituitary stalk may be implicated [14]. Autopsy studies demonstrating necrotic pituitary tissue support this theory. Autoimmune reactions activated as a result of inflammatory cascades following diffuse brain injury have also been postulated as contributing factors [2]. Other mechanical causes of injury, including compression from edema, elevated intracranial pressure (ICP), and depressed or displaced fractures have been suggested [15]. It is thought that the reason hypogonadotropic hypogonadism and growth hormone deficiency are the most

© Springer International Publishing AG, part of Springer Nature 2018
S. D. Timmons (ed.), *Controversies in Severe Traumatic Brain Injury Management*,
https://doi.org/10.1007/978-3-319-89477-5_8

Table 1 Evaluation and treatment algorithm for common hormone dysfunctions in TBI

Hormone derangement	Clinical symptoms	Laboratory findings	Management options
Hypogonadotropic hypogonadism	Fatigue Depressed mood Weight gain Decreased libido (men) Amenorrhea (women)	↓ Testosterone LH FSH	Testosterone replacement therapy
Growth hormone deficiency	Fatigue Anxiety Depression Elevated triglycerides Elevated LDL levels Reduced bone density Decreased exercise Tolerance Delayed puberty (pediatric population)	↓ GH IGF-1	Recombinant GH
Hypothalamic storming (dysautonomia, paroxysmal sympathetic hyperactivity)	Tachycardia Tachypnea Hyperthermia Dystonia Diaphoresis Hypertension	——	Symptomatic: Beta-blockade Opioids Bromocriptine

LH luteinizing hormone, *FSH* follicle-stimulating hormone, *LDL* low-density lipoprotein, *GH* growth hormone, *IGF-1* insulin-like growth factor 1

common hormone dysfunctions in TBI may be that somatotrophic and gonadotrophic cells are located laterally within the anterior pituitary, making them more vulnerable to ischemic and compressive damage [16]. However, there are instances of pituitary dysfunction following mild TBI, specifically in cases where no significant radiographic injury is seen.

Individual Hormone Deficiencies

Hypogonadotropic Hypogonadism

Secondary, or hypogonadotropic, hypogonadism (HH) is the most common hormone dysfunction in TBI patients, both in the short- and long-term periods. It occurs in nearly 100% of patients in

the acute phase of TBI and becomes persistent (PHH) in 37% [14]. It is described in 1.4–29% of patients overall [8, 14, 15] and manifests in decreased testosterone levels. Patients with HH have also been demonstrated to have decreased estradiol levels. It is postulated that, given estradiol's role in neuroprotection and neuroplasticity, these decreased levels may contribute to poor cognitive function in TBI patients [14], and progesterone has been explored as a potential therapy for TBI, with good preclinical results but poor results in two large clinical trials (SYNAPSE and PRoTECT III) [17, 18].

The symptoms of HH may overlap with the neuropsychological symptoms affecting many TBI patients. These include decreased energy, depressed mood/apathy, weight gain, decreased libido (men), and amenorrhea (women).

Evaluation of HH includes serum testosterone, luteinizing hormone (LH), and follicle-stimulating hormone (FSH) levels. Despite theories regarding estradiol levels and cognitive outcomes, it is not clear if laboratory evaluation is routinely necessary for clinical assessment and management.

Growth Hormone

Growth hormone (GH) deficiency has been reported in 9–25% of individuals with mild TBI [1, 3, 9, 10, 19–21]. Patients with GH deficiency may demonstrate cognitive dysfunction greater than counterparts with TBI and normal GH [9], and some studies have demonstrated increased depression and decreased energy levels in patients with TBI and GH deficiency [22].

The symptoms of GH deficiency vary widely and may overlap with the neuropsychological symptoms affecting many TBI patients, including fatigue, anxiety, and depression. Other symptoms include elevated triglyceride and low-density lipoprotein (LDL) levels, reduced bone density, and decreased exercise tolerance. In the pediatric population, symptoms include increased adiposity (particularly around the face and abdomen), decreased growth rate, and delayed or absent puberty.

Evaluation of GH deficiency includes measurement of insulin-like growth factor 1 (IGF-1) level and a stimulation test: the glucagon tolerance test, growth hormone releasing hormone-arginine test, and insulin tolerance test are all acceptable methods for laboratory evaluation and may be used based on institutional availability or clinician preference [2, 23].

Other Hormone Derangements

In addition to the hormone imbalances described in detail above, patients with TBI have been shown to have hyperprolactinemia [24, 25], which is more commonly noted in severe TBI. Patients are also noted to have decreased levels of thyroid-stimulating hormone (TSH) [24, 25], which may lead to sluggish metabolism, weight gain, and fatigue. The presence of hypothyroidism in TBI patients leads to a compensatory increase in thyrotropin-releasing hormone (TRH), which in turn may stimulate release of prolactin. It is postulated that the presence of hyperprolactinemia in TBI patients may be due to direct injury of the pituitary and stalk or a result of increased TRH release in response to hypothyroidism in severe brain injury [26].

Hypothalamic Storm

Hypothalamic storming was first described by Wilder Penfield in a patient with a tumor compressing the hypothalamus [27]. In the period immediately following severe TBI, hypothalamic storming (also referred to as dysautonomia, sympathetic storm, diencephalic seizure, or more recently paroxysmal sympathetic hyperactivity) may occur in up to 1/3 of patients [28], causing rapid and severe changes in physiologic parameters and metabolic function. These changes may be life-threatening in this population if not anticipated, with early and effective recognition and intervention. The pathophysiology driving this sympathetic overactivity is incompletely understood.

Patients may demonstrate tachycardia, tachypnea, hyperthermia, dystonia, diaphoresis, and hypertension. In some patients, specific stimuli may be identified as triggers to these episodes, allowing clinicians to minimize their occurrence or to preemptively treat the patient to mitigate or avoid a sympathetic storm.

Treatment is largely symptomatic, aimed at preventing prolonged symptoms and reducing the risk of secondary brain injury from prolonged derangements in physiologic parameters. Bromocriptine, an agent commonly used in the treatment of prolactin-secreting tumors, has been used successfully to mitigate hyperthermia and hypertension by acting as a dopamine receptor agonist at the hypothalamus [29, 30], but other agents are typically employed first. (See chapter

"Optimal Treatment of Dysautonomia" for discussion in further detail.)

It is important to note that in patients with multisystem traumas and prolonged intensive care unit (ICU) stays, these individual symptoms may be indicative of other underlying pathologies, including sepsis, pulmonary embolus/deep venous thrombosis, hemodynamic instability, or myocardial infarction. The diagnosis of hypothalamic storm should only be made if other potential etiologies are considered and ruled out through clinical and laboratory testing. Some authors have suggested a structured method for diagnosis including requiring 5 of 7 clinical findings consistent with sympathetic storm [31] or requiring episodes on multiple consecutive days [32] to ensure accuracy of diagnosis.

Fluid Balance Derangements

TBI may disrupt pathways from the hypothalamus and pituitary, leading to a range of potential fluid balance derangements, including the syndrome of inappropriate antidiuretic hormone secretion (SIADH), cerebral salt wasting (CSW), and central diabetes insipidus (CDI) (Table 2).

SIADH

SIADH is a common fluid imbalance seen in TBI patients and tends to develop in the acute setting within a week of injury. It is important to distinguish SIADH from CSW, as hyponatremia is a common laboratory finding in both disorders, but the treatments are diametrically opposed. Patients with SIADH demonstrate hyponatremia and normovolemia or hypervolemia. Management requires fluid and free water restriction to correct the electrolyte imbalance, which may be complicated in TBI patients requiring multiple infusions. In many institutions, concentrating the medications may be possible, which will help reduce the overall volume given. In patients who are symptomatic from hyponatremia, or those who require an elevated serum sodium for management of ICP, loop diuretics in conjunction with saline infusions may help correct hyponatremia, and hyperosmolar sodium solutions may be used to further correct the hyponatremia. Although the electrolyte changes in TBI patients are acute, the risk of central pontine myelinolysis should be kept in mind when addressing hyponatremia aggressively.

Table 2 Fluid balance derangements in TBI

Fluid balance derangement	Etiology	Laboratory findings	Management
SIADH	↑ ADH	Hyponatremia Normovolemia or hypervolemia	Fluid and free water restriction Loop diuretics Hypertonic saline (Severe or symptomatic hyponatremia)
CSW		Hyponatremia Hypovolemia	Fluid resuscitation: Normal saline (Mild, asymptomatic) Hypertonic saline (Severe, symptomatic, and/or patients with hypernatremic goals for ICP management)
CDI	↓ ADH	Hypernatremia Hypovolemia	Desmopressin (Intranasal or intravenous) Vasopressin-releasing medications (chlorpropamide, carbamazepine, and clofibrate) Thiazide diuretics Avoid dehydration (PO or IV fluid)

SIADH syndrome of inappropriate antidiuretic hormone secretion, CSW cerebral salt wasting, CDI central diabetes insipidus, ADH antidiuretic hormone secretion, ICP intracranial pressure, PO per os, IV intravenous

Cerebral Salt Wasting

CSW occurs within the first week post-injury and generally resolves in 2–4 weeks, although some patients may exhibit symptoms for a few months [33–35]. It is postulated that CSW occurs after TBI as a result of damage to the hypothalamic-pituitary axis, leading to increased dopamine release and sympathetic activation, which has downstream influences on renal processing of fluid and sodium, although the precise mechanisms are incompletely understood [33].

These patients demonstrate hypovolemia and hyponatremia, both of which pose significant risk to patients with TBI. Particularly in moderate to severe TBI, maintaining volume status is imperative for cerebral perfusion, while normonatremia or even hypernatremia may be an electrolyte goal aimed at managing cerebral edema and thereby intracranial pressure. Management of CSW requires restoration of normovolemia and maintenance of normonatremia; in mild cases normal saline may be adequate for restoration of these parameters, but in more severe CSW, or cases where sodium goals are hypernatremic, the use of hyperosmolar sodium solutions may be most appropriate.

Central Diabetes Insipidus

Nearly 25% of TBI patients are diagnosed with CDI in the immediate post-injury phase, although less than 10% demonstrate chronic or long-term symptoms [36–38]. The etiology of this fluid imbalance is damage to the hypothalamic-pituitary axis, leading to a deficiency of vasopressin/antidiuretic hormone. These patients demonstrate polydipsia (if clinical condition permits PO intake), excessive thirst, and polyuria with dilute urine. In patients with low Glasgow Coma Scale (GCS), those requiring ongoing intubation, and those unable to take PO fluids, assessing these signs and symptoms may be challenging. These patients may become severely dehydrated if volume status is not maintained with either PO intake or intravenous (IV) fluids.

The primary mode of treatment involves desmopressin, a synthetic vasopressin analog that may be given intravenously or intranasally. Additional medications include thiazide diuretics, which mitigate polyuria by increasing proximal tubule reabsorption, and vasopressin-releasing medications such as chlorpropamide, carbamazepine, and clofibrate. However, these medications have limited efficacy in patients with CDI, and should not be considered as first-line therapies.

Management and Complications

A thorough endocrine evaluation should be conducted in patients with moderate to severe TBI both in the acute phase and during routine follow-up, as some hormone dysfunctions may resolve without replacement therapy or further intervention [2, 8].

A handful of prospective studies have demonstrated that at 1 year following the initial TBI pituitary function improves in a significant percentage of patients, there are persistent deficits in many, and some patients develop new or worsening hormone dysfunction [2]. It is hypothesized that chronic hormone dysfunction may be related to autoimmunity [2], although further research is needed to establish the role of antibodies in developing or compounding hormone dysfunction in TBI patients.

Effect on Rehabilitation Capacity/ Facility Needs

The symptoms of many hormone dysfunctions include decreased energy and depressed mood, both of which may be factors in patients' ability to participate in the rehabilitation programs necessary after moderate to severe TBI, particularly in instances where multisystem trauma requires significant physical therapy. Beyond depressed mood, patients with GH deficiency have been described as having worse cognitive deficits than counterparts with similar TBI and normally functioning hormone axes [39]. This may impact both overall quality of life and ability to participate meaningfully in an intensive rehabilitation program [40].

Patients with GH deficiency have a higher-than-average body mass index (BMI) [9, 23], and specifically increased abdominal adiposity has been reported in patients with low IGF-1 levels secondary to GH deficiency [2, 41, 42]. Although limited information is available about how this directly impacts the prognosis of patients with TBI, individuals with an elevated BMI are likely to be less participatory in rehabilitation programs and to develop a multitude of additional health issues that may impact overall quality of life [40]. In addition, patients with GH deficiency have elevated total cholesterol, LDL, and triglyceride levels [2], potentially contributing to overall long-term health issues, namely, increased cardiovascular and cerebral infarction risk.

Special Considerations in the Pediatric Population

The overall incidence of pituitary dysfunction following TBI is now known to be far more common than was previously believed. Over the past decade, groups have evaluated the incidence of hormone dysfunction, particularly GH deficiency, in the pediatric TBI population, finding that treatment with GH replacement improved overall growth rate [13, 43]. Given the importance of adequate hormone levels and function during development, thorough endocrine evaluation and intervention is necessary in children and adolescents following TBI. Monitoring the height velocity in growing children may be a surrogate marker for growth hormone levels [44].

Special Considerations in the Military Population

In addition to the non-blast-related TBI affecting their civilian counterparts, military personnel are at increasing risk of blast TBI (bTBI). The common use of IEDs in recent conflicts in Iraq and Afghanistan has led bTBI to be described as a "signature injury" of these arenas [11, 12].

The physical and psychological health of active-duty personnel and combat veterans is complex, and the long-term consequences of bTBI may cloud the clinical picture and further complicate the coordination and provision of adequate healthcare.

Recent studies have demonstrated improvement in a variety of symptoms attributed to posttraumatic TBI complications with administration of hormone replacement therapy [11]. The authors of these studies recommend thorough initial and interval endocrine panels to fully assess hormone dysfunction in all military personnel affected by bTBI [11]; as hormone dysfunction appears similar in bTBI and non-blast-related TBI, extending this recommendation to military personnel experiencing TBI regardless of etiology may be prudent.

Future Directions for Research

Some preliminary research has been conducted regarding the role of autoimmunity in pituitary hormone deficiencies following TBI [2], with increased hormone dysfunction seen in patients with anti-hypothalamus and anti-pituitary antibodies. However, additional studies on a larger scale will be necessary to determine the precise role autoimmunity may play in acute and chronic hormone dysfunction following TBI.

The UK BIOSAP study reveals the need for adequate diagnosis, treatment, and long-term psychosocial and hormone therapy support for combat veterans sustaining bTBI with consequent pituitary hormone deficiencies as sequelae [11].

Conclusions

Hormone dysfunction is an important, yet under-recognized, consequence of TBI in the acute and chronic clinical setting. The effects of the most common hormone deficits may be vague and complicated by the myriad of other physical and psychological issues facing patients affected by TBI. Recognition of these hormone dysfunctions is paramount, as adequate pharmacologic management may improve overall quality of life and allow more effective treatment of concomitant ailments.

References

1. Ulfarsson T, Arnar Gudnason G, Rosén T, Blomstrand C, Sunnerhagen KS, Lundgren-Nilsson A, et al. Pituitary function and functional outcome in adults after severe traumatic brain injury: the long-term perspective. J Neurotrauma. 2013;30(4):271–80.

2. Tanriverdi F, Schneider HJ, Aimaretti G, Masel BE, Casanueva FF, Kelestimur F. Pituitary dysfunction after traumatic brain injury: a clinical and pathophysiological approach. Endocr Rev. 2015;36(3):305–42.

3. Agha A, Rogers B, Sherlock M, O'Kelly P, Tormey W, Phillips J, et al. Anterior pituitary dysfunction in survivors of traumatic brain injury. J Clin Endocrinol Metab. 2004;89(10):4929–36.

4. Casanueva FF, Leal A, Koltowska-Häggström M, Jonsson P, Góth MI. Traumatic brain injury as a relevant cause of growth hormone deficiency in adults: a KIMS-based study. Arch Phys Med Rehabil. 2005;86(3):463–8.

5. Leal-Cerro A, Flores JM, Rincon M, Murillo F, Pujol M, Garcia-Pesquera F, et al. Prevalence of hypopituitarism and growth hormone deficiency in adults long-term after severe traumatic brain injury. Clin Endocrinol (Oxf). 2005;62(5):525–32.

6. Popovic V, Aimaretti G, Casanueva FF, Ghigo E. Hypopituitarism following traumatic brain injury. Front Horm Res. 2005;33:33–44.

7. Popovic V, Aimaretti G, Casanueva FF, Ghigo E. Hypopituitarism following traumatic brain injury (TBI): call for attention. J Endocrinol Invest. 2005;28(5 Suppl):61–4.

8. Tanriverdi F, Senyurek H, Unluhizarci K, Selcuklu A, Casanueva FF, Kelestimur F. High risk of hypopituitarism after traumatic brain injury: a prospective investigation of anterior pituitary function in the acute phase and 12 months after trauma. J Clin Endocrinol Metab. 2006;91(6):2105–11.

9. Ioachimescu AG, Hampstead BM, Moore A, Burgess E, Phillips LS. Growth hormone deficiency after mild combat-related traumatic brain injury. Pituitary. 2015;18(4):535–41.

10. Kelly DF, Chaloner C, Evans D, Mathews A, Cohan P, Wang C, et al. Prevalence of pituitary hormone dysfunction, metabolic syndrome, and impaired quality of life in retired professional football players: a prospective study. J Neurotrauma. 2014;31(13):1161–71.

11. Baxter D, Sharp DJ, Feeney C, Papadopoulou D, Ham TE, Jilka S, et al. Pituitary dysfunction after blast traumatic brain injury: the UK BIOSAP study. Ann Neurol. 2013;74(4):527–36.

12. Benzinger TL, Brody D, Cardin S, Curley KC, Mintun MA, Mun SK, et al. Blast-related brain injury: imaging for clinical and research applications: report of the 2008 St. Louis workshop. J Neurotrauma. 2009;26(12):2127–44.

13. Acerini CL, Tasker RC. Neuroendocrine consequences of traumatic brain injury. J Pediatr Endocrinol Metab. 2008;21(7):611–9.

14. Wagner AK, Brett CA, McCullough EH, Niyonkuru C, Loucks TL, Dixon CE, et al. Persistent hypogonadism influences estradiol synthesis, cognition and outcome in males after severe TBI. Brain Inj. 2012;26(10):1226–42.

15. Agha A, Thompson CJ. High risk of hypogonadism after traumatic brain injury: clinical implications. Pituitary. 2005;8(3–4):245–9.

16. Richmond E, Rogol AD. Traumatic brain injury: endocrine consequences in children and adults. Endocrine. 2014;45(1):3–8.

17. Skolnick BE, Maas AI, Narayan RK, van der Hoop RG, MacAllister T, Ward JD, et al. A clinical trial of progesterone for severe traumatic brain injury. N Engl J Med. 2014;371(26):2467–76.

18. Wright DW, Yeatts S, Silbergleit R, Palesch YY, Hertzberg VS, Frankel M, Goldstein FC, Caveney AF, Howlett-Smith H, Bengelink EM, Manley GT, Merck LH, Janis LS, Barsan WG, Investigators NETT. Very early administration of progesterone for acute traumatic brain injury. N Engl J Med. 2014;371(26):2457–66.

19. Bavisetty S, McArthur DL, Dusick JR, Wang C, Cohan P, Boscardin WJ, et al. Chronic hypopituitarism after traumatic brain injury: risk assessment and relationship to outcome. Neurosurgery. 2008;62(5):1080–93; discussion 1093–84.

20. Lieberman SA, Oberoi AL, Gilkison CR, Masel BE, Urban RJ. Prevalence of neuroendocrine dysfunction in patients recovering from traumatic brain injury. J Clin Endocrinol Metab. 2001;86(6):2752–6.

21. Aimaretti G, Ambrosio MR, Di Somma C, Gasperi M, Cannavò S, Scaroni C, et al. Residual pituitary function after brain injury-induced hypopituitarism: a prospective 12-month study. J Clin Endocrinol Metab. 2005;90(11):6085–92.

22. van Liempt S, Vermetten E, Lentjes E, Arends J, Westenberg H. Decreased nocturnal growth hormone secretion and sleep fragmentation in combat-related posttraumatic stress disorder; potential predictors of impaired memory consolidation. Psychoneuroendocrinology. 2011;36(9):1361–9.

23. Toogood A, Brabant G, Maiter D, Jonsson B, Feldt-Rasmussen U, Koltowska-Haggstrom M, et al. Similar clinical features among patients with severe adult growth hormone deficiency diagnosed with insulin tolerance test or arginine or glucagon stimulation tests. Endocr Pract. 2012;18(3):325–34.

24. Bondanelli M, Ambrosio M, Zatelli MC, De Marinis L, degli Uberti EC. Hypopituitarism after traumatic brain injury. Eur J Endocrinol. 2005;152(5):679–91.

25. Benvenga S, Campenní A, Ruggeri RM, Trimarchi F. Clinical review 113: hypopituitarism secondary to head trauma. J Clin Endocrinol Metab. 2000;85(4):1353–61.

26. Matsuura H, Nakazawa S, Wakabayashi I. Thyrotropin-releasing hormone provocative release of prolactin and thyrotropin in acute head injury. Neurosurgery. 1985;16(6):791–5.

27. Penfield W. Diencephalic autonomic epilepsy. Arch Neurol Psychiatry. 1929;22:358–74.
28. Lemke DM. Riding out the storm: sympathetic storming after traumatic brain injury. J Neurosci Nurs. 2004;36(1):4–9.
29. Scott JS, Ockey RR, Holmes GE, Varghese G. Autonomic dysfunction associated with locked-in syndrome in a child. Am J Phys Med Rehabil. 1997;76(3):200–3.
30. Russo RN, O'Flaherty S. Bromocriptine for the management of autonomic dysfunction after severe traumatic brain injury. J Paediatr Child Health. 2000;36(3):283–5.
31. Baguley IJ, Cameron ID, Green AM, Slewa-Younan S, Marosszeky JE, Gurka JA. Pharmacological management of dysautonomia following traumatic brain injury. Brain Inj. 2004;18(5):409–17.
32. Blackman JA, Patrick PD, Buck ML, Rust RS. Paroxysmal autonomic instability with dystonia after brain injury. Arch Neurol. 2004;61(3):321–8.
33. Leonard J, Garrett RE, Salottolo K, Slone DS, Mains CW, Carrick MM, et al. Cerebral salt wasting after traumatic brain injury: a review of the literature. Scand J Trauma Resusc Emerg Med. 2015;23:98.
34. Moro N, Katayama Y, Igarashi T, Mori T, Kawamata T, Kojima J. Hyponatremia in patients with traumatic brain injury: incidence, mechanism, and response to sodium supplementation or retention therapy with hydrocortisone. Surg Neurol. 2007;68(4):387–93.
35. Lohani S, Devkota UP. Hyponatremia in patients with traumatic brain injury: etiology, incidence, and severity correlation. World Neurosurg. 2011;76(3–4):355–60.
36. Agha A, Sherlock M, Phillips J, Tormey W, Thompson CJ. The natural history of post-traumatic neurohypophysial dysfunction. Eur J Endocrinol. 2005;152(3):371–7.
37. Agha A, Thornton E, O'Kelly P, Tormey W, Phillips J, Thompson CJ. Posterior pituitary dysfunction after traumatic brain injury. J Clin Endocrinol Metab. 2004;89(12):5987–92.
38. Diamandis T, Gonzales-Portillo C, Gonzales-Portillo GS, Staples M, Borlongan MC, Hernandez D, et al. Diabetes insipidus contributes to traumatic brain injury pathology via cd36 neuroinflammation. Med Hypotheses. 2013;81(5):936–9.
39. Popovic V, Pekic S, Pavlovic D, Maric N, Jasovic-Gasic M, Djurovic B, et al. Hypopituitarism as a consequence of traumatic brain injury (TBI) and its possible relation with cognitive disabilities and mental distress. J Endocrinol Invest. 2004;27(11):1048–54.
40. Nourollahi S, Wille J, Weiß V, Wedekind C, Lippert-Grüner M. Quality-of-life in patients with post-traumatic hypopituitarism. Brain Inj. 2014;28(11):1425–9.
41. Herrmann BL, Rehder J, Kahlke S, Wiedemayer H, Doerfler A, Ischebeck W, et al. Hypopituitarism following severe traumatic brain injury. Exp Clin Endocrinol Diabetes. 2006;114(6):316–21.
42. Kleindienst A, Brabant G, Bock C, Maser-Gluth C, Buchfelder M. Neuroendocrine function following traumatic brain injury and subsequent intensive care treatment: a prospective longitudinal evaluation. J Neurotrauma. 2009;26(9):1435–46.
43. Acerini CL. Head-injury-induced pituitary dysfunction. An old curiosity rediscovered. Arch Dis Child. 2008;93(5):364–5.
44. Bellone S, Einaudi S, Caputo M, Prodam F, Busti A, Belcastro S, et al. Measurement of height velocity is an useful marker for monitoring pituitary function in patients who had traumatic brain injury. Pituitary. 2013;16(4):499–506.

Management to Optimal Parameters: Euboxia?

Kyle Mueller, Anthony Conte, Rocky Felbaum, Randy Bell, Shelly D. Timmons, and Rocco Armonda

Introduction

Critical care management of patients with traumatic brain injury (TBI) has seen significant improvements over the last several decades. As technology has improved, increasing volumes of data on patient parameters are now available to the clinician, leading to management questions as to what the optimal parameters should be in order to improve outcomes. These parameters should not be viewed in isolation but should be assessed collectively when treating TBI patients.

K. Mueller, MD (✉) · A. Conte, MD · R. Felbaum, MD
Department of Neurosurgery, Georgetown University Hospital, Washington, DC, USA

R. Bell, MD
Department of Neurosurgery, Walter Reed National Military Medical Center, Bethesda, MD, USA

S. D. Timmons, MD, PhD, FACS, FAANS
Department of Neurosurgery, Penn State University Milton S. Hershey Medical Center,
Hershey, PA, USA
e-mail: stimmons@mac.com

R. Armonda, MD
Department of Neurosurgery, Georgetown University Hospital, Washington Hospital Center,
Washington, DC, USA

Hematology

Complete Blood Count

A complete blood count (CBC) should be performed on all patients with significant TBI upon arrival to the hospital. The results assign values to the three cell lines in blood, red blood cells (RBC), white blood cells (WBC), and platelets, among other findings. These parameters can be altered by trauma, and their management will be discussed in sequence.

The normal WBC count in adults ranges from 3.5 to 10.5 thousand cells/μL. White blood cells are involved in the physiological response to inflammation, which can be traumatic or infectious in nature. In the acute traumatic setting, the WBC can increase as a physiological response to tissue injury sustained from the inciting event [1]. This response usually normalizes over the following days; however, initial levels may serve as a marker of severity of TBI, with higher levels correlating with greater severity [2]. The acute phase response is due to increased endogenous levels of catecholamines and cortisol due to physiological stress. Exogenous administration of steroids medications can also cause an elevation in the WBC count; however, corticosteroid medications are not used in the treatment of TBI. The Corticosteroid Randomisation After Significant Head Injury (CRASH) trial did not show any improvement in outcomes in severe TBI (sTBI) patients and was

© Springer International Publishing AG, part of Springer Nature 2018
S. D. Timmons (ed.), *Controversies in Severe Traumatic Brain Injury Management*,
https://doi.org/10.1007/978-3-319-89477-5_9

associated with increased mortality [3, 4]. As such, current guidelines have a level 1 recommendation that steroids are contraindicated in the initial management of TBI patients.

Many severe TBI patients have prolonged hospitalizations, with extended intensive care unit (ICU) time, as well as prolonged ventilatory support. In addition, many sTBI patients sustain polytrauma. The combination of these factors makes these patients at a higher risk for developing an infection and possibly leading to sepsis [5]. The WBC count can be used to aid physicians in detecting systemic inflammatory response syndrome (SIRS) and is considered together with the patient's vital signs such as heart rate, blood pressure, and temperature, to make this diagnosis and guide treatment. The WBC count also serves as a marker of infection that can be trended during treatment and to help prevent the development of septic shock.

The RBC's impact on physiology is clinically reported as the hemoglobin (Hgb) and hematocrit (Hct). The normal Hgb and Hct vary among male and females but are generally 14–18 g/dL and 39–50% for males and 12–16 g/dL and 35–45% for females, respectively. The RBC is an oxygen carrier and is thus important for brain tissue oxygenation. As such, Hgb and Hct represent potential treatment parameters to optimize, in order to reduce secondary injury to cerebral tissue. Anemia, can be a "second insult," is frequent in patients with TBI and has been associated with poor outcome, [6] via reduced cerebral oxygenation [7]. Improved cerebral oxygenation has been shown to improve patient outcomes with TBI [8, 9].

Transfusion targets in medicine have by and large fallen under two strategies: restrictive and liberal. Restrictive strategies most often utilize a threshold of 7 g/dL, whereas liberal strategies typically target 10 g/dL. Some studies of general critically ill patients have shown that more restrictive strategies may improve survival compared with liberal strategies, presumably due to avoiding the risks associated with blood transfusions [10]. The population of patients in studies assessing optimal transfusion thresholds underrepresent those with acute neurological conditions such as TBI, [11] limiting the generalizability of this practice to neu-

rotrauma patients. Some studies have not found any difference in mortality with various transfusion strategies when specific TBI populations are assessed [12]. Despite the findings in critically ill patients, concern lingers that hemoglobin concentrations as low as 7 g/dL may not be tolerated in patients with severe TBI due to the potential for end-organ damage. Some reviews have still advocated a liberal transfusion strategy in this population [13], and a recent survey of practitioners demonstrated considerable variation in transfusion practices in patients with TBI [14] because there exists a paucity of data on the topic. Therefore, no consensus has been reached on how best to optimize Hgb and Hct in TBI, be it with restrictive or liberal transfusion strategies [15–18]. Further studies are needed in specific TBI subpopulations to identify which TBI patients may benefit from more liberal transfusion strategies. Brain tissue oxygenation monitoring may be used in future trials to better evaluate the optimal Hgb and Hct ranges, by helping define which patients will benefit from transfusion and balancing the treatment goals of improving cerebral oxygenation while limiting risks of transfusions [19]. (For further detailed discussion, see chapter "Treatment of Anemia".)

Platelets, produced by the fragmentation of megakaryocytes from bone marrow, are the third component of the CBC of importance in TBI management. The main contribution of platelets to hemostasis is to initiate blood clotting at the site of disrupted endothelium. Platelets defects may be either quantitative (too few) or qualitative (dysfunctional). The normal range is 150,000 to 450,000/mL. Prior to elective surgical procedures, surgeons frequently optimize the platelet count to >100,000 so as to reduce the chance of both intraoperative and postoperative bleeding. As the platelet count declines incrementally below 100,000, the chance for spontaneous bleeding increases. A high proportion of severe TBI patients have traumatic intracranial hemorrhage (ICH). There has been an association of thrombocytopenia below 100,000 and increased mortality as well as increased progression of traumatic ICH [20]. Further research is needed to assess specific quantifiable platelet count ranges to target in order to improve outcomes, but clinically, treatment is based upon procedural and surgical need, imaging progression, and a variety of other factors, including the presence of other coagulopathies, spleen injury, and transfusion requirements overall. The practice of maintaining a count of >100,000 is reasonable even with the paucity of clinical evidence. Animal models have suggested that platelet dysfunction occurs as a result of acute TBI, [21] and there is ample literature in humans to support this. As such, it is important not only to assess platelet count but also platelet function as more reliable and sophisticated assays become available.

The effect of coagulopathy on increasing mortality in TBI patients has been evaluated in the literature [22]. Coagulopathy is influenced not only by platelets but other clotting pathways that can be evaluated with activated partial thromboplastin time (PTT), prothrombin time (PT), and the international normalized ratio (INR). Abnormal initial coagulation studies have been associated with progression of ICH, which can lead to poor outcomes [23]. Other injuries may contribute to derangements in clotting studies, including hepatic injury and fluid resuscitation most commonly.

Thromboelastography (TEG) is a technique that can give a better evaluation of the coagulation status of a patient as opposed to traditional blood tests. Future studies may utilize this as a way to guide targeted therapy in TBI patients, especially those with ICH [24–26]. (For a detailed discussion of the pathophysiology of trauma-induced coagulopathy and testing mechanisms, see chapter "Management of Traumatic Brain Injury in the Face of Antithrombotic Medication Therapy".) In general, for TBI, the closer to normal values for CBC parameters of WBC, Hgb, Hct, and platelet count, as well as PT and PTT, the less likely there are to be significant downstream consequences of cerebral secondary injury.

Electrolytes

Sodium

Sodium is the major extracellular cation in the body with a normal range of 135–145 mmol/L. It is intimately associated with the normal water balance of the body and can be deranged by a variety of conditions caused by TBI, including cerebral salt wasting (CSW) and the syndrome of inappropriate antidiuretic hormone secretion (SIADH). As such, sodium is an aggressively monitored and oft-targeted electrolyte in the management of TBI patients.

Symptoms of hyponatremia may mimic those of TBI, including nausea and vomiting, headache, confusion, fatigue/lethargy, irritability, muscle weakness or spasms, and even coma if profound. Furthermore, hyponatremia may contribute to seizures, to which TBI patients are already prone, and the combination may make them difficult to control, especially in chronic alcohol abusers, worsening ultimate outcome. In the setting of severe TBI, progressively worsening hyponatremia can lead to increased pericontusional edema and may contribute to increasing hematoma volume (as illustrated in Fig. 1), both of which can also lead to worse outcomes. The full mechanism of hematoma expansion is still being elucidated but is likely due to a combination of osmotic effect as well as a reduction in blood viscosity.

Hyponatremia is therefore to be avoided, and a proper work-up for etiology is critical, because the treatments for iatrogenic hyponatremia, CSW, and SIADH are all different. Iatrogenic hyponatremia is treated by adjusting fluid concentrations and volumes. Whereas CSW is due to renal loss of both electrolytes and volume and must be treated with volume replacement with isotonic fluids (typically normal saline), SIADH is treated initially with volume restriction. In general, unless hyperosmolar euvolemic therapy is being employed, normal serum sodium levels should be goals of therapy. In those patients presenting with severe hyponatremia upon admission, care must be taken not to correct the sodium too rapidly, which can contribute to central pontine myelinolysis, particularly in chronic alcohol abusers.

The main symptom of hypernatremia is thirst, which of course cannot be gauged in the comatose patient, and is of little clinical consequence as long as input is controlled. While extreme hypernatremia can lead to confusion, seizures, or

Fig. 1 A 24-year-old male s/p assault. (**a**) Initial computed tomography (CT) head showing multiple contusions, admission sodium of 141. (**b**) Repeat CT showing blossoming contusions, patient intact with repeat sodium level of 137. (**c**) Patient with declining Glaucoma Coma Scale (GCS) requiring intubation, repeat CT showing worsening contusions with cerebral edema, emergent external ventricular drain (EVD) placed, repeat sodium level of 132. (**d**) Post-EVD CT showing global cerebral edema with loss of gray-white matter differentiation, repeat sodium level of 129; patient aggressively treated with 3% NaCl, hypothermia, phenobarbital coma, and cerebrospinal fluid (CSF) diversion

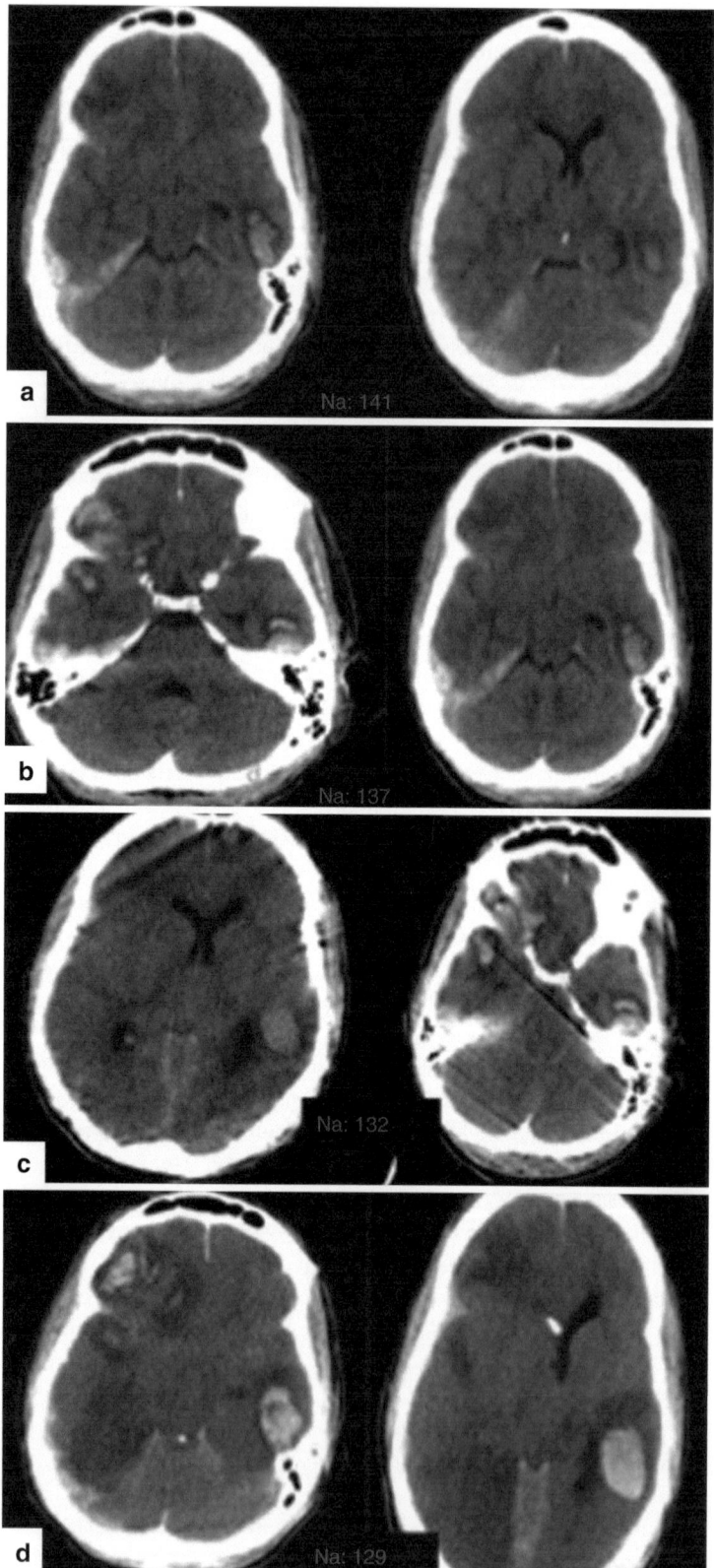

coma, and neuromuscular excitability and hyper-reflexia, these typically occur with non-iatrogenic chronic hypernatremia or extremely high values of serum sodium.

Artificial elevation of serum sodium may be employed (especially in younger healthier patients) as part of hyperosmolar euvolemic therapy, which is frequently used to treat cerebral edema (general or peri-contusional) after sTBI. This therapy is implemented via administration of various combinations of diuretics, concentrated salt solutions, and other fluid management techniques. Furthermore, hypertonic saline (HTS) is often employed in sTBI as a mechanism of reducing intracranial pressure (ICP) by reducing tissue fluid through osmotic intravascular gradients. In several small studies, HTS has been shown to reduce ICP when used as a first-line agent [27–29]. As no robust evidence suggests that using HTS prophylactically improves outcomes, the use of hypertonic saline, normal saline, diuretics, and other measures to achieve certain sodium and osmolarity values should be conceptualized and used as a treatment for edema and not a preventive strategy. Those with TBI and no significant tissue edema would not be presumed to significantly benefit. However, there is some evidence that HTS improves microscopic blood flow and may therefore confer additional benefit by reducing secondary ischemia in injured tissue, even when significant edema is not present.

In many neurocritical care units across the United States, a target of greater than 150 mmol/L is frequently used. Serum osmolarity values are normally 275–295 mosm/kg and generally are kept <320 mosm/kg, although higher values may be tolerated by some patients. The formulation and mode of HTS administration is a subject of frequent controversy. While animal and human data both suggest that bolus administration is more effective [30], it may be used as a bolus or a continuous drip in a variety of concentrations. HTS is available for either in most hospitals in 2 and 3% concentrations. Higher concentrations up to 23.4% are also available and are typically used in small volume boluses to treat elevated ICP [31].

When employing any form of hyperosmolar euvolemic therapy, it is important to monitor the degree of each parameter. Overshooting target levels to majorly elevated sodium levels and severe hyperosmolarity can have deleterious effects as well, including seizures and renal injury. Both serial serum sodium and serum osmolarity levels should therefore be monitored in order to limit drug or HTS administration when target goals are reached and to guide volume adjustments to maintain target levels. Severe hypernatremia ("overshooting the mark") is more common with continuous infusions, and this technique should be used with caution in patients who have significant third spacing of fluids. Volume status must be estimated in a continuous fashion and attention paid to avoidance of hypovolemia (resulting in decreased cerebral and renal perfusion) and hypervolemia (leading to cerebral, pulmonary, and other tissue edema and even cardiac failure).

When osmotherapy is considered, the ideal agent should be able to reduce ICP and cerebral tissue edema while maintaining cerebral perfusion pressure (CPP). Mannitol is a mainstay drug used in the treatment of sTBI. It is an osmotic diuretic used to rapidly reduce tissue edema (and thereby ICP), but it has other mechanisms of action as well, including increasing blood viscosity to enhance CBF [30]. Care must be taken with repeated administration, however, so as not to deplete the intravascular volume or to cause leaking of mannitol into cerebral tissues via broken down blood-brain barrier, thereby reversing the osmotic gradient and worsening cerebral edema. HTS has the benefit of helping to maintain euvolemia and cerebral perfusion while reducing edema [32, 33]. The future of hyperosmolar therapy will focus on identifying which situations call for which agent or agents and their optimal means of administration (i.e., concentrations and bolus vs. continuous infusion for HTS) and enhancing understanding of precise mechanisms of action.

See also chapter "Fluid and Electrolyte Management: Hyperosmolar Euvolemia and the Use of Hypertonic Saline for Intracranial Hypertension" for additional detailed discussion of fluid and electrolyte disturbances in TBI.

Magnesium

Magnesium has an important role in homeostatic regulation of the pathways involved in the delayed secondary phase of brain injury [34]. A depletion of magnesium has been observed in brain tissue in animals and in blood of humans after brain injury. During normal physiological processes, magnesium is a noncompetitive inhibitor of the N-Methyl-D-aspartate (NMDA) receptor, which is an important regulator of calcium influx. In turn, calcium influx is related to several secondary cellular processes that lead to neuronal cell death and degeneration after TBI [35].

Currently, only animal models have shown the neuroprotective effects of magnesium therapy, with little to support translation to outcomes in humans [36]. Some data do suggest that ionized magnesium could be a clinically useful predictor of late outcomes after brain injury, [37] but it is still not clear from the literature whether there is therapeutic benefit to targeting serum magnesium levels, due to conflicting effects on mortality and outcomes [38, 39]. Some studies have shown that a neuroprotective effect may become apparent when magnesium therapy is synergistic with other treatment modalities [40]. Future studies are needed to clarify what role, if any, magnesium as a therapeutic has in the management of acute TBI.

Regardless, maintaining normal magnesium levels is important, as hypomagnesemia can cause many signs and symptoms that can be confused with high ICP and TBI, including lethargy; nausea and vomiting; motor weakness, spasms, and incoordination; numbness and paresthesias; hyperreflexia; tremors; involuntary eye movements; and dysphagia, and it can also contribute to a lower seizure threshold. Other symptoms of confusion, impaired cognition, irritability, anxiety, and behavioral disturbances can manifest as ICU delirium. Finally, associated metabolic and cardiovascular effects can confound ICU management, including diarrhea; derangements in glucose, calcium, or potassium; and irregular cardiac rhythms and tachycardia.

Hypermagnesemia may result in nausea and vomiting, hyporeflexia, muscle weakness including respiratory muscles, hypotension, bradycardia, and cardiac arrest.

Potassium

Potassium plays a key role in neural signaling, and much of our understanding of the significance of serum levels is imputed from knowledge of how potassium impacts neurophysiological and intracellular processes, about which a great deal is known.

Some studies have suggested TBI patients are more prone to developing hypokalemia, [41] and as such potassium levels should be carefully monitored, not only because of potassium's central nervous system (CNS) effects but also because of the impact of potassium on other ions. Refractory hypokalemia is often observed in patients with marked magnesium deficiency.

Hyperkalemia can also lead to cardiac side effects, including dysrhythmias that can be catastrophic. Other symptoms of nausea and vomiting, paresthesias, muscle paralysis, and respiratory problems may complicate ICU management.

Hypokalemia can also cause neuromuscular paralysis (including respiratory musculature), nausea and vomiting, constipation, and even rhabdomyolysis.

Phosphorus

Hypophosphatemia is prevalent in ICU care, as critically ill patients often have many conditions that predispose them to hypophosphatemia, including inadequate nutrition, diabetic ketoacidosis, respiratory alkalosis, alcoholism, and gastrointestinal losses. Low phosphorus levels may impact WBC, RBC, and platelet function. Hypophosphatemia may also cause muscle weakness (including respiratory failure), confusion, ataxia, seizures, and coma, as well as cardiac dysrhythmias and cardiomyopathy.

Hyperphosphatemia is uncommon due to efficient renal excretion even in the face of high intake and is primarily related to chronic renal failure/chronic kidney disease.

Calcium

Calcium plays a major role in cellular signaling, modulation of neurotransmitters, and intracellular metabolism. The roles of calcium are well-characterized in terms of cellular firing in neurons and hyperexcitability, as well as in secondary injury from excitotoxicity and other negative sequelae of traumatic brain injury. Theoretically at least, it is important to keep calcium levels in the normal range, as a result. Trials of calcium channel blockade in TBI have not yielded results in terms of neuroprotection, but these studies may have had methodological challenges preventing effects on mortality or functional outcomes from being observed, with only limited evidence of benefit from the selective calcium channel blocker nimodipine specifically in patients with traumatic subarachnoid hemorrhage [42].

Electrophysiology

Cortical Spreading Depression

Cortical spreading depression (also known as spreading cortical depolarizations [CSDs]) is slowly propagating cortical waves (2–5 mm/min) that were originally described by A. P. Leao in the 1940s [43, 44]. They represent pathological events that recur acutely in the cerebral gray matter of patients with TBI and other acute brain injuries and can result in further secondary injury [45–47]. During depolarizations, there is a breakdown of ion gradients that propagates a signaling cascade, in turn causing an increased metabolic burden and reduced cerebral perfusion. This increasing supply-demand mismatch contributes to further secondary ischemic injury [48]. Ultimately, spreading depressions cause a persistent loss of cellular function [49].

These depolarizations can be monitored clinically at the bedside with electroencephalography (EEG) both with scalp and subdural recordings [50]. Spreading depolarizations can have widespread hemispheric propagation, which can be a marker of ongoing secondary injury. Persistent

isoelectricity of the cortex (flatline) is induced by spreading depolarizations and does not precede it. They are a dominant electrophysiological pathology in TBI and occur with an incidence as high as 60% [50]. There has been no association of the occurrence of spreading depressions with measures of injury severity, but recently, they have been independently associated with unfavorable extended Glasgow Outcome Scale (GOS) scores at 6 months after controlling for conventional prognostic variables [51].

Spreading depression monitoring provides a measure of neuronal pathophysiologic processes that is independent of other clinical monitoring variables and could be targeted for patient management and/or neuroprotection. Future studies should seek to evaluate the impact of various treatment regimens on CSDs, expand the number of patients undergoing monitoring for CSDs, and provide more data regarding the impact of CSDs on long-term outcomes.

Nutrition Replacement and Metabolic Needs

The optimization of nutritional status in patients with severe traumatic brain injury plays a vital role in recovery and prevention of secondary injury. Patients with severe TBI will often maintain a hypermetabolic state secondary to stress-mediated hormones and pro-inflammatory cytokine release from trauma. This hypermetabolic state may lead to upward of 200% increase in normal resting energy expenditure [52, 53]. Historical data suggests a mean metabolic expenditure of 140–160% in severe TBI patients [54]. Hypercatabolism of proteins and other nutrients makes meeting adequate nutrition requirements in these patients a challenge that must be met by considering the composition of nutritional replacement, the timing of initiation of replacement, the delivery method, and the critical neurological interventions and treatments that may increase energy expenditure. Failure to meet these nutritional requirements may result in increased incidence of pneumonia, multi-organ failure, poor wound healing, and sepsis [55]. In a retrospective cohort study of 797 TBI patients, for every 10 kcal/kg decrease in nutritional support in the first 5–7 days post-injury, there was an associated 30–40% incremental increased mortality risk [56]. The impact of failure to meet nutritional goals on long-term recovery is unknown but is presumed to be high. Unfortunately, nutrition requirements are often overlooked when dealing with the enormously complex care structure of a patient with severe traumatic brain injury.

Practitioners must have an understanding of the increased energy requirements caused by the elevated cerebral metabolic rate following TBI. Attempts to control metabolic energy expenditure (i.e., sedation, neuromuscular blockade, barbiturate coma) may only decrease demand by 10–15% [53]. Therefore, nutrition goals must be adjusted to prevent long-term malnutrition and its associated complications.

There is a long history of nutritional replacement research in the trauma critical care literature [57]. Recognition that early replacement decreases complications in trauma patients in general has been widespread since the 1980s to 1990s. It should be assumed that TBI patients fall under the same rubric, as evidenced by the aforementioned study showing a two- and fourfold increase in mortality rates for TBI patients in which nutrition was withheld in the first 5 and 7 days post-injury, respectively, even when controlled for severity of injury and neurologic impairment [56]. Another trial comparing 145 severe TBI patients receiving enteral nutrition in the first 48 h after injury with 152 demographically matched patients not receiving enteral nutrition until after 48 h [58] demonstrated survival rates and GCS scores that were significantly improved in the early nutrition group at 7 days and 1 month. A recent randomized controlled trial comparing initiation of nutrition at the 48-h post-injury mark did not show differences in morbidity or ventilator-associated pneumonia rates; however, both improved thyroid hormone profiles and lower cortisol concentrations were observed in the early enteral feeding group [59]. Early feeding replenishes glucose and macronutrient stores that are rapidly depleted by an increased cerebral metabolic rate and post-traumatic stress response, mediated by increased

levels of catecholamines, cortisol, and pro-inflammatory cytokines, [56] among other postulated mechanisms. (For impact see chapter "Nutrition: Time to Revisit?" for further detailed discussion, including route of administration.)

Additional nutritional supplementation in the form of probiotics, vitamins, and minerals may also serve a role in the management of the TBI patient. Probiotic supplements have been shown to lower pro-inflammatory cytokines in TBI patients, with the potential to decrease the risk of nosocomial infections and shorten ICU stays [60]. Zinc, vitamin C, vitamin E, and magnesium replacement therapies may all serve roles in preventing secondary cortical injury and cell death in TBI patients, yet many of these studies have yet to provide conclusive evidence [61–64]. Key questions will include the impact of deficiencies of these elements, optimal replacement, and serum level follow-up strategies.

Glucose

One of the most important secondary insults that can affect TBI prognosis is hyperglycemia [65, 66]. The main source of energy for the human brain is glucose [67]. Transporters in the blood-brain barrier (BBB), GLUT-1 and GLUT-3, regulate glucose movement into the neural cells [68, 69]. These transporters are implicated in a glucose-lactate synthesis pathway. Tissue lactic acidosis plays a pivotal role in neuronal excitotoxicity and secondary neuronal injury with a variety of mechanisms being postulated [70, 71], ultimately resulting in metabolism via the glycolytic pathway—a dysfunctional energy state [72, 73].

Ongoing hyperglycemia and altered glucose metabolism has been associated with higher TBI mortality rates in clinical trials [74–76] and a lower likelihood of a favorable outcome [65, 77]. This is particularly problematic, as patients with severe TBI have been shown to have greater admission blood glucose levels than patients with mild TBI [78].

Although consensus on the optimal glucose levels in patients with TBI has not yet been reached, [79, 80] for the practicing clinician managing severe TBI patients, incorporating close monitoring of serum glucose is important, as is implementing fairly normal target glucose ranges, avoiding hypoglycemia, and avoiding significant hyperglycemia above 200 mg/dL. Ways of modulating glucose levels include initiating enteric nutrition as soon as possible, [81, 82] utilizing enteral nutrition with small amounts of carbohydrates, [83, 84] and limiting the amount of intravenous (IV) glucose administered in IV solutions, in addition to insulin therapy.

Acid-Base Balance and the Arterial Blood Gas

PaCO$_2$

Arterial carbon dioxide levels directly correlate with arteriolar diameters in the cerebral vasculature and therefore determine at least to some extent the degree of cerebral blood flow (CBF) to the injured brain [85]. Lower levels of CO$_2$ (induced by hyperventilation or otherwise) cause a decline in perivascular pH and, via chemoreceptors, contraction of the vascular musculature leading to decreases in cerebral blood flow, cerebral blood volume, and eventually intracranial pressure. Higher carbon dioxide (CO$_2$) (hypercarbia) levels will lead to higher pH and vasodilation and increased cerebral blood flow (CBF) (hyperemia), which may further exacerbate cerebral edema. While moderate, short-term hypocapnia can be beneficial in lowering ICP, prolonged and/or severe hypocapnia leads to prolonged vasoconstriction and reduced CBF, contributing to cerebral ischemia and infarction. It is therefore recommended to maintain normocapnia at a PaCO$_2$ of 35–40, utilizing hyperventilation and moderate hypocapnia as a temporary measure in the setting of acute ICP increases or herniation [86].

PaO$_2$

Numerous studies have shown that the duration and number of hypoxic episodes, whether in the prehospital or hospital setting, correlate with a poor prognosis [87–90]. Persistent hypoxemia further exacerbates cerebral ischemia and secondary insult to critically injured brain [91]. Early intubation in the field to reduce hypoxic events and prehospital resuscitation efforts to prevent hypotension have been recognized by the trauma community as vitally important to the treatment of the TBI patient because hypoxia and hypotension dramatically increase mortality with more than additive effects if both occur [92]. Close monitoring of arterial oxygen levels should be employed to prevent secondary cerebral injury, ensuring PaO$_2$ is maintained above 60 mmHg, and in the absence of PaO$_2$, oxygen saturations should be maintained in the normal range.

Acid-Base Balance

Acid-base abnormalities are a marker of tissue perfusion, hypoxia, and predict overall morbidity and mortality in patients with systemic trauma. While a plethora of data exist in the general trauma literature on the influence of acid-base imbalance on mortality, roles in isolated brain trauma are less well defined. Pediatric data correlates the presence of a mixed respiratory and metabolic acidosis with increased mortality rates when compared with children with a compensatory metabolic alkalosis [93]. A similar study in adults did not show increased mortality rates with increasing base deficits, though base deficits were associated with lower Glasgow Coma Scores [94]. Mean arterial pH of TBI patients correlates with outcome [95]; however, arterial pH levels may not correlate with brain tissue pH levels [95, 96]. Brain tissue acidosis has been associated with a decline in mitochondrial ATP generation and an increase in free radical formation, potentiating neuronal cell death. Brain tissue monitoring has shown that TBI patients with poor outcomes tend to have lower brain tissue pH, higher lactate, and higher CO$_2$ levels, with the most pronounced effects in the first 24 h following injury [95].

Arterial acid-base derangements should be addressed promptly by the trauma, neurosurgical, and neurocritical care teams due to their association with mortality and overall outcomes, though more data is needed on correlation of systemic derangements on cerebral tissue and how to modify the latter.

Temperature, Avoidance of Hyperthermia

Targeted temperature management (TTM) is currently a goal that is implemented in most neurointensive care units. The goal is to prevent second insult episodes of rapid or episodic temperature elevations that can result in secondary injury cascades after traumatic brain injury [97–104].

As many as 50% of TBI patients develop temperatures above 38.5 °C while in the ICU, with at least 2/3 of patients experiencing more than one fever episode [105]. Although infection is a primary concern, fever in TBI patients may be due to a disruption in endogenous pyrogen release from a deranged hypothalamic set point [106]. Multiple prior studies have indicated that fever following TBI is highly associated with worse outcomes. In particular, early fever confers an approximately twofold increased relative risk of a poor outcome, worse with every 1 °C elevation [107]. Elevated core temperature exacerbates the cycle of neuronal excitotoxicity by promoting blood-brain barrier breakdown, production of more free radicals, and degradation of important cellular repair pathways [108, 109]. Further, elevated temperature can lead to increased ICP and reduced brain tissue oxygenation, as demonstrated in Fig. 2.

While a great deal of clinical research has been targeted toward therapeutic hypothermia based upon promising preclinical results, individual clinical studies have found conflicting results regarding the benefit of therapeutic hypothermia in severe TBI patients [105, 110, 111]. Larger trials have not been able to establish concrete findings [112, 113]. On the other hand, other studies have found no difference or even worse outcomes in a hypothermia group versus a normothermia group [106, 114]. A Cochrane Database meta-analysis of hypothermia revealed no overall benefit of hypothermia in severe TBI [115]. Several large-scale clinical trials have been performed. The National Acute Brain Injury Study: Hypothermia (NABISH) trial showed no benefit in the hypothermia group [106]. Although center differences in critical care management may have impacted the NABISH trial, a second NABISH trial with tighter clinical protocols also proved negative, as did the Japanese Brain Hypothermia (B-HYPO) trial [114]. And, more recently, although the European Study of Therapeutic Hypothermia (32–35 °C) trial found no functional outcomes improvements from hypothermia (32–35 °C), it did effectively reduce ICP [116].

Nonetheless, some important findings have been noted. For example, in a separate analysis of the patients enrolled in the B-HYPO trial, aggressive fever control management with normothermia (euthermia) significantly reduced TBI-mediated mortality compared to the mild therapeutic hypothermia group [108]. In a recent systematic review, targeted normothermia was associated with better outcomes in TBI [117]. In a separate study comparing normothermia to moderate hypothermia in TBI patients, an analysis of patients found that fever control with a goal temperature of 35.5–37.0 °C had a statistically significant 9.7% versus 34.0% reduction in mortality compared to a moderate hypothermia group [115]. A plethora of other data exist supporting fever avoidance and targeted euthermia [30].

In aiming to achieve normothermia, it is important to note that brain temperature exceeds body core temperature with a peak gap >2 °C [107, 118]. Normothermia can be achieved using multiple modalities. These can include acetaminophen, indomethacin, cooling blankets, rapid cold saline infusion, and cold gastric lavage [30, 114]. In more severely affected patients, achieving normothermia can be attained through endovascular cooling via subclavian vein access or through controlled external gel-coated cooling pads. More studies are needed to identify the optimal duration of induced normothermia, brain-directed temperature goals, localized brain cooling, and the relation of outcomes to fever burden in TBI patients.

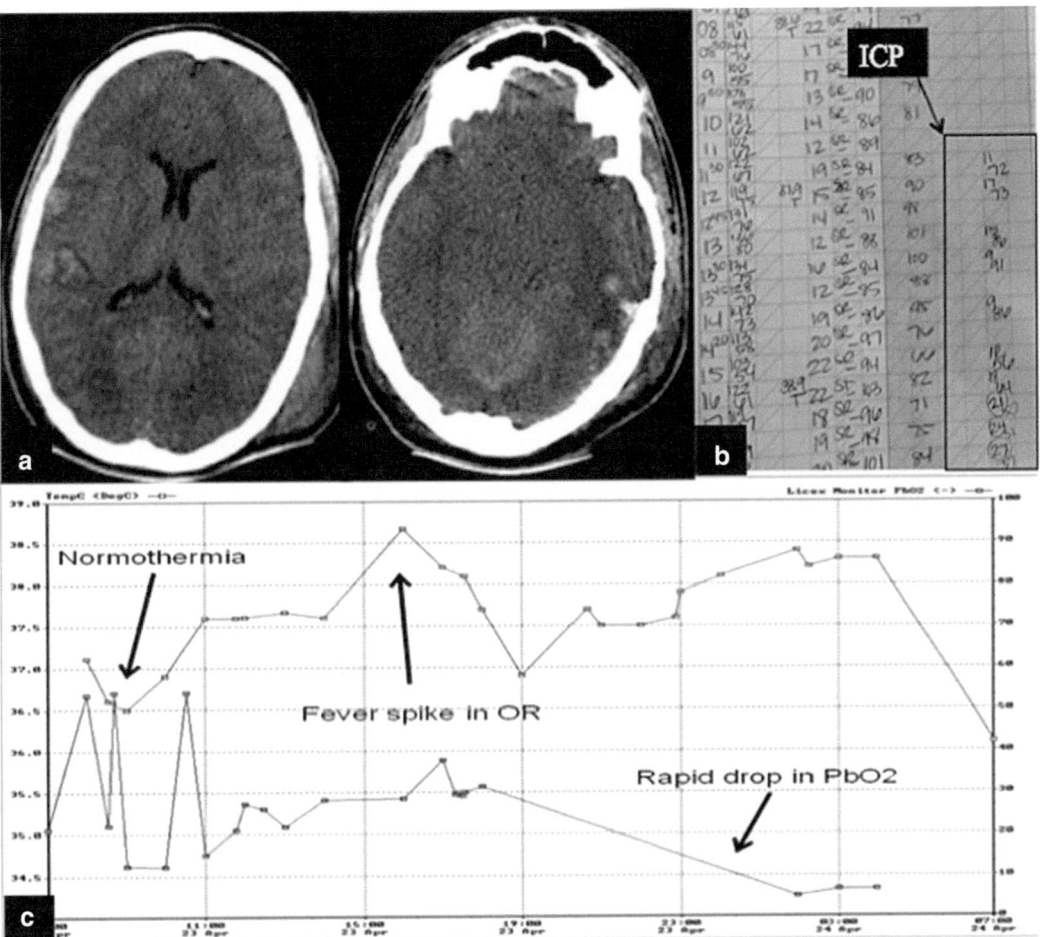

Fig. 2 A 27-year-old male s/p motor vehicle collision (MVC) with multiple frontal and temporal contusions. (**a**) Initial computed tomography (CT) head demonstrating multiple contusions and a left scalp hematoma. Licox monitor and external ventricular drain (EVD) placed for low Glaucoma Coma Score (GCS) and severity of injury. (**b**) Patient with spiking fevers correlating with sustained intracranial pressures (ICPs) over 20 mmHg; repeat CT (not shown) with blossoming contusions and midline shift. (**c**) Patient taken emergently for hemicraniectomy. Licox showing decreased brain tissue oxygenation correlating with temperature spikes

Conclusions

The management of TBI has significantly evolved over the last several decades. With the advancements in technology and research, more information is now available to treating physicians. Optimal management of a variety of parameters is complex, and a single approach to every patient is unlikely to be of benefit. Physicians now more than ever are being exposed to a large volume of clinical data with relatively little evidence to guide management directed at outcomes improvement. Further research will be beneficial, but in the meanwhile, adhering to basic medical management principles; avoiding significant laboratory derangements; avoiding secondary insults such as anemia, coagulopathy, electrolyte abnormalities, seizures, and the like; and ultimately tailoring therapy to each patient's physiology will provide the optimal environment for brain healing after injury.

References

1. Hartl R, Medary MB, Ruge M, Arfors KE, Ghajar J. Early white blood cell dynamics after traumatic brain injury: effects on the cerebral microcirculation. J Cereb Blood Flow Metab. 1997;17(11):1210–20.
2. Rovlias A, Kotsou S. The blood leukocyte count and its prognostic significance in severe head injury. Surg Neurol. 2001;55(4):190–6.
3. Roberts I, Yates D, Sandercock P, Farrell B, Wasserberg J, Lomas G, et al. CRASH trial collaborators. Effect of intravenous corticosteroids on death within 14 days in 10008 adults with clinically significant head injury (MRC CRASH trial): randomised placebo-controlled trial. Lancet. 2004;364(9442):1321–8.
4. Edwards P, Arango M, Balica L, Cottingham R, El-Sayed H, Farrell B, et al. CRASH trial collaborators. Final results of MRC CRASH, a randomised placebo-controlled trial of intravenous corticosteroid in adults with head injury-outcomes at 6 months. Lancet. 2005;365(9475):1957–9.
5. Kourbeti IS, Vakis AF, Papadakis JA, Karabetsos DA, Bertsias G, Fillipou M, et al. Infections in traumatic brain injury patients. Clin Microbiol Infect. 2012;18(4):359–64.
6. Salim A, Hadjizacharia P, DuBose J, Brown C, Inaba K, Chan L, et al. Role of anemia in traumatic brain injury. J Am Coll Surg. 2008;207(3):398–406.
7. Zygun DA, Nortje J, Hutchinson PJ, Timofeev I, Menon DK, Gupta AK. The effect of red blood cell transfusion on cerebral oxygenation and metabolism after severe traumatic brain injury. Crit Care Med. 2009;37(3):1074–8.
8. Spiotta AM, Stiefel MF, Gracias VH, Garuffe AM, Kofke WA, Maloney-Wilensky E, et al. Brain tissue oxygen-directed management and outcome in patients with severe traumatic brain injury. J Neurosurg. 2010;113(3):571–80.
9. Narotam PK, Morrison JF, Nathoo N. Brain tissue oxygen monitoring in traumatic brain injury and major trauma: outcome analysis of a brain tissue oxygen-directed therapy. J Neurosurg. 2009;111(4):672–82.
10. Hebert PC, Wells G, Blajchman MA, Marshall J, Martin C, Pagliarello G, et al. A multicenter, randomized, controlled clinical trial of transfusion requirements in critical care. Transfusion Requirements in Critical Care Investigators, Canadian Critical Care Trials Group. N Engl J Med. 1999;340(6):409–17.
11. Corwin HL, Gettinger A, Pearl RG, Fink MP, Levy MM, Abraham E, et al. The CRIT Study: anemia and blood transfusion in the critically ill—current clinical practice in the United States. Crit Care Med. 2004;32(1):39–52.
12. McIntyre LA, Fergusson DA, Hutchison JS, Pagliarello G, Marshall JC, Yetisir E, et al. Effect of a liberal versus restrictive transfusion strategy on mortality in patients with moderate to severe head injury. Neurocrit Care. 2006;5(1):4–9.
13. Boutin A, Chassé M, Shemilt M, Lauzier F, Moore L, Zarychanski R, et al. Red blood cell transfusion in patients with traumatic brain injury: a systematic review protocol. Syst Rev. 2014;3:66.
14. Sena MJ, Rivers RM, Muizelaar JP, Battistella FD, Utter GH. Transfusion practices for acute traumatic brain injury: a survey of physicians at US trauma centers. Intensive Care Med. 2009;35(3):480–8.
15. Desjardins P, Turgeon AF, Tremblay MH, Lauzier F, Zarychanski R, Boutin A, et al. Hemoglobin levels and transfusions in neurocritically ill patients: a systematic review of comparative studies. Crit Care. 2012;16(2):R54.
16. Utter GH, Shahlaie K, Zwienenberg-Lee M, Muizelaar JP. Anemia in the setting of traumatic brain injury: the arguments for and against liberal transfusion. J Neurotrauma. 2011;28(1):155–65.
17. Warner MA, O'Keeffe T, Bhavsar P, Shringer R, Moore C, Harper C, et al. Transfusions and long-term functional outcomes in traumatic brain injury. J Neurosurg. 2010;113(3):539–46.
18. Lelubre C, Bouzat P, Crippa IA, Taccone FS. Anemia management after acute brain injury. Crit Care. 2016;20:152.
19. Oddo M, Levine JM, Kumar M, Iglesias K, Frangos S, Maloney-Wilensky E, et al. Anemia and brain oxygen after severe traumatic brain injury. Intensive Care Med. 2012;38(9):1497–504.
20. Schnuriger B, Inaba K, Abdelsayed GA, Lustenberger T, Eberle BM, Barmparas G, et al. The impact of platelets on the progression of traumatic intracranial hemorrhage. J Trauma. 2010;68(4):881–5.
21. Donahue DL, Beck J, Fritz B, Davis P, Sandoval-Cooper MJ, Thomas SG, et al. Early platelet dysfunction in a rodent model of blunt traumatic brain injury reflects the acute traumatic coagulopathy found in humans. J Neurotrauma. 2014;31(4):404–10.
22. Halpern CH, Reilly PM, Turtz AR, Stein SC. Traumatic coagulopathy: the effect of brain injury. J Neurotrauma. 2008;25:997–1001.
23. Allard CB, Scarpelini S, Rhind SG, Baker AJ, Shek PN, Tien H, et al. Abnormal coagulation tests are associated with progression of traumatic intracranial hemorrhage. J Trauma. 2009;67(5):959–67.
24. Johansson PI, Sørensen AM, Larsen CF, Windeløv NA, Stensballe J, Perner A, et al. Low hemorrhage-related mortality in trauma patients in a Level I trauma center employing transfusion packages and early thromboelastography-directed hemostatic resuscitation with plasma and platelets. Transfusion. 2013;53(12):3088–99.
25. Holcomb JB, Minei KM, Scerbo ML, Radwan ZA, Wade CE, Kozar RA, et al. Admission rapid thrombelastography can replace conventional coagulation tests in the emergency department: experience with 1974 consecutive trauma patients. Ann Surg. 2012;256(3):476–86.
26. Walsh M, Fritz S, Hake D, Son M, Greve S, Jbara M, et al. Targeted thromboelastographic (TEG) blood component and pharmacologic hemostatic therapy

in traumatic and acquired coagulopathy. Curr Drug Targets. 2016;17(8):954–70.

27. Horn P, Münch E, Vajkoczy P, Herrmann P, Quintel M, Schilling L, et al. Hypertonic saline solution for control of elevated intracranial pressure in patients with exhausted response to mannitol and barbiturates. Neurol Res. 1999;21(8):758–64.

28. Oddo M, Levine JM, Frangos S, Carrera E, Maloney-Wilensky E, Pascual JL, et al. Effect of mannitol and hypertonic saline on cerebral oxygenation in patients with severe traumatic brain injury and refractory intracranial hypertension. J Neurol Neurosurg Psychiatry. 2009;80(8):916–20.

29. Rockswold GL, Solid CA, Paredes-Andrade E, Rockswold SB, Jancik JT, Quickel RR. Hypertonic saline and its effect on intracranial pressure, cerebral perfusion pressure, and brain tissue oxygen. Neurosurgery. 2009;65(6):1035–41; discussion 1041–2.

30. Timmons SD. Current trends in neurotrauma care. Crit Care Med. 2010;38(9 Suppl):S431–44.

31. Kerwin AJ, Schinco MA, Tepas JJ 3rd, Renfro WH, Vitarbo EA, Muehlberger M. The use of 23.4% hypertonic saline for the management of elevated intracranial pressure in patients with severe traumatic brain injury: a pilot study. J Trauma. 2009;67(2):277–82.

32. Ropper AH. Hyperosmolar therapy for raised intracranial pressure. N Engl J Med. 2012;367:746–52.

33. Doyle JA, Davis DP, Hoyt DB. The use of hypertonic saline in the treatment of traumatic brain injury. J Trauma. 2001;50(2):367–83.

34. van den Heuvel C, Vink R. The role of magnesium in traumatic brain injury. Clin Calcium. 2004;14:9–14.

35. Garfinkel L, Garfinkel D. Magnesium regulation of the glycolytic pathway and the enzymes involved. Magnesium. 1985;4:60–72.

36. Lifshitz J, Friberg H, Neumar RW, Raghupathi R, Welsh FA, Janmey P, et al. Structural and functional damage sustained by mitochondria after traumatic brain injury in the rat: evidence for differentially sensitive populations in the cortex and hippocampus. J Cereb Blood Flow Metab. 2003;23:219–31.

37. Memon ZI, Altura BT, Benjamin JL, Cracco RQ, Altura BM. Predictive value of serum ionized but not total magnesium levels in head injuries. Scand J Clin Lab Invest. 1995;55:671–7.

38. Temkin NR, Anderson GD, Winn HR, Ellenbogen RG, Britz GW, Schuster J, et al. Magnesium sulfate for neuroprotection after traumatic brain injury: a randomised controlled trial. Lancet Neurol. 2007;6:29–38.

39. Dhandapani SS, Gupta A, Vivekanandhan S, Sharma BS, Mahapatra AK. Randomized controlled trial of magnesium sulphate in severe closed traumatic brain injury. Indian J Neurotrauma. 2008;5:27–33.

40. Sen AP, Gulati A. Use of magnesium in traumatic brain injury. Neurotherapeutics. 2010;7(1):91–9.

41. Wu X, Lu X, Lu X, Yu J, Sun Y, Du Z, et al. Prevalence of severe hypokalemia in patients with traumatic brain injury. Injury. 2015;46(1):35–41.

42. Langham J, Goldfrad C, Teasdale G, Shaw D, Rowan K. Calcium channel blockers for acute traumatic brain injury. Cochrane Database Syst Rev. 2003;(4):CD000565.

43. Leao AAP. Spreading depression of activity in the cerebral cortex. J Neurophysiol. 1944;7:359–90.

44. Leao AAP. Further observations on the spreading depression of activity in the cerebral cortex. J Neurophysiol. 1947;10:409–14.

45. Fabricius M, Fuhr S, Bhatia R, Boutelle M, Hashemi P, Strong AJ, et al. Cortical spreading depression and peri-infarct depolarization in acutely injured human cerebral cortex. Brain. 2006;129:778–90.

46. Hartings JA, Strong AJ, Fabricius M, Manning A, Bhatia R, Dreier JP, et al. Co-Operative Study of Brain Injury Depolarizations. Spreading depolarizations and late secondary insults after traumatic brain injury. J Neurotrauma. 2009;26:1857–66.

47. Dohmen C, Sakowitz OW, Fabricius M, Bosche B, Reithmeier T, Ernestus RI, et al. Spreading depolarizations occur in human ischemic stroke with high incidence. Ann Neurol. 2008;63(6):720–8.

48. Lauritzen M, Dreier JP, Fabricius M, Hartings JA, Graf R, Strong AJ. Clinical relevance of cortical spreading depression in neurological disorders: migraine, malignant stroke, subarachnoid and intracranial hemorrhage, and traumatic brain injury. J Cereb Blood Flow Metab. 2011;31:17–35.

49. Hartings JA, Watanabe T, Bullock MR, Okonkwo DO, Fabricius M, Woitzik J, et al. Co-Operative Study on Brain Injury Depolarizations. Spreading depolarizations have prolonged direct current shifts and are associated with poor outcome in brain trauma. Brain. 2011;134(pt 5):1529–40.

50. Hartings JA, Wilson JA, Hinzman JM, Pollandt S, Dreier JP, DiNapoli V, et al. Spreading depression in continuous electroencephalography of brain trauma. Ann Neurol. 2014;76(5):681–94.

51. Hartings JA, Bullock MR, Okonkwo DO, Murray LS, Murray GD, Fabricius M, et al. Co-Operative Study on Brain Injury Depolarisations. Spreading depolarisations and outcome after traumatic brain injury: a prospective observational study. Lancet Neurol. 2011;10:1058–64.

52. Wilson RF, Tyburski JG. Metabolic responses and nutritional therapy in patients with severe head injuries. J Head Trauma Rehabil. 1998;13:11–27.

53. Osuka A, Uno T, Nakanishi J, Hinokiyama H. Energy expenditure in patients with severe head injury: controlled normothermia with sedation and neuromuscular blockade. J Crit Care. 2013;28(2):218.e9–13.

54. Costello L, Lithander F, Gruen R, Williams L. Nutrition therapy in the optimization of health outcomes in adult patients with moderate to severe traumatic brain injury: findings from a scoping review. Injury. 2014;45:1834–41.

55. Marik P, Zaloga G. Early enteric nutrition in critically ill patients: a systemic review. Crit Care Med. 2001;29(12):2264–70.

56. Hartl R, Gerber LM, Ni Q, Ghajar J. Effect of early nutrition on deaths due to severe traumatic brain injury. J Neurosurg. 2008;109(1):50–6.

57. Timmons SD. How soon should patients receive nutrition? How much, which formulation, and by which route? In: Valadka AB, Andrews BT, editors. Neurotrauma: evidence based answers to common questions. New York, Stuttgart: Thieme; 2005.

58. Chiang Y, Chao D, Chu S, Lin H, Huang S, Yeh Y, et al. Early enteral nutrition and clinical outcomes of severe traumatic brain injury patients in acute stage: a multi-center cohort study. J Neurotrauma. 2012;29(1):75–80.

59. Chourdakis M, Kraus M, Tzellos T, Sardeli C, Peftoulidou M, Vassilakos D, et al. Effect of early compared with delayed enteral nutrition on endocrine function in patients with traumatic brain injury: an open-labeled randomized trial. J Parenter Enteral Nutr. 2012;36(1):108–16.

60. Tan M, Zhu JC, Du J, Zhang LM, Yin HH. Effects of probiotics on serum levels of Th1/Th2 cytokine and clinical outcomes in severe traumatic brain-injured patients: a prospective randomized pilot study. Crit Care. 2011;15(6):R290–300.

61. Cope EC, Morris DR, Levenson CW. Improving treatments and outcomes: an emerging role for zinc in traumatic brain injury. Nutr Rev. 2012;70(7):410–3.

62. Vizzini A, Aranda-Michel J. Nutritional support in head injury. Nutrition. 2011;27(2):129–32.

63. Razmkon A, Sadidi A, Sherafat-Kazemzadeh E, Mehrafshan A, Jamali M, Malekpour B, et al. Administration of vitamin C and vitamin E in severe head injury: a randomized double-blind controlled trial. Clin Neurosurg. 2011;58:133–7.

64. Stippler M, Fischer MR, Puccio AM, Wisniewski SR, Carson-Walter EB, Dixon CE, et al. Serum and cerebrospinal fluid magnesium in severe traumatic brain injury outcome. J Neurotrauma. 2007;24(8):1347–54.

65. Rovlias A, Kotsou S. The influence of hyperglycemia on neurological outcome in patients with severe head injury. Neurosurgery. 2000;46(2):335–42; discussion 342–3.

66. Cochran A, Scaife ER, Hansen KW, Downey EC. Hyperglycemia and outcomes from pediatric traumatic brain injury. J Trauma Inj Infect Crit Care. 2003;55:1035–8.

67. Falkowska A, Gutowska I, Goschorska M, Nowacki P, Chlubek D, Baranowska-Bosiacka I. Energy metabolism of the brain, including the cooperation between astrocytes and neurons, especially in the context of glycogen metabolism. Int J Mol Sci. 2015;16:25959–81.

68. Simpson IA, Carruthers A, Vannucci SJ. Supply and demand in cerebral energy metabolism: the role of nutrient transporters. J Cereb Blood Flow Metab. 2007;27:1766–91.

69. Güemes M, Rahman SA, Hussain K. What is a normal blood glucose? Arch Dis Child. 2016;101(6):569–74.

70. Bavisetty S, McArthur D. Chronic hypopituitarism after traumatic brain injury: risk assessment and relationship to outcome. Neurosurgery. 2008;62:1080–94.

71. Sorensen L, Siddall PJ, Trenell MI, Yue DK. Differences in metabolites in pain-processing brain regions in patients with diabetes and painful neuropathy. Diabetes Care. 2008;31:980–1.

72. Muizelaar JP, Ward JD, Marmarou A, Newlon PG, Wachi A. Cerebral blood flow and metabolism in severely head-injured children. J Neurosurg. 1989;71:72–6.

73. Kim GS, Jung JE, Narasimhan P, Sakata H, Chan PH. Induction of thioredoxin-interacting protein is mediated by oxidative stress, calcium, and glucose after brain injury in mice. Neurobiol Dis. 2012;46:440–9.

74. Jeremitsky E, Omert LA, Dunham CM, Wilberger J, Rodriguez A. The impact of hyperglycemia on patients with severe brain injury. Ratio. 2005;58:47–50.

75. Salim A, Hadjizacharia P, Dubose J, Brown C, Inaba K, Chan LS, et al. Persistent hyperglycemia in severe traumatic brain injury: an independent predictor of outcome. Am Surg. 2009;75:25–9.

76. Chong SL, Harjanto S, Testoni D, Ng ZM, Low CYD, Lee KP, et al. Early hyperglycemia in pediatric traumatic brain injury predicts for mortality, prolonged duration of mechanical ventilation, and intensive care stay. Int J Endocrinol. 2015;2015:719476.

77. Seyed Saadat SM, Bidabadi E, Seyed Saadat SN, Mashouf M, Salamat F, Yousefzadeh S. Association of persistent hyperglycemia with outcome of severe traumatic brain injury in pediatric population. Childs Nerv Syst. 2012;28:1773–7.

78. Alexiou GA, Lianos G, Fotakopoulos G, Michos E, Pachatouridis D, Voulgaris S. Admission glucose and coagulopathy occurrence in patients with traumatic brain injury. Brain Inj. 2014;28:438–41.

79. Meier R, Béchir M, Ludwig S, Sommerfeld J, Keel M, Steiger P, et al. Differential temporal profile of lowered blood glucose levels (3.5 to 6.5 mmol/l versus 5 to 8 mmol/l) in patients with severe traumatic brain injury. Crit Care. 2008;12:R98.

80. Van den Berghe G, Wouters P, Weekers F, Verwaest C, Bruyninckx F, Schetz M, et al. Intensive insulin therapy in critically ill patients. N Engl J Med. 2001;345:1359–67.

81. Rapp RP, Young B, Twyman D, Bivins BA, Haack D, Tibbs PA, et al. The favorable effect of early parenteral feeding on survival in head-injured patients. J Neurosurg. 1983;58:906–12.

82. Finfer S, Chittock DR, Su SY-S, Blair D, Foster D, Dhingra V, et al. Intensive versus conventional glucose control in critically ill patients. N Engl J Med. 2009;360:1283–97.

83. Bilotta F, Rosa G. Glycemia management in critical care patients. World J Diabetes. 2012;3:130–4.

84. Oddo M, Schmidt JM, Carrera E, Badjatia N, Connolly ES, Presciutti M, et al. Impact of tight glycemic control on cerebral glucose metabolism after severe brain injury: a microdialysis study. Crit Care Med. 2008;36:3233–8.

85. Muizelaar JP, van der Poel H, Li Z, Kontos H, Levasseur J. Pial arterial vessel diameter and CO_2

reactivity during prolonged hyperventilation in the rabbit. J Neurosurg. 1988;63:923–7.

86. Carney N, Totten AM, O'Reilly C, Ullman JS, Hawryluk GWJ, Bell MJ, et al. Brain Trauma Foundation. Guidelines for the management of severe traumatic brain injury. 4th ed. 2016. https://braintrauma.org/uploads/03/12/Guidelines_for_Management_of_Severe_TBI_4th_Edition.pdf. Accessed 1 Mar 2018.

87. Robertson CS. Desaturation episodes after severe head injury: influence on outcome. Acta Neurochir Suppl (Wien). 1993;59:98–101.

88. Winchel RJ, Hoyt DB. Endotracheal intubation in the field improves survival in patients with severe head injury. Arch Surg. 1997;132:592–7.

89. Stochetti N, Furlan A, Volta F. Hypoxemia and arterial hypotension at the accident scene in head injury. J Trauma. 1996;40:764–7.

90. Moppett I. Traumatic brain injury: assessment, resuscitation, and early management. Br J Anaesth. 2007;99(1):18–31.

91. Chesnut RM, Marshall LF, Klauber MR. The role of secondary brain injury in determining outcome from severe head injury. J Trauma. 1993;34:216–22.

92. Davis DP, Meade W, Sise MJ, Kennedy F, Simon F, Tominaga G, et al. Both hypoxemia and extreme hyperoxemia may be detrimental in patients with severe traumatic brain injury. J Neurotrauma. 2009;26(12):2217–23.

93. Rahimi S, Bidabadi E, Mashouf M, Saadat S. Prognostic value of arterial blood gas disturbances for in-hospital mortality in pediatric patients with severe traumatic brain injury. Acta Neurochir. 2014;156:187–92.

94. Zehtabchi S, Sinert R, Soghoian S, Liu Y, Carmody K, Shah L, et al. Identifying traumatic brain injury in patients with isolated head trauma: are arterial lactate and base deficit as helpful as in polytrauma. Emerg Med J. 2007;24:333–5.

95. Clausen T, Khaldi A, Zauner A, Reinert M, Doppenberg E, Menzel M, et al. Cerebral acid-base homeostasis after severe traumatic brain injury. J Neurosurg. 2005;103:597–607.

96. Shallwani H, Waqas M, Waheed S, Siddiqui M, Froz A, Bari ME. Does base deficit predict mortality in patients with severe traumatic brain injury. Int J Surg. 2015;22:125–30.

97. Rincon F, Hunter K, Schorr C, Dellinger RP, Zanotti-Cavazzoni S. The epidemiology of spontaneous fever and hypothermia on admission of brain injury patients to intensive care units: a multicenter cohort study. J Neurosurg. 2014;121:950–60.

98. Thompson HJ, Pinto-Martin J, Bullock MR. Neurogenic fever after traumatic brain injury: an epidemiological study. J Neurol Neurosurg Psychiatry. 2003;74:614–9.

99. Bao L, Chen D, Ding L, Ling W, Xu F. Fever burden is an independent predictor for prognosis of traumatic brain injury. PLoS One. 2014;9(3):e90956.

100. Dietrich WD. Therapeutic hypothermia for spinal cord injury. Crit Care Med. 2009;37:S238–42.

101. Dietrich WD, Bramlett HM. Hyperthermia and central nervous system injury. Prog Brain Res. 2007;162:201–17.

102. Gaither JB, Chikani V, Spaite DW, Smith JJ, Curry M, Mhayamaguru M, et al. Association between elevated initial trauma center body temperature and non-mortality outcomes following major traumatic brain injury. Circulation. 2015;132(Suppl 3):A16144.

103. Natale JE, Joseph JG, Helfaer MA, Shaffner DH. Early hyperthermia after traumatic brain injury in children: risk factors, influence on length of stay, and effect on short-term neurologic status. Crit Care Med. 2000;28:2608–15.

104. Sakuma J, Suzuki K, Sasaki T, Matsumoto M, Oinuma M, Kawakami M, et al. Monitoring and preventing blood flow insufficiency due to clip rotation after the treatment of internal carotid artery aneurysms. J Neurosurg. 2004;100:960–2.

105. Clifton GL, Miller ER, Choi SC, Levin HS, McCauley S, Smith KR Jr, et al. Lack of effect of induction of hypothermia after acute brain injury. N Engl J Med. 2001;344:556–63.

106. Clifton GL, Valadka A, Zygun D, Coffey CS, Drever P, Fourwinds S, et al. Very early hypothermia induction in patients with severe brain injury (the National Acute Brain Injury Study: Hypothermia II): a randomised trial. Lancet Neurol. 2011;10:131–9.

107. Hutchison JS, Ward RE, Lacroix J, Hébert PC, Barnes MA, Bohn DJ, et al. Hypothermia therapy after traumatic brain injury in children. N Engl J Med. 2008;358:2447–56.

108. Hifumi T, Kuroda Y, Kawakita K, Yamashita S, Oda Y, Dohi K, et al. Fever control management is preferable to mild therapeutic hypothermia in traumatic brain injury patients with abbreviated injury scale 3-4: a multicenter, randomized controlled trial. J Neurotrauma. 2016;33(11):1047–53.

109. Dietrich WD, Bramlett HM. Therapeutic hypothermia and targeted temperature management in traumatic brain injury: clinical challenges for successful translation. Brain Res. 2016;1640:94–103.

110. Beca J, McSharry B, Erickson S, Yung M, Schibler A, Slater A, et al. Hypothermia for traumatic brain injury in children-a phase II randomized controlled trial. Crit Care Med. 2015;43:1458–66.

111. Adelson PD, Ragheb J, Muizelaar JP, Kanev P, Brockmeyer D, Beers SR, et al. Phase II clinical trial of moderate hypothermia after severe traumatic brain injury in children. Neurosurgery. 2005;56:740–53.

112. Polderman KH. Induced hypothermia and fever control for prevention and treatment of neurological injuries. Lancet. 2008;371:1955–69.

113. Suehiro E, Koizumi H, Kunitsugu I, Fujisawa H, Suzuki M. Survey of brain temperature management in patients with traumatic brain injury in the Japan neurotrauma data bank. J Neurotrauma. 2014;31:315–20.

114. Maekawa T, Yamashita S, Nagao S, Hayashi N, Ohashi Y. Prolonged mild therapeutic hypothermia versus fever control with tight hemodynamic monitoring and slow rewarming in patients with severe traumatic brain injury: a randomized controlled trial. J Neurotrauma. 2015;32:422–9.

115. Marion DW, Regasa LE. Revisiting therapeutic hypothermia for severe traumatic brain injury... again. Crit Care. 2014;18:160.

116. Andrews PJ, Sinclair HL, Battison CG, Polderman KH, Citerio G, Mascia L, et al. Eurotherm3235Trial collaborators. European society of intensive care medicine study of therapeutic hypothermia (32-35 °C) for intracranial pressure reduction after traumatic brain injury (the Eurotherm3235Trial). Trials. 2011;12:8.

117. Madden LK, DeVon HA. A systematic review of the effects of body temperature on outcome after adult traumatic brain injury. J Neurosci Nurs. 2015;47:190–203.

118. Rumana CS, Gopinath SP, Uzura M, Valadka AB, Robertson CS. Brain temperature exceeds systemic temperature in head-injured patients. Crit Care Med. 1998;26:562–7.

Nutrition: Time to Revisit?

Rani Patal and Guy Rosenthal

Introduction

Traumatic brain injury (TBI) constitutes a serious public health and socioeconomic problem as it remains the leading cause of death and long-term disability in people younger than 40 years worldwide. Moreover, TBI is expected to surpass many diseases as the major cause of death and disability by the year 2020 [1]. Traumatic brain injury incites a chain reaction of pathophysiological events that can have an adverse impact on the integrity of axons, cell membranes, ion channels, mitochondria, and cellular function. Cerebral metabolism and the delivery of substrates to the brain are also affected. TBI leads to a cascade resulting in a release of excitatory amino acids, the production of free radicals, and cellular ion imbalance. A process of neuroinflammation also occurs after TBI. Severe TBI leads to a disruption of the normal cerebral metabolic state, and TBI patients enter a hypercatabolic state that increases systemic and cerebral energy requirements. Adequate nutritional support is therefore a crucial part of the care of severe TBI patients.

Proper management of nutrition in severe TBI patients is important because it influences clinical outcomes. A large study has demonstrated that every 10-kcal/kg decrease in caloric intake was associated with a 30–40% increase in mortality rates adjusted for injury severity [2]. Achieving adequate nutritional support for TBI patients has long been a clinical challenge.

Enteral feeding is generally preferred over parenteral feeding as the former better maintains gut integrity and also reduces the risk of sepsis. However, there are still situations in which parenteral feeding should be used. The preferred route for enteral feeding remains a matter of debate. Some clinicians prefer using the percutaneous gastrostomy (PEG) relatively early during the hospitalization course, while others prefer deferring it to a later phase. Other controversies include the exact timing by which enteral feeding should begin, by what post-injury day full caloric replacement should be achieved, and if it is necessary to insist on transpyloric feeding exclusively. Uncertainty also remains on how tightly serum glucose should be controlled and on the role of nutritional supplements.

In this chapter we discuss these controversies in nutritional support of severe TBI patients, as follows: the optimal timing of enteral feeding after injury, the preferred method of enteral feeding, enteral versus parenteral nutrition, glucose control, and the role of vitamins and supplements. In each section we review key studies relevant to each topic and review their implications and remaining uncertainties.

R. Patal, MD · G. Rosenthal, MD (✉)
Department of Neurosurgery, Hadassah-Hebrew University Medical Center, Jerusalem, Israel
e-mail: rosenthalg@neurosurg.ucsf.edu,
ROSENTHALG@HADASSAH.ORG.IL

© Springer International Publishing AG, part of Springer Nature 2018
S. D. Timmons (ed.), *Controversies in Severe Traumatic Brain Injury Management*,
https://doi.org/10.1007/978-3-319-89477-5_10

The Optimal Timing of Enteral Feeding After Injury

Many studies have demonstrated the benefits of early feeding on outcome in trauma patients in general and severe TBI patients in particular. Härtl et al. conducted a large study based on 797 patients with severe TBI [2]. Patients who were not fed within 5 and 7 days after TBI had a twofold and fourfold increased likelihood of death within the first 2 weeks of injury, respectively. These results were statistically significant and held up even after controlling for factors known to affect mortality, including age, pupillary status, initial Glasgow Coma Scale (GCS), arterial hypotension, and computed tomography (CT) scan findings. In addition, they demonstrated that every 10-kcal/kg decrease in caloric intake was associated with a 30–40% increase in mortality rates adjusted for injury severity. The benefits of early enteral feeding also extend to reduced complication rates in severe TBI patients. Lepelletier et al. conducted a retrospective cohort study on 161 patients with severe TBI [3]. They demonstrated that early enteral feeding (>2000 Kcal before day 5) is a protective factor (OR = 0.33, 95% confidence interval [CI]: 0.21–0.85) for early onset ventilator-associated pneumonia, which in turn was significantly associated with a longer duration of mechanical ventilation and a longer sedation duration. Dhandapani et al. conducted a prospective study on 67 hospitalized patients with severe TBI [4]. Eighty percent of patients fed before 3 days had favorable outcome at 3 months compared to 43% among those fed later (OR = 5.29, 95% CI 1.03–27.03, $p = 0.04$). The difference between those fed before 3 days and 4–7 days was not significant at 6 months, even though patients fed before 7 days still had significantly higher favorable outcome compared to those fed after 7 days (OR 7.69, $p = 0.002$). Multivariate analysis for unfavorable outcome at 6 months showed significance of $p = 0.03$ for feeding after 3 days and $p = 0.01$ for feeding after 7 days.

The rate at which feeding is increased and caloric requirements are met also seems to be important in severe TBI patients. Taylor et al. performed a prospective randomized study on 82 patients with head injury who required mechanical ventilation [5]. Patients were randomized to two groups. The first received standard enteral nutrition (SEN), whereby feeding was gradually increased from 15 mL/h up to the estimated energy and nitrogen requirements. The second group received enhanced enteral nutrition (EEN), whereby the feeding rate that met the estimated energy and nitrogen requirements was given from the first post-injury day. Patients in the EEN group had a higher percentage of energy ($p = 0.0008$) and nitrogen ($p < 0.0001$) requirements met by enteral nutrition in the first week after injury. Neurologic outcome at 6 months was similar between groups, but there was a tendency for more EEN patients to have a good neurologic outcome at 3 months compared to SEN patients (61% vs. 39%, $p = 0.08$). Fewer EEN patients had an infective complication (61% vs. 85%, $p = 0.02$), and fewer had two or more complications (37% vs. 61%, $p = 0.046$) compared with SEN patients.

Early enteral nutrition may also have measurable benefits on endocrine function. Chourdakis et al. conducted a prospective randomized study on 59 TBI patients [6]. Twenty-five patients received delayed enteral feeding (DEF), and thirty-four patients received early (within 24–48 h) enteral feeding (EEF). The effect on the endocrine function of patients with TBI was investigated. Levels of thyroid-stimulating hormone, free triiodothyronine, free thyroxine, and testosterone (in males) of DEF patients declined in comparison to intensive care unit (ICU) admission day levels. The decrease of hormonal values was less pronounced in the EEF group. Cortisol concentrations rose in the DEF group; a lesser hormonal change was found in the EEF group. Deaths during the study for the DEF group and EEF group were two and three, respectively. EEF may exert beneficial effects on the hormonal profile of TBI patients. However, there was no significant difference in infections, hyperglycemia, or other complications in this study.

In summary, these studies clearly demonstrate that starting feeding early is associated with better outcomes and lower rates of complications. However, these studies used different time cutoffs when comparing early versus delayed feeding, making it difficult to identify a precise time point by which feeding must be initiated. The study by Härtl and colleagues suggests that full nutritional replacement should be achieved by days 5–7 post-injury and that doing so has a beneficial effect on mortality [2]. Clearly, enteral feeding should be started as soon as it is feasible to do so, and a policy of "the earlier the better" is supported by the existing literature. Importantly, these studies indicate that in addition to improved mortality, a decrease in rates of complications, especially infectious complications, can be expected with early enteral nutrition.

The Preferred Method of Enteral Feeding

Several studies evaluated the benefits of a transpyloric feeding over prepyloric feeding in TBI patients. Acosta-Escribano et al. conducted a prospective randomized study on 104 TBI patients [7]. Patients were randomized to transpyloric feeding (TPF, 50 patients) or gastric feeding (GF, 54 patients) groups. They received the same dietary formulas. The TPF group had a significant lower incidence of pneumonia: 16 patients (34%) versus 31 patients (55%) (OR = 0.3, 95% CI 0.1–0.7, $p = 0.01$). There were no significant differences in other nosocomial infections. The TPF group received higher amounts of feedings compared to the GF group (92% vs. 84%, $p < 0.01$) and had lower incidence of increased gastric residuals (OR = 0.2, 95% CI 0.04–0.6, $p = 0.003$). A smaller study by Grahm and colleagues randomized 32 TBI patients with GCS scores less than 10 to a group fed by transpyloric feeding (TPF) and a group that were fed by the gastric route (GF) [8]. The TPF group had nasojejunal feeding tubes placed fluoroscopically, and these patients received nutritional support equal to their measured resting energy expenditure within 36 h of injury. Patients in the GF group were fed when bowel sounds could be heard on auscultation. The mean resting energy expenditure, serum albumin, glucose, lymphocyte count, body weight, and total nitrogen loss were similar for both groups. With transpyloric feedings, daily caloric (TPF = 2102 kcal versus GF = 1100 kcal), nitrogen intake (TPF = 11.1 g versus GF = 5.6 g), and daily nitrogen balance (TPF = −4.3 g versus GF = −11.8 g) improved. The incidence of bacterial infections (TPF = 3 versus GF = 14) and days of ICU hospitalization (TPF = 6 versus GF = 10) were significantly reduced.

Other studies have used the gastric route for feeding but utilized early placement of a percutaneous gastrostomy (PEG) rather than a nasogastric tube to deliver nutrition. Klodell et al. evaluated the safety and effectiveness of gastric enteral nutrition by PEG in TBI patients [9]. They retrospectively analyzed 118 patients with moderate and severe TBI. Their management strategy included routine PEG by post-injury day 4. PEG was performed and gastric feeding instituted within a mean of 3.6 days following admission. PEG tubes were placed in 97% (114 of 118) of the cohort. No complications related to PEG placement were reported. Overall, 111 of 114 (97%) patients with PEGs were able to tolerate enteral nutrition via this route. Two patients required endoscopic conversion to gastrojejunostomy, because of gastroparesis with high gastric residuals. No patient required conversion to parenteral nutrition. Seventy-seven percent of patients achieved the goal rate of feeding by the fourth day of nutritional support. Five patients (4%) had aspiration related to initiation of enteral nutrition and subsequently developed pneumonia. Four of these patients had PEG tubes at the time of the aspiration event.

In summary, these studies have generally demonstrated a lower incidence of infectious complications in patients fed via the transpyloric route as opposed to the gastric route. A lower incidence of bacterial infections in general [8] and of pneumonia in particular [7] has been described. The small number of patients in all these studies makes it difficult to draw definitive conclusions, since all are underpowered to truly assess complication rates in comparison to possible benefit. The existing evidence is not sufficient to recommend transpyloric feeding for all TBI patients. However, it seems reasonable to use transpyloric feeding when possible.

Enteral vs. Parenteral Nutrition

Several studies evaluated the influence of parenteral feeding in TBI patients on outcome parameters, complications rates, and nutritional parameters. Young et al. conducted a prospective randomized study on 51 patients with TBI with a GCS of 4–10 [10]. They were randomized to receive total parenteral nutrition (TPN) or enteral nutrition (EN). Patients were studied from hospital admission to 18 days post-injury. The TPN group received a significantly higher cumulative mean intake of protein and caloric balance than the EN group. Nitrogen balance was significantly more negative in the EN group during the first week post-injury. The incidence of pneumonia, urinary tract infections, septic shock, and infections was not significantly different between the groups. A study by Borzotta et al. showed similar results regarding complications rates, but with no advantage in terms of meeting nutritional goals [11]. They conducted a prospective randomized study on 38 patients. Twenty-one (21) patients received parenteral feeding, and twenty-seven received jejunal feeding with identical formulations. Both routes were equally effective at meeting nutritional goals. The mean resting energy expenditure rose to 2400 ± 531 kcal/day in both groups and remained at 135–146% of predicted energy expenditure over 4 weeks. Infections were equally frequent: 1.86 episodes/TPN patient versus 1.89 episodes/EN patient. Similarly, Hadley et al. conducted a prospective randomized study on 45 patients with TBI comparing TPN versus EN [12]. TPN patients had significantly higher mean daily nitrogen intakes and mean daily nitrogen losses than the EN patients; however, no significant differences were found with respect to maintenance of serum albumin levels, weight loss, the incidence of infection, nitrogen balance, and final outcome.

In a small prospective randomized study by Rapp et al., an advantage in mortality rates was seen in patients given TPN when comparing the effects of early parenteral nutrition with delayed enteral nutrition upon the outcome of TBI patients [13]. There were 38 patients, of whom 18 were randomized to the delayed enteral nutrition group and 20 to the early parenteral nutrition group. The mortality rate within 18 days of injury of the delayed enteral nutrition patients was 44%, whereas no patient in the early parenteral nutrition group died within this period ($p < 0.0001$). However, the results of this study may have been influenced more by the delay in initiating enteral nutrition than in any effect of TPN per se, especially given later work on the timing of nutritional supplementation.

TPN does not seem to positively influence cerebral physiological parameters in a beneficial manner in comparison to enteral nutrition. A study by Young et al. evaluated the influence of TPN on intracranial pressure (ICP), in addition to outcome [14]. They conducted a prospective randomized study in 96 severely brain-injured patients. They were randomly assigned to receive TPN or EN and were studied from hospital admission until 18 days post-injury. TPN was started within 48 h post-injury, and the EN was started when tolerated. Peak daily ICP was not significantly different on admission and over time. Intracranial pressure was greater than 20 mmHg in 75% of TPN patients and in 73% of EN patients.

In conclusion, these studies indicate that in severe TBI patients, there is no substantial benefit to TPN in comparison to enteral nutrition in those patients who tolerate enteral feeding. Moreover, the rates of nosocomial infections, including pneumonia, are not reduced by the use of TPN. In general, TPN should be reserved for patients who are unable to tolerate enteral nutrition.

Glucose Control

Some studies have demonstrated benefit of intensive insulin therapy; others have not. Studies have also demonstrated the risks involved when very tight glucose control is sought, specifically induced hypoglycemia. In 2009, Yang and colleagues found lower infection rates and to some extent better functional outcome in patients treated with tight glucose control [15]. They conducted a prospective randomized study on 240 patients with severe TBI. A total of 121 patients were assigned to the intensive glucose control group and received continuous insulin infusion to maintain glucose levels between 4.4 mmol/L (80 mg/dL) and 6.1 mmol/L (110 mg/dL). Some 119 patients were assigned to the conventional treatment group and were not given insulin unless glucose levels were greater than 11.1 mmol/L (200 mg/dL). Both in-hospital and overall mortality rates at 6 months were similar in the two groups. However, good neurological outcome (Glasgow Outcome Scale of 4 or 5 at 6 months post-injury) was better in the intensive insulin therapy group (34 of 117, 29%) than that in the conventional therapy group (26 of 116, 22%, $p < 0.05$). In addition, the infection rate was higher in patients who received conventional insulin therapy compared with patients who received intensive insulin therapy (46% vs. 31%; $p < 0.05$), and length of stay in the intensive care unit was shorter in the intensive insulin control group (4.2 days vs. 5.6 days, $p < 0.05$), indicating a benefit for intensive insulin therapy and tight glucose control.

While the study by Yang and colleagues demonstrates encouraging results, several other investigations have not demonstrated clear benefit for tight glucose control and have noted worrying rates of hypoglycemia. In 2008, Bilotta et al. reported a prospective randomized study on 97 patients with severe TBI [16]. The patients were randomly assigned to either conventional or intensive glucose control. In the conventional group, insulin was infused when blood glucose levels exceeded 220 mg/dL (12.2 mmol/L), while in the intensive glucose control group, insulin was infused to maintain blood glucose between 80 and 120 mg/dL (4.4–6.7 mmol/L). There was no difference in mortality, functional outcome measured by Glasgow Outcome Scale at 6 months post-injury, or rates of infection in the ICU between the two groups. The only advantage for intensive glucose control was in a shorter ICU stay (7.3 vs. 10.0 days; $p < 0.05$). However, episodes of hypoglycemia (defined as blood glucose <80 mg/dL or 4.4 mmol/L) were significantly more frequent in patients receiving intensive insulin therapy. Other studies have confirmed a worrying increased frequency of hypoglycemic

episodes with intensive glucose control. In 2010, Coester and colleagues reported a prospective randomized study of 88 patients with severe non-penetrating TBI [17]. Forty-two (42) patients were assigned to intensive glucose control to maintain blood glucose between 80 and 110 mg/dL (4.4–6.1 mmol/L) with continuous insulin infusion. Forty-six (46) patients were assigned to conventional glucose control to maintain blood glucose below 180 mg/dL (10 mmol/L) with subcutaneous insulin and insulin infusion only if blood glucose levels exceeded 220 mg/dL (12.2 mmol/L). The authors found no difference in neurologic outcomes, incidence of sepsis, or ICU days between the two groups. However, the percentage of patients that endured an episode of hypoglycemia was substantially higher in the intensive glucose control group (82% versus 18%, $p < 0.001$), indicating a meaningful risk of potentially inducing harm.

Although these studies used different protocols for controlling glucose and different outcome measures, in all, the reported improvements in outcome from intensive glucose control are inconsistent and limited. In contrast, episodes of documented hypoglycemia seem to be substantially higher in patients treated with intensive glucose control. The potential to cause harm when implementing a tight glucose control in severe TBI patients due to induced hypoglycemia needs to be taken into account when deciding on ICU management protocols. While some centers may have special expertise in implementing a program of tight glucose control, the majority of centers that do not should employ caution. Therefore, for most centers, a policy of conventional glucose control in the ICU for severe TBI patients is recommended in order to avoid the possibility of inducing hypoglycemia with its severe consequences for the injured brain.

Vitamins and Supplements

There is very scant evidence regarding feeding patients with specific nutritional supplements or specific types of nutritional formula. Painter et al. reported lower rates of infectious complications in patients receiving immune-enhanced nutrition (IEN), a protein-rich formulation supplemented with arginine, glutamine, and omega-3 fatty acids [18]. They conducted a retrospective study on 240 patients with severe TBI. In all, 126 patients received an IEN formulation, and 114 patients received a standard formulation (SF). Patients receiving IEN were found to have lower rates of blood stream infections (10.3% vs. 19.3%, $p < 0.05$). However, IEN patients spent longer in the ICU (11.2 vs. 9.4, $p = 0.02$) and on ventilators (11.1 vs. 7.6, $p = 0.001$). Both groups had similar rates of all-cause mortality and hospital length of stay.

Nutritional supplementation with zinc has also been evaluated in severe TBI patients. Young et al. conducted a randomized, prospective, double-blind controlled study on 68 patients with severe TBI to evaluate the effects of supplemental zinc versus standard nutrition [19]. There was a trend toward a higher mortality rate at 1 month post-injury in the control group compared with the zinc-supplemented group (26% versus 12%, $p = 0.09$), but this difference did not attain statistical significance.

In conclusion, there is very little evidence about the influence of any specific type of nutritional supplement on outcome in severe TBI patients. Therefore, no concrete recommendations can be made regarding specific nutritional supplementation at this time.

Conclusions

Time to Revisit? Directions for Future Research

This brief survey of the literature on nutrition in severe TBI patients makes it clear that many unanswered questions remain regarding proper nutritional support in TBI patients. Current evidence does clearly suggest that the earlier nutritional support is initiated, and the earlier caloric replacement goals are achieved, the better. However, we have very little data in the literature to indicate how often we actually achieve these goals in clinical practice. The little evidence that exists suggests that we are not achieving nutri-

tional targets in a satisfactory manner. Zarbock and colleagues found that in patients admitted to the neurosurgical intensive care unit, the maximum daily mean amount of calories given in the first week post-injury was 1100 kcal, which constituted only 55% of the caloric goal [20]. Large prospective observational registry studies are needed to assess to what extent the targets we set for nutritional support are actually being attained in daily practice and what factors prevent us from reaching these goals.

Comparative effectiveness research, which seeks to assess the impact of different treatment strategies on outcomes without altering the current practice of any single center, is gaining favor in TBI research. It is advantageous in that each center maintains its usual treatment protocols and markers of outcome are followed between centers, taking into account the different population profiles and injury severities between centers. This approach may be particularly beneficial in evaluating different nutritional support strategies between centers. Rates of achieving full caloric replacement, complication rates including infection rates, and functional outcome measures could be evaluated between centers that employ different nutritional support strategies in order to assess which strategies are the most effective.

Further important questions that need to be answered include how we can achieve better glucose control without inducing hypoglycemia and whether any specific nutritional supplementation can help improve outcome and recovery in severe TBI patients. It is clear that we have much work to do in order to optimize our nutritional support strategies for severe TBI patients. It will take a multidisciplinary effort of neurosurgeons, ICU physicians, nursing, and nutritional specialists to achieve progress on this important front.

Key Points

- Feeding should be started as soon as feasible after injury and certainly within 5–7 days post-injury with a goal of attaining full caloric replacement as fast as tolerated, since achieving this goal is associated with decreased mortality and lower rates of complications.

- There is not enough evidence to recommend transpyloric feeding for all patients. However, it seems reasonable to use transpyloric feeding when possible in order to decrease the incidence of infection and pneumonia.
- The use of TPN should be reserved for patients who are intolerant of enteral nutrition.
- A policy of conventional glucose control to maintain blood glucose below 180 mg/dL (10 mmol/L) with subcutaneous insulin is recommended. Insulin infusion should be initiated only if blood glucose levels exceeded 220 mg/dL (12.2 mmol/L).
- To date there is not enough evidence to support a specific type of enhanced nutrition rather than standard formulations.

References

1. Lopez AD, Murray CCJL. The global burden of disease, 1990–2020. Nat Med. 1998;4:1241–3.
2. Härtl R, Gerber LM, Ni Q, Ghajar J. Effect of early nutrition on deaths due to severe traumatic brain injury. J Neurosurg. 2008;109:50–6.
3. Lepelletier D, Roquilly A, Demeure dit latte D, Mahe PJ, Loutrel O, Champin P, et al. Retrospective analysis of the risk factors and pathogens associated with early-onset ventilator-associated pneumonia in surgical-ICU head-trauma patients. J Neurosurg Anesthesiol. 2010,22.32–7.
4. Dhandapani S, Dhandapani M, Agarwal M, Chutani AM, Subbiah V, Sharma BS, et al. The prognostic significance of the timing of total enteral feeding in traumatic brain injury. Surg Neurol Int. 2012;3:31.
5. Taylor SJ, Fettes SB, Jewkes C, Nelson RJ. Prospective, randomized, controlled trial to determine the effect of early enhanced enteral nutrition on clinical outcome in mechanically ventilated patients suffering head injury. Crit Care Med. 1999;27:2525–31.
6. Chourdakis M, Kraus MM, Tzellos T, Sardeli C, Peftoulidou M, Vassilakos D, et al. Effect of early compared with delayed enteral nutrition on endocrine function in patients with traumatic brain injury: an open-labeled randomized trial. JPEN J Parenter Enteral Nutr. 2012;36:108–16.
7. Acosta-Escribano J, Fernández-Vivas M, Grau Carmona T, Caturla-Such J, Garcia-Martinez M, Menendez-Mainer A, et al. Gastric versus transpyloric feeding in severe traumatic brain injury: a prospective, randomized trial. Intensive Care Med. 2010;36:1532–9.
8. Grahm TW, Zadrozny DB, Harrington T. The benefits of early jejunal hyperalimentation in the head-injured patient. Neurosurgery. 1989;25:729–35.
9. Klodell CT, Carroll M, Carrillo EH, Spain DA. Routine intragastric feeding following traumatic brain injury is safe and well tolerated. Am J Surg. 2000;179:168–71.
10. Young B, Ott L, Twyman D, Norton J, Rapp R, Tibbs P, et al. The effect of nutritional support on outcome from severe head injury. J Neurosurg. 1987;67(5):668–76.
11. Borzotta AP, Pennings J, Papasadero B, Paxton J, Mardesic S, Borzotta R, et al. Enteral versus parenteral nutrition after severe closed head injury. J Trauma. 1994;37(3):459–68.
12. Hadley MN, Grahm TW, Harrington T, Schiller WR, McDermott MK, Posillico DB. Nutritional support and neurotrauma: a critical review of early nutrition in forty-five acute head injury patients. Neurosurgery. 1986;19(3):367–73.
13. Rapp RP, Young B, Twyman D, Bivins BA, Haack D, Tibbs PA, et al. The favorable effect of early parenteral feeding on survival in head-injured patients. J Neurosurg. 1983;58(6):906–12.
14. Young B, Ott L, Haack D, Twyman D, Combs D, Oexmann JB, et al. Effect of total parenteral nutrition upon intracranial pressure in severe head injury. J Neurosurg. 1987;67(1):76–80.
15. Yang M, Guo Q, Zhang X, Sun S, Wang Y, Zhao L, et al. Intensive insulin therapy on infection rate, days in NICU, in-hospital mortality and neurological outcome in severe traumatic brain injury patients: a randomized controlled trial. Int J Nurs Stud. 2009;46(6):753–8.
16. Bilotta F, Caramia R, Cernak I, Paoloni FP, Doronzio A, Cuzzone V, et al. Intensive insulin therapy after severe traumatic brain injury: a randomized clinical trial. Neurocrit Care. 2008;9(2):159–66.
17. Coester A, Neumann CR, Schmidt MI. Intensive insulin therapy in severe traumatic brain injury: a randomized trial. J Trauma. 2010;68:904–11.
18. Painter TJ, Rickerds J, Alban RF. Immune enhancing nutrition in traumatic brain injury—a preliminary study. Int J Surg. 2015;21:70–4.
19. Young B, Ott L, Kasarskis E, Rapp R, Moles K, Dempsey RJ, et al. Zinc supplementation is associated with improved neurologic recovery rate and visceral protein levels of patients with severe closed head injury. J Neurotrauma. 1996;13(1):25–34.
20. Zarbock SD, Steinke D, Hatton J, Magnuson B, Smith KM, Cook AM. Successful enteral nutritional support in the neurocritical care unit. Neurocrit Care. 2008;9:210–6.

Deep Vein Thrombosis and Venous Thromboembolism Prophylaxis in Traumatic Brain Injury: Current Treatment Options and Controversies

Timothy J. Kovanda and Richard B. Rodgers

Introduction

Fear of hemorrhage has historically led neurosurgeons to avoid the use of anticoagulants, and thus chemical deep vein thrombosis (DVT) prophylaxis, in patients undergoing both elective and nonelective procedures. This trepidation is exacerbated in patients with traumatic brain injury (TBI) due to the possible need for emergent surgical intervention and concern for worsening intracranial hemorrhage. These concerns are justified. In a retrospective cohort study performed by Kwiatt et al., TBI patients treated prophylactically with low-molecular-weight heparin (LMWH) were more likely to demonstrate progression of intracranial hemorrhage on repeat imaging than those who were not given this medication [1]. Patients receiving LMWH in this study were also more likely to require neurosurgical intervention for hemorrhage progression [1].

T. J. Kovanda, MD
Department of Neurological Surgery,
Indiana University School of Medicine,
Indianapolis, IN, USA
e-mail: tkovanda@iupui.edu

R. B. Rodgers, MD, FAANS, FACS (✉)
Department of Neurological Surgery,
Indiana University School of Medicine, Goodman
Campbell Brain and Spine, Indianapolis, IN, USA
e-mail: rrodgers@goodmancampbell.com

Still, the risk of DVT and venous thromboembolism (VTE) in patients with TBI cannot be ignored. The overall incidence of DVT in isolated TBI is estimated to be 25% [2], while the incidence in moderate to severe TBI is just over 30% [3]. Finally, in trauma patients with an Injury Severity Score (ISS) > 8, DVT incidence is 58% [4]. Patients with TBI are prone to develop disseminated intravascular coagulation, are frequently immobile, and are often subject to long surgical procedures—all factors that predispose them to DVT [5]. Other risk factors associated with an increased risk of DVT in moderate to severe TBI include multisystem trauma, male gender, lower extremity injury, age $\geq$ 55 years, subarachnoid hemorrhage, and an ISS $\geq$ 15 [3]. Additionally, TBI itself is known to be an independent risk factor for the development of DVT, leading to a threefold to fourfold increase in DVT risk [6]. Finally, risk of DVT/VTE is known to correlate directly with severity of head injury, suggesting that patients suffering from severe TBI may benefit from DVT screening while hospitalized [7]. Current hospital reporting requirements mandate assessment of VTE risk factors and appropriate prophylaxis documentation. Potential repercussions for noncompliance only increase the importance of the issue [8].

Conflicting views regarding the risks and benefits of DVT/VTE prophylaxis have led the Brain Trauma Foundation to make the following Level

© Springer International Publishing AG, part of Springer Nature 2018
S. D. Timmons (ed.), *Controversies in Severe Traumatic Brain Injury Management*,
https://doi.org/10.1007/978-3-319-89477-5_11

III recommendations regarding the use of DVT/VTE prophylaxis in severe TBI [9]:

- Low-molecular-weight heparin (LMWH) or low-dose unfractioned heparin may be used in combination with mechanical prophylaxis. However, there is an increased risk for expansion of intracranial hemorrhage.
- In addition to compression stockings, pharmacologic prophylaxis may be considered if the brain injury is stable, and the benefit is considered to outweigh the risk of increased intracranial hemorrhage.
- There is insufficient evidence to support recommendations regarding the preferred agent, dose, or timing of pharmacologic prophylaxis for deep vein thrombosis.

We will review the options for DVT screening and DVT/VTE prophylaxis and include a proposed algorithm for the use of DVT prophylaxis in traumatic brain injury patients, as used in our institution.

Deep Vein Thrombosis Screening in Traumatic Brain Injury Patients

There is an ongoing debate regarding DVT screening in trauma patients. This debate has centered around the use of venous Doppler ultrasound for screening, as D-dimer assays are known to have lower-than-expected negative predictive rates early after trauma [10]. The American College of Chest Physicians currently recommends against routine venous compression ultrasound for DVT surveillance in major trauma patients, including patients with TBI [11]. In a retrospective review of DVT incidence in trauma patients, Jawa et al. found no significant difference in DVT detection rates after implementation of a DVT screening protocol for high-risk trauma patients [12]. Although DVT detection rates did not differ, there was a fivefold increase in the number of ultrasound scans performed, leading to higher costs [12]. This study had several limitations, including its retrospective nature and lack of uniformity in testing after implementation of the protocol, as not all patients meeting criteria were screened [12]. In another retrospective analysis, Dietch et al. found that use of lower extremity ultrasound for DVT screening was associated with higher rates of DVT diagnosis but not a reduction in pulmonary embolus (PE) incidence, suggesting screening may result in the diagnosis and treatment of clinically insignificant DVTs [13].

Others have argued for the use of duplex ultrasound DVT screening in trauma patients. In a retrospective review, Azarbal et al. found that 40/162 (15.2%) trauma patients admitted to the intensive care unit (ICU) had lower extremity DVTs as diagnosed on weekly surveillance duplex ultrasound [14]. The authors found no significant difference in DVT rates between low-risk patients receiving LMWH and high-risk patients who did not receive chemical prophylaxis. Thirty percent of all DVTs in the study were diagnosed within 1 week of admission. Based on these results, Azarbal et al. recommended early and continued screening for DVTs in critically ill trauma patients [14].

Few studies have specifically addressed the question of whether TBI patients should undergo routine screening for DVT. Meythaler et al. found that 8.5% of patients admitted to their brain injury rehab unit over a 21-month period had a lower extremity DVT as diagnosed by color Doppler ultrasound [15]. The authors argued that screening this patient population for DVTs on admission to rehab is more cost-effective than other potentially lifesaving screening programs, such as breast cancer and colorectal cancer screening [15]. However, this study included both traumatic and non-traumatic "brain injury" patients and did not address whether screening was beneficial or cost-effective during acute hospitalization after TBI. Dermody et al. sought to evaluate the efficacy of DVT screening in neurosurgical patients. In the study, 174 consecutive neurosurgical patients who were expected to be non-ambulatory for 7 or more days received weekly venous duplex ultrasound testing until discharge or until they became ambulatory [16]. Forty patients (23%) tested positive for a DVT [16]. Chemical prophylaxis in this study was determined by surgeon preference. Of the patients who received unfractionated heparin or LMWH, 19.3% were found to have a DVT, whereas DVTs were identified in 41.4% of patients who did not receive chemical DVT prophylaxis. Although chemical DVT prophylaxis significantly reduced the risk of DVT, the risk remained high in all neurosurgical patients. Based on these findings, the authors argued for routine DVT screening using venous duplex ultrasound in neurosurgical patients while maximizing DVT prophylaxis using chemical and mechanical means [16]. This study included TBI patients, but it was not specific to this population.

Mechanical Deep Vein Thrombosis Prophylaxis

While multiple studies have been done on the efficacy of mechanical DVT prophylaxis in general, only one available study addresses the effectiveness of mechanical DVT prophylaxis specifically in TBI patients. Knudson et al. performed a prospective, randomized controlled trial comparing different prophylaxis options in trauma patients [17]. Patients were separated into three groups based on type of injuries sustained. Group 1 consisted of general trauma patients who could be treated with either low-dose heparin (5000 units subcutaneously every 12 h) or sequential compression devices (SCDs) and thromboembolic deterrent (TED) hose. Patients in this group were randomized to one of three treatment arms: low-dose heparin, SCDs, or no prophylaxis. Group 2 consisted of trauma patients who could not wear SCDs or TED hose due to lower extremity fractures or severe soft tissue injury. Patients in this group were randomized to low-dose heparin or no prophylaxis. Group 3 consisted of 65 patients in whom low-dose heparin was contraindicated (patients with severe head or spinal cord injuries) and who were randomized to one of two treatment arms: SCDs or no prophylaxis. Twenty-six patients received SCDs, and 39 patients received no DVT prophylaxis. In this group, patients with SCDs had lower rates of DVT/PE when compared with the control arm (5 vs. 0, $p = 0.057$) [17]. Still, this outcome

only approached significance. Therefore, the study does not truly demonstrate efficacy of mechanical prophylaxis in neurotrauma patients. In Groups 1 and 2, neither low-dose heparin nor SCDs afforded protection against DVT/PE [17]. Although Group 3 in this study consisted of neurotrauma patients, it was not specific to TBI.

More evidence supporting the use of SCDs is found in the general medical literature. In a meta-analysis comparing the effectiveness of intermittent pneumatic compression (IPC) with no DVT prophylaxis, Urbankova et al. found that IPC lowered DVT rates by 60% [18]. The analysis included 15 randomized controlled trial of IPC vs. no prophylaxis (2270 patients total). PE rates were not significantly different between the two groups [18]. The study included neurosurgical patients but was not specific to trauma or neurosurgical populations.

Two studies have assessed the effectiveness of IPC in neurosurgical patients. In a randomized controlled trial assessing the effectiveness of IPC vs. no prophylaxis, Turpie et al. found that IPC reduced the incidence of DVT from 18.4% (9/49) to 1.9% (1/53) [19]. The findings of this study were supported by another randomized controlled trial performed by Skillman et al., demonstrating a significant decrease in DVT incidence with IPC [20]. Both of these studies were included in the previously mentioned meta-analysis. Given the paucity of information regarding mechanical DVT prophylaxis in TBI populations and taking into account the minimal morbidity associated with IPC, the benefit of mechanical DVT prophylaxis is inferred, and IPC is currently commonplace for TBI patients.

Chemical Deep Vein Thrombosis Prophylaxis

Different studies have evaluated the effectiveness of chemical DVT/VTE prophylaxis in TBI. In a retrospective review of TBI patients, Kwiatt et al. found a significantly lower incidence of DVT in patients receiving LMWH than patients who did not receive chemical prophylaxis [1]. Authors of this study were not specifically looking for DVTs, leading to different rates of venous duplex ultrasound testing. Forty-two percent of patients in the LMWH group had ultrasounds performed, while only 11% of control patients received ultrasounds. This same study demonstrated a higher risk of hemorrhage progression in TBI patients receiving LMWH.

Mohseni et al. performed a retrospective matched case-control study comparing chemical DVT/VTE prophylaxis (unfractionated heparin or LMWH) with no chemical prophylaxis [21]. The authors found a 3.5-fold increase in the incidence of DVT for patients who did not receive chemical prophylaxis [21]. Similar findings were produced by a retrospective cohort study performed by Scudday et al. [22]. No comparison between unfractionated heparin and LMWH was made in either study.

A retrospective cohort study performed by Daley et al. showed opposing results [23]. In this study, authors found no significant difference in DVT/VTE rates in patients who received prophylactic LMWH after trauma craniotomy when compared to patients who did not receive prophylaxis. The mean time to initiation of LMWH was 11 days in this study, which most would consider to be late in the acute TBI treatment course.

Based on these studies and inferences from trauma literature, most neurosurgeons agree that TBI patients benefit from chemical DVT prophylaxis; but the type of prophylaxis, timing of prophylaxis, and dosing management remain topics of debate. We review the most commonly utilized chemical DVT/VTE prophylaxis options as follows. We discuss the limitations and benefits of each and provide a brief review of the literature as it relates to timing/initiation of prophylaxis.

Low-Dose, Unfractionated Heparin

Heparin is an anticoagulant that binds antithrombin and leads to the inactivation of thrombin and factor Xa [24]. The inactivation of thrombin prevents fibrin formation and inhibits activation of platelets and multiple clotting factors, leading to the anticoagulant effect [24]. For DVT/VTE prophylaxis, 5000 units of unfractionated heparin are dosed subcutaneously every 8–12 h. Major side effects include bleeding and heparin-induced thrombocytopenia (HIT). When hemorrhage occurs, protamine sulfate can be used to reverse the effects of heparin.

HIT occurs in two forms. Type I is a nonimmune-mediated reaction to heparin causing a reduction in platelet count, likely from direct effects on platelet activation. Onset is within 2 days of initiation of therapy, and it is usually self-limited even without stopping heparin. Type II HIT (sometimes termed HITT or heparin-induced thrombocytopenia and thrombosis) is an immune-mediated response resulting in formation of heparin-platelet factor IV complexes. Onset is typically after 4 days of initiation of therapy and can result in life- and limb-threatening thrombosis. Signs and symptoms include a precipitous drop in platelet count (>50% of baseline even if nadir is normal); systemic symptoms of purpura, rash, chills, fever, shortness of breath, or chest pain; and thrombotic events including DVT, PE, or even myocardial infarction, cerebral infarction, and limb necrosis if severe. Diagnosis is confirmed with laboratory testing for the antibody. Heparin must be stopped immediately, and treatment of thrombotic complications is with other anticoagulants (Fig. 1) [25].

Multiple studies have demonstrated efficacy for low-dose unfractionated subcutaneous heparin in lowering rates of DVT/VTE in surgical patients by as much as 70% [26, 27]. This benefit is not as clear in trauma patients. As previously mentioned, a randomized controlled trial performed by Knudson et al. did not demonstrate significant benefit for low-dose heparin over no DVT prophylaxis in general trauma patients [17]. This finding was supported by a meta-analysis demonstrating no significant decrease in DVT rates for low-dose unfractionated heparin when compared to no prophylaxis [28]. It remains uncertain whether this therapy is ineffective in trauma patients or whether it simply has not been sufficiently investigated in this subpopulation.

	Score = 2	Score = 1	Score = 0
Thrombocytopenia Compare the highest platelet count within the sequence of declining platelet counts with the lowest count to determine the % of platelet fall. (Select only 1 option)	○ >50% platelet fall AND nadir of ≥ 20 AND no surgery within preceding 3 days	○ >50% platelet fall BUT surgery within preceding 3 days OR ○ any combination of platelet fall and nadir that does not fit criteria for Score 2 or Score 0 (eg, 30-50% platelet fall or nadir 10-19)	○ < 30% platelet fall ○ any platelet fall with nadir< 10
<u>T</u>**iming (of platelet count fall or thrombosis*)** Day 0 = first day of most recent heparin exposure (Select only 1 option)	○ platelet fall day 5-10 after start of heparin ○ platelet fall within 1 day of start of heparin AND exposure to heparin within past 5-30 days	○ consistent with platelet fall days 5-10 but not clear (eg, missing counts) ○ platelet fall within 1 day of start of heparin AND exposure to heparin in past 31-100 days ○ platelet fall after day 10	○ platelet fall ≤ day 4 without exposure to heparin in past 100 days
<u>T</u>**hrombosis (or other clinical sequelae)** (Select only 1 option)	○ confirmed new thrombosis (venous or arterial) ○ skin necrosis at injection site ○ anaphylactoid reaction to IV heparin bolus ○ adrenal hemorrhage	○ recurrent venous thrombosis in a patient receiving therapeutic anticoagulants ○ suspected thrombosis (awaiting confirmation with imaging) ○ erythematous skin lesions at heparin injection sites	○ thrombosis not suspected
o<u>T</u>**her cause for Thrombocytopenia**** (Select only 1 option)	○ no alternative explanation for platelet fall is evident	**Possible other cause is evident:** ○ sepsis without proven microbial source ○ thrombocytopenia associated with initiation of ventilator ○ other	**Probable other cause present:** ○ within 72 h of surgery ○ confirmed bacteremia/ fungemia ○ chemotherapy or radiation within past 20 days ○ DIC due to non-HIT cause ○ posttransfusion purpura (PTP) ○ platelet count < 20 AND given a drug implicated in causing D-ITP(see list) ○ non-necrotizing skin lesions at LMWH injection site (presumes DTH) ○ other

> **Drugs implicated in drug-induced immune thrombocytopenia (D-ITP)**
>
> **Relatively Common:** glycoprotein IIb/IIIa antagonists (abciximab, eptifibatide, tirofiban); quinine, quinidine, sulfa antibiotics, carbamazepine, vancomycin
> **Less Common:** actinomycin, amitriptyline, amoxicillin/piperacillin/nafcillin, cephalosporins (cefazolin, ceftazidime, ceftriaxone), celecoxib, ciprofloxacin, esomeprazole, fexofenadine, fentanyl, fucidic acid, furosemide, gold salts, levofloxacin, metronidazole, naproxen, oxaliplatin, phenytoin, propranolol, propoxyphene, ranitidine, rifampin, suramin, trimethoprim. Note: This is a partial list.

Fig. 1 4Ts score. *Asterisk* Timing of clinical sequelae, such as thrombocytopenia, thrombosis, or skin lesions. *Double asterisk* Two points if necrotizing heparin-induced skin lesions even if thrombocytopenia not present. Reprinted with permission from Linkins L-A, Dans AL, Moores LK, Bona R, Davidson BL, Schulman S, et al. Treatment and Prevention of Heparin-Induced Thrombocytopenia. Antithrombotic Therapy and Prevention of Thrombosis, 9th ed: American College of Chest Physicians Evidence-Based Clinical Practice Guidelines. Chest. 2012;141(2)(Suppl):e495S–e530S

Low-Molecular-Weight Heparin

Low-molecular-weight heparins (LMWH) are a product of the depolymerization of unfractionated heparin. This process decreases the size of unfractionated heparin, leading to increased inactivation of factor Xa [29]. (See also chapter "Management of Traumatic Brain Injury in the Face of Antithrombotic Medication Therapy" for a detailed discussion.)

Two major side effects should be considered when using LMWH for chemical DVT prophylaxis:

hemorrhage and heparin-induced thrombocytopenia (HIT). In a retrospective review, Kwiatt et al. found that LMWH led to higher rates of hemorrhage progression after blunt TBI [1]. When hemorrhage occurs, protamine sulfate incompletely reverses the effects of LMWH. Protamine sulfate administration results in only partial reversal of the increased antifactor Xa activity found in LMWH [29, 30]. HIT rates are lower in patients treated with LMWH when compared to unfractionated heparin [31].

In a multicenter, randomized controlled trial of elective neurosurgical patients, compression stockings with 40 mg of enoxaparin given subcutaneously once daily for at least 7 days starting within 24 h after surgery led to significantly lower DVT rates than compression stockings alone (32% vs. 17%, $p = 0.004$) [32]. No significant difference in bleeding risk was identified in this study.

Appropriate dosing of LMWH remains a topic of debate. Malinoski et al. demonstrated that standard trauma dosing of enoxaparin (30 mg subcutaneously twice daily) can result in low plasma antifactor Xa levels [33]. They also found that low levels of antifactor Xa were associated with increased risk of DVT when compared to patients who had normal antifactor Xa levels after receiving enoxaparin for DVT prophylaxis [33]. Based on these results, the authors suggested using adjusted-dose LMWH in surgical intensive care unit patients. However, neurosurgical trauma patients were not included in this study due to concern for elevated bleeding risk. Studies have also suggested a benefit to monitoring thrombin-antithrombin complex or D-dimer levels as a marker of coagulation activation, which in turn can be used to adjust LMWH dosing appropriately [34, 35].

Unfractionated Heparin vs. Low-Molecular-Weight Heparin

As previously mentioned, the efficacy of unfractionated heparin for chemical DVT prophylaxis in trauma has been questioned in recent years. For this reason, a prospective, randomized controlled trial was performed to directly compare the effects of LMWH with unfractionated heparin in trauma patients. In this study, the authors found that LMWH (30 mg enoxaparin every 12 h) led to significantly lower DVT rates than unfractionated heparin (5000 units every 12 h) (31% vs. 44%, $p = 0.014$) [36]. However, patients with intracranial bleeding as noted on head computed tomography (CT) were again excluded from this study.

As is a theme with the topic of DVT/VTE prophylaxis, effects in TBI patients are inferred due to lack of literature specific to this patient population.

Due to the limited reversal with protamine sulfate and the longer half-life of LMWH, many neurosurgeons still prefer low-dose unfractionated heparin for chemical DVT prophylaxis in TBI, at least in the initial stages after injury.

Fondaparinux

In patients with a heparin allergy or a history of HIT, both LMWH and unfractionated heparin are contraindicated. In this select patient population, DVT prophylaxis with low-dose subcutaneous fondaparinux may be considered. Fondaparinux is a synthetic medication that binds antithrombin and increases inhibition of factor Xa [37]. This treatment gained favor with orthopedic surgeons after a double-blinded randomized controlled trial demonstrated superiority of 2.5 mg of subcutaneous fondaparinux given once daily over once-daily enoxaparin (40 mg subcutaneously) for prevention of DVT/VTE after hip fracture surgery [38]. Another double-blinded randomized controlled trial produced similar results for patients undergoing elective knee surgery [39]. It should be noted that a meta-analysis of four double-blinded randomized controlled trial demonstrated an increased risk of bleeding with fondaparinux when compared with enoxaparin [40].

In the trauma population, Lu et al. performed a prospective observational study of high-risk patients demonstrating that 2.5 mg of subcutaneous fondaparinux given once daily was both safe and effective [41]. The incidence of DVT in patients receiving this medication was 1.2% (1/80 patients). TBI patients were included in this study. Treatment with fondaparinux did not lead to any major bleeding issues or episodes of thrombocytopenia.

The long half-life of fondaparinux (17–21 h) allows for once-daily dosing but means the drug is slow to clear should major bleeding occur [37]. If bleeding occurs, no specific reversal agent is available; however, prothrombin complex concentrates (PCCs) or recombinant factor VIIa may help [37]. (See chapter "Management of Traumatic Brain Injury in the Face of Antithrombotic Medication Therapy" for further detailed discussion.)

Timing of Chemical Deep Vein Thrombosis Prophylaxis

Most neurosurgeons agree that chemical DVT prophylaxis is beneficial in TBI patients, but when to initiate therapy remains open to discussion. In a retrospective analysis comparing early vs. late administration of unfractionated heparin for DVT prophylaxis after severe TBI, Kim et al. did not find a significant increase in bleeding complications with early administration of low-dose heparin (within 72 h of admission) [42]. No significant differences in rates of DVT were noted in this study either, however [42].

Due to lack of uniformity regarding initiation of chemical DVT prophylaxis after TBI, two studies have evaluated the use of protocols to standardize treatment. In a retrospective cohort study evaluating the efficacy of a protocol for instituting DVT prophylaxis after TBI, Farooqui et al. found that initiating chemical DVT prophylaxis (5000 units of unfractionated heparin three times daily or 30 mg enoxaparin twice daily) at least 24 h after injury with demonstrated stability of injury on head CT led to decreased rates of DVT [43]. There was no significant difference in the number of patients with worsening intracranial injuries. Average time to initiation of chemical DVT prophylaxis was significantly longer prior to initiation of the protocol (159 vs. 61 h). In a similar retrospective cohort study, Nickele et al. found that the use of a protocol was effective in improving rates of patients placed on chemical DVT prophylaxis after TBI at their institution [44]. However, there were no outcome differences noted, as there was no significant difference in likelihood of hemorrhage expansion or DVT/PE rates.

Our Practice

At our institution, neurosurgeons work closely with trauma surgeons to determine optimal management strategies for each patient. When possible, our TBI DVT prophylaxis protocol is followed. As demonstrated in the previously described studies, we have found anecdotally that implementation of a protocol leads to higher chemical prophylaxis treatment rates and earlier initiation of treatment.

Figure 2 illustrates our institution's TBI chemical DVT prophylaxis protocol. Enoxaparin

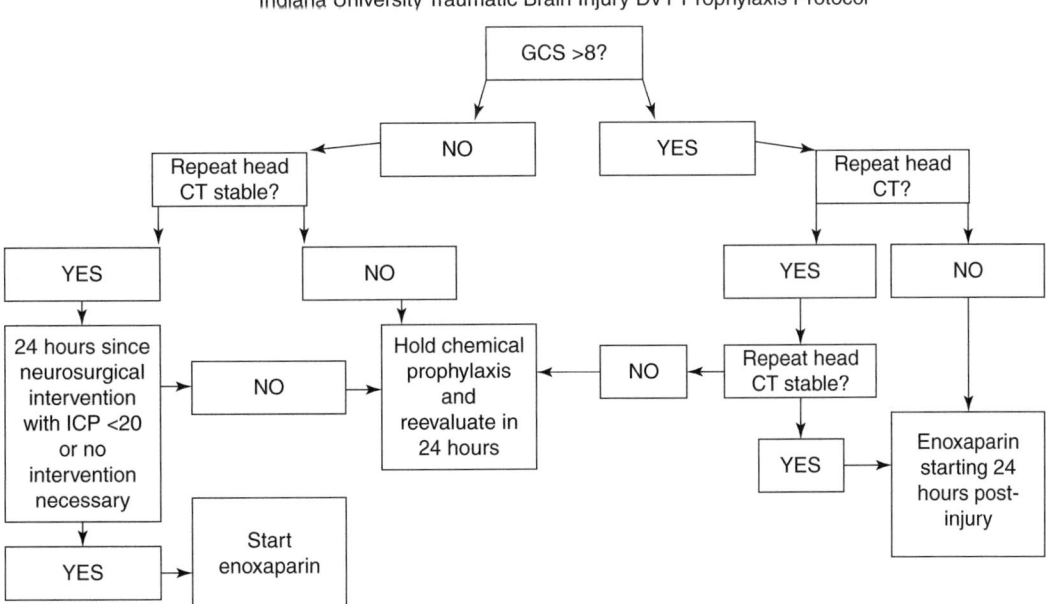

Fig. 2 Indiana University traumatic brain injury DVT prophylaxis protocol

Table 1 Chemical DVT prophylaxis—special circumstances

Chronic renal insufficiency (CrCl < 30 mL/min)—enoxaparin 30 mg subcutaneously Q24H
Hemodialysis or acute renal failure—unfractionated heparin 5000 units subcutaneously Q8H
Obesity (weight > 120 kg)—enoxaparin 40 mg subcutaneously Q12H
Heparin allergy or history of HIT—fondaparinux 2.5 mg subcutaneously Q24H (contraindicated if CrCl < 30 mL/min)

(30 mg subcutaneously every 12 h) is our medication of choice given its demonstrated superiority over unfractionated heparin in the trauma population [36]. Other treatment options are considered under special circumstances (Table 1). Our algorithm is divided into two groups, based on severity of TBI.

For patients with a Glasgow Coma Score (GCS) of >8, enoxaparin is started 24 h post-injury under two circumstances: (1) if a repeat head CT demonstrates stability of the intracranial injury and (2) if a repeat head CT is not clinically indicated. In patients with a GCS ≤ 8 (severe TBI), a head CT demonstrating stability of the intracranial bleed is required prior to initiation of the therapy. Furthermore, in patients with severe TBI, we built in a 72-h window post-injury that allows for surgical intervention should it be warranted prior to initiation of enoxaparin. If the neurosurgical team does not feel the patient is a surgical candidate, the patient has already undergone neurosurgical intervention, or intracranial pressure (ICP) is less than 20 mmHg (if monitored), enoxaparin may be started prior to the 72-h period. If head CT demonstrates progression of injury under any circumstance, chemical prophylaxis is held, and the patient is reevaluated 24 h later for consideration for prophylaxis initiation. Antifactor Xa levels are monitored and enoxaparin dosing is adjusted as needed. All patients are treated with intermittent pneumatic compression sleeves with or without compression stockings unless contraindicated.

Conclusions

Future Directions

Patients suffering from TBI are at high risk for the development of DVT/VTE. When intracranial injuries are stable and no contraindication exists, chemical and mechanical prophylaxes are effective measures in lowering the incidence of DVT/VTE. Continued work is needed to optimize prophylaxis within this patient population. Type of treatment, dosing, and time to initiation of therapy remain controversial and will require further study. Institutional implementation of a protocol may improve prophylactic treatment (vis-à-vis timing and rates) and thus patient outcomes, but more evidence is needed to link the two.

References

1. Kwiatt ME, Patel MS, Ross SE, Lachant MT, MacNew HG, Ochsner MG, et al. Is low-molecular-weight heparin safe for venous thromboembolism prophylaxis in patients with traumatic brain injury? A Western Trauma Association multicenter study. J Trauma Acute Care Surg. 2012;73(3):625–8.
2. Denson K, Morgan D, Cunningham R, Nigliazzo A, Brackett D, Lane M, et al. Incidence of venous thromboembolism in patients with traumatic brain injury. Am J Surg. 2007;193(3):380–3; discussion 383–4.
3. Ekeh AP, Dominguez KM, Markert RJ, McCarthy MC. Incidence and risk factors for deep venous thrombosis after moderate and severe brain injury. J Trauma. 2010;68(4):912–5.
4. Geerts WH, Code KI, Jay RM, Chen E, Szalai JP. A prospective study of venous thromboembolism after major trauma. N Engl J Med. 1994;331(24):1601–6.
5. Byrne JP, Mason SA, Gomez D, Hoeft C, Subacius H, Xiong W, et al. Timing of pharmacologic venous thromboembolism prophylaxis in severe traumatic brain injury: a Propensity-Matched Cohort Study. J Am Coll Surg. 2016;223(4):621–31.e5.
6. Reiff DA, Haricharan RN, Bullington NM, Griffin RL, Jr MGG, Rue LW III. Traumatic brain injury is associated with the development of deep vein thrombosis independent of pharmacological prophylaxis. J Trauma. 2009;66(5):1436–40.
7. Van Gent JM, Bandle J, Calvo RY, Zander AL, Olson EJ, Shackford SR, et al. Isolated traumatic brain injury and venous thromboembolism. J Trauma Acute Care Surg. 2014;77(2):238–42.

8. The Joint Commission. Specifications manual for national hospital inpatient quality measures, version 5.1. Retrieved from: www.jointcommission.org. Accessed 12/1/16.

9. Carney N, Totten AM, O'Reilly C, Ullman JS, Hawryluk GW, Bell MJ, et al. Guidelines for the management of severe traumatic brain injury, fourth edition. Neurosurgery. 2017;80(1):6–15.

10. Wahl WL, Ahrns KS, Zajkowski PJ, Brandt MM, Proctor M, Arbabi S, et al. Normal D-dimer levels do not exclude thrombotic complications in trauma patients. Surgery. 2003;134(4):529–32; discussion 332–3.

11. Guyatt GH, Akl EA, Crowther M, Gutterman DD, Schuunemann HJ. Executive summary: antithrombotic therapy and prevention of thrombosis, 9th ed: American College of Chest Physicians Evidence-Based Clinical Practice Guidelines. Chest. 2012;141(2 Suppl):7s–47s.

12. Jawa RS, Warren K, Young D, Wagner M, Nelson L, Yetter D, et al. Venous thromboembolic disease in trauma and surveillance ultrasonography. J Surg Res. 2011;167(1):24–31.

13. Dietch ZC, Edwards BL, Thames M, Shah PM, Williams MD, Sawyer RG. Rate of lower-extremity ultrasonography in trauma patients is associated with rate of deep venous thrombosis but not pulmonary embolism. Surgery. 2015;158(2):379–85.

14. Azarbal A, Rowell S, Lewis J, Urankar R, Moseley S, Landry G, et al. Duplex ultrasound screening detects high rates of deep vein thromboses in critically ill trauma patients. J Vasc Surg. 2011;54(3):743–7; discussion 747–8

15. Meythaler JM, DeVivo MJ, Hayne JB. Cost-effectiveness of routine screening for proximal deep venous thrombosis in acquired brain injury patients admitted to rehabilitation. Arch Phys Med Rehabil. 1996;77(1):1–5.

16. Dermody M, Alessi-Chinetti J, Iafrati MD, Estes JM. The utility of screening for deep venous thrombosis in asymptomatic, non-ambulatory neurosurgical patients. J Vasc Surg. 2011;53(5):1309–15.

17. Knudson MM, Lewis FR, Clinton A, Atkinson K, Megerman J. Prevention of venous thromboembolism in trauma patients. J Trauma. 1994;37(3):480–7.

18. Urbankova J, Quiroz R, Kucher N, Goldhaber SZ. Intermittent pneumatic compression and deep vein thrombosis prevention. A meta-analysis in postoperative patients. Thromb Haemost. 2005;94(6):1181–5.

19. Turpie AG, Gallus A, Beattie WS, Hirsh J. Prevention of venous thrombosis in patients with intracranial disease by intermittent pneumatic compression of the calf. Neurology. 1977;27(5):435–8.

20. Skillman JJ, Collins RE, Coe NP, Goldstein BS, Shapiro RM, Zervas NT, et al. Prevention of deep vein thrombosis in neurosurgical patients: a controlled, randomized trial of external pneumatic compression boots. Surgery. 1978;83(3):354–8.

21. Mohseni S, Talving P, Lam L, Chan LS, Ives C, Demetriades D. Venous thromboembolic events in isolated severe traumatic brain injury. J Emerg Trauma Shock. 2012;5(1):11–5.

22. Scudday T, Brasel K, Webb T, Codner P, Somberg L, Weigelt J, et al. Safety and efficacy of prophylactic anticoagulation in patients with traumatic brain injury. J Am Coll Surg. 2011;213(1):148–53; discussion 153–4

23. Daley MJ, Ali S, Brown CV. Late venous thromboembolism prophylaxis after craniotomy in acute traumatic brain injury. Am Surg. 2015;81(2):207–11.

24. Hirsh J, Anand SS, Halperin JL, Fuster V. Mechanism of action and pharmacology of unfractionated heparin. Arterioscler Thromb Vasc Biol. 2001;21(7):1094–6.

25. Linkins L-A, Dans AL, Moores LK, Bona R, Davidson BL, Schulman S, et al. Treatment and prevention of heparin-induced thrombocytopenia. Antithrombotic therapy and prevention of thrombosis, 9th ed: American College of Chest Physicians Evidence-Based Clinical Practice Guidelines. Chest. 2012;141(2 Suppl):e495S–530S.

26. Collins R, Scrimgeour A, Yusuf S, Peto R. Reduction in fatal pulmonary embolism and venous thrombosis by perioperative administration of subcutaneous heparin. Overview of results of randomized trials in general, orthopedic, and urologic surgery. N Engl J Med. 1988;318(18):1162–73.

27. Gruber UF, Duckert F, Fridrich R, Rem J, Torhorst J. Prevention of fatal postoperative pulmonary embolism by low-dose heparin. Lancet (London, England). 1977;1(8017):898.

28. Velmahos GC, Kern J, Chan LS, Oder D, Murray JA, Shekelle P. Prevention of venous thromboembolism after injury: an evidence-based report--part I: analysis of risk factors and evaluation of the role of vena caval filters. J Trauma. 2000;49(1):132–8; discussion 139.

29. Weitz JI. Low-molecular-weight heparins. N Engl J Med. 1997;337(10):688–98.

30. Holst J, Lindblad B, Bergqvist D, Garre K, Nielsen H, Hedner U, et al. Protamine neutralization of intravenous and subcutaneous low-molecular-weight heparin (tinzaparin, Logiparin). An experimental investigation in healthy volunteers. Blood Coagul Fibrinolysis. 1994;5(5):795–803.

31. Warkentin TE, Levine MN, Hirsh J, Horsewood P, Roberts RS, Gent M, et al. Heparin-induced thrombocytopenia in patients treated with low-molecular-weight heparin or unfractionated heparin. N Engl J Med. 1995;332(20):1330–5.

32. Agnelli G, Piovella F, Buoncristiani P, Severi P, Pini M, D'Angelo A, et al. Enoxaparin plus compression stockings compared with compression stockings alone in the prevention of venous thromboembolism after elective neurosurgery. N Engl J Med. 1998;339(2):80–5.

33. Malinoski D, Jafari F, Ewing T, Ardary C, Conniff H, Baje M, et al. Standard prophylactic enoxaparin dosing leads to inadequate anti-Xa levels and increased deep venous thrombosis rates in critically ill trauma and surgical patients. J Trauma. 2010;68(4): 874–80.

34. Peetz D, Hafner G, Hansen M, Mayer A, Rippin G, Rommens PM, et al. Dose-adjusted thrombosis prophylaxis in trauma surgery according to levels of D-Dimer. Thromb Res. 2000;98(6):473–83.

35. Mayer A, Hansen M, Peetz D, Hafner G, Vogel N, Prellwitz W, et al. [Prevention of thromboembolism in trauma surgery by dose adjustment of low molecular weight heparin depending on levels of TAT and D-dimer]. Unfallchirurg. 2003;106(12):1020–8.

36. Geerts WH, Jay RM, Code KI, Chen E, Szalai JP, Saibil EA, et al. A comparison of low-dose heparin with low-molecular-weight heparin as prophylaxis against venous thromboembolism after major trauma. N Engl J Med. 1996;335(10):701–7.

37. de Oliveira Manoel AL, Goffi A, Zampieri FG, Turkel-Parrella D, Duggal A, Marotta TR, et al. The critical care management of spontaneous intracranial hemorrhage: a contemporary review. Crit Care (London England). 2016;20:272.

38. Eriksson BI, Bauer KA, Lassen MR, Turpie AG. Fondaparinux compared with enoxaparin for the prevention of venous thromboembolism after hip-fracture surgery. N Engl J Med. 2001;345(18):1298–304.

39. Bauer KA, Eriksson BI, Lassen MR, Turpie AG. Fondaparinux compared with enoxaparin for the prevention of venous thromboembolism after elective major knee surgery. N Engl J Med. 2001;345(18):1305–10.

40. Turpie AG, Bauer KA, Eriksson BI, Lassen MR. Fondaparinux vs enoxaparin for the prevention of venous thromboembolism in major orthopedic surgery: a meta-analysis of 4 randomized double-blind studies. Arch Intern Med. 2002;162(16):1833–40.

41. Lu JP, Knudson MM, Bir N, Kallet R, Atkinson K. Fondaparinux for prevention of venous thromboembolism in high-risk trauma patients: a pilot study. J Am Coll Surg. 2009;209(5):589–94.

42. Kim J, Gearhart MM, Zurick A, Zuccarello M, James L, Luchette FA. Preliminary report on the safety of heparin for deep venous thrombosis prophylaxis after severe head injury. J Trauma. 2002;53(1):38–42; discussion 43

43. Farooqui A, Hiser B, Barnes SL, Litofsky NS. Safety and efficacy of early thromboembolism chemoprophylaxis after intracranial hemorrhage from traumatic brain injury. J Neurosurg. 2013;119(6):1576–82.

44. Nickele CM, Kamps TK, Medow JE. Safety of a DVT chemoprophylaxis protocol following traumatic brain injury: a single center quality improvement initiative. Neurocrit Care. 2013;18(2):184–92.

Treatment of Anemia

Peter Le Roux

Introduction

Traumatic brain injury (TBI) is the most common cause of death and long-term disability among young adults and children in developed (and many developing) countries [1]. In the United States, the annual incidence of TBI is greater than 1.5 million; this includes about 235,000 hospitalizations and 50,000 deaths [2] with large direct and indirect costs to society. Part of this poor outcome is associated with the evolution of secondary brain injury since the acutely injured brain is vulnerable to secondary insults that can exacerbate outcome. Hence TBI care has two broad management goals. First, the damage triggered at the time of the "primary" insult needs to be addressed; e.g., space-occupying lesions must be evacuated and efforts made to control cerebral edema and intracranial pressure (ICP). Second, clinicians also must attempt to attenuate any subsequent physiologic derangements that can contribute to additional, "secondary" cerebral damage that can reduce the chance of a favorable recovery. Among these insults are hypotension, hypoxia, hypo- and hypercapnia, hypo- and hyperglycemia, anemia, and disturbed temperature regulation to name a few [3–5].

In patients with severe TBI, there is a known relationship between brain hypoxia and poor outcome [6], and maintaining adequate oxygenation through resuscitation is an important component in TBI management [5, 7]. Because brain oxygen delivery (DO_2) depends, in part, on the concentration of circulating hemoglobin (Hgb), anemia is a major potential cause of secondary brain injury. Although anemia can be corrected easily with red blood cell transfusion (RBCT), there is a well-described association between RBCT, adverse events, and worse outcome in critical care. Therefore, the decision to transfuse should only be made after clinicians have considered whether RBCT is physiologically necessary and balance this consideration with an awareness of the potentially deleterious effects of allogeneic blood products. In addition, decisions about transfusion in TBI patients may need to consider more than Hgb concentrations alone [8, 9].

While the existing evidence demonstrates that a restrictive transfusion strategy (hemoglobin ~7 g/dL) in general critical care patients without serious cardiac disease is similar to more liberal strategies [10–14], the optimal Hgb and transfusion trigger for patients with TBI (and other acute brain injury, e.g., subarachnoid hemorrhage [SAH] and stroke) has still to be fully elucidated, and there is great variance in how these patients are transfused [15, 16], with convincing arguments being made for both liberal (Hgb ~10 g/dL) and restrictive RBCT strategies [17, 18]. In this chapter we will review

P. Le Roux, MD, FACS
Department of Neurosurgery, The Brain and Spine
Center, Lankenau Medical Center,
Wynnewood, PA, USA
e-mail: LeRouxP@MLHS.ORG

© Springer International Publishing AG, part of Springer Nature 2018
S. D. Timmons (ed.), *Controversies in Severe Traumatic Brain Injury Management*,
https://doi.org/10.1007/978-3-319-89477-5_12

117

anemia in TBI, the pathophysiology of anemia, the effects of anemia on outcome, the physiology of transfusion, and the relationship between RBCT and outcome. The role of hematopoiesis-stimulating agents and hemoglobin-based blood substitutes will be briefly considered, and the chapter will conclude with a suggested approach to anemia management in TBI. Coagulation, coagulopathy, and the administration of other blood products (e.g., platelets or coagulation factors) are beyond the scope of this chapter.

Epidemiology

The World Health Organization (WHO) defines anemia as an Hgb concentration less than 12 g/dL in females or less than 13 g/dL in males [17, 19]. Multicenter cohort studies have found anemia to be one of the most common medical complications in critically ill patients [20, 21]. Hgb concentrations in these patients tend to decrease at a rate of about 0.5 g/dL/day [22]. The etiology of this decline is multifactorial and includes blood loss, hemodilution attributable to large volume resuscitation, frequent phlebotomy, and the effects of systemic inflammation on endogenous erythropoietin production and bone marrow function [17, 20–23] (Table 1).

Studies that report the prevalence of anemia specifically in TBI patients vary somewhat in their inclusion criteria (isolated TBI vs. polytrauma, Glasgow Coma Scale [GCS] ≤8 vs. other), definitions of "significant" anemia (Hgb 8–10 g/dL), and the timing of Hgb measurements (admission only vs. repeated over time) [24–31]. Nevertheless, the cumulative data suggests that clinically relevant

Hgb reductions eventually occur in 22–69% of patients with moderate to severe TBI. Up to 50% of patients have at least one Hgb <10 g/dL at admission or during their intensive care unit (ICU) stay [18, 25, 32, 33]. These same studies suggest that RBCTs are administered in approximately one-third to one-half of patients. The likelihood of anemia and of RBCT is highest among patients with more severely impaired consciousness, longer length of stay, concomitant extracranial injuries, and in those who undergo surgical procedures [33].

Pathophysiology of Anemia

When Hgb decreases, and particularly when anemia develops, there is a decrease in the oxygen content of arterial blood (CaO_2). In healthy individuals several mechanisms compensate for this anemia-induced CaO_2 decrease, including an increase in heart rate, stroke volume, and cardiac output and a decrease in blood viscosity. Viscosity changes are complex and are, in large part, a function of hematocrit (Hct). There are a variety of adaptive mechanisms (Table 2).

Following acute brain injury, the primary concern with anemia is its effect on DO_2 and how the brain compensates for this [17, 18, 34, 35]. Delivery of O_2 to the brain depends upon cerebral blood flow (CBF) (and therefore is affected by cerebral autoregulation), Hgb concentration, the degree to which Hgb is saturated with oxygen, and the relatively small amount of O_2 dissolved in blood, according to the following equation:

Table 1 Pathophysiology of anemia in traumatic brain injury

• Multifactorial
• Primary blood losses (e.g., trauma, surgery, gastrointestinal bleeding)
• Blood losses related to minor procedures or phlebotomy
• Hemodilution secondary to fluid resuscitation
• Altered red blood cell (RBC) production
• Reduced RBC half-life
• Reduced eyrthropoetin

Table 2 Adaptation to anemia

• ↑Cardiac output
– Heart rate and left ventricular stroke volume
• ↑Microcirculatory density
• ↑Red cell synthesis of 2,3-DPG
– Shift to the right of the oxyhemoglobin dissociation curve (aids oxygen unloading)
• ↑Oxygen extraction
• Reduced blood visocity
– Reduces endothelial shear stress
– Promotes venous return
• Vasodilitation—enhanced nitric oxide (NO) production

$$DO_2 \left(mL\, O_2/min \right)$$
$$= \left[\text{cerebral blood flow} \left(L/min \right) \times Hgb \left(g/L \right) \times \text{oxygen saturation} \left(\% \right) \times 1.39 \left(mL\, O_2/g\, Hgb \right) \right]$$
$$+ \left(0.003 \times P_a O_2 \right)$$

Ischemia occurs when DO_2 is inadequate to meet the cerebral metabolic rate for oxygen ($CMRO_2$). If the Hgb concentration decreases sufficiently, ischemia eventually will develop. However, in healthy adults, the degree of Hgb reduction must be relatively large before this occurs. In experiments of healthy volunteers exposed to extreme isovolemic hemodilution, neurocognitive dysfunction is detected when Hgb concentrations fall below 7 g/dL [36]. These abnormalities can be reversed by RBCT or delivery of supplemental O_2 [37].

When Hgb reductions are more modest, natural compensatory mechanisms help ensure that DO_2 remains sufficient to meet $CMRO_2$:

1. *Anemia consistently increases CBF*—The major determinants of CBF include cerebral perfusion pressure (CPP), blood viscosity, and the caliber of cerebral blood vessels, as predicted by the Hagen-Poiseuille equation:
   Flow = π(pi) r^4 Δ(Delta)P/(8η[eta] L)
   where r = radius, P = pressure, L = length, and η(eta) = viscosity.
   Each of these three factors is modified by Hgb reductions. Anemia causes sympathetic stimulation, leading to systemic vasoconstriction and an increased cardiac output, thereby increasing blood pressure and CPP [38]. The reduced Hgb concentration decreases viscosity and so may increase microcirculatory flow. Anemia also induces a cascade of biochemical events, such as increased production of nitric oxide in the cerebral circulation and upregulation of cerebral β(beta)$_2$ receptors, which in turn leads to cerebral vasodilatation [39].
2. Cerebral DO_2 typically exceeds $CMRO_2$ by a wide margin, thereby maintaining a protective "buffer." When Hgb declines, cerebral O_2 extraction fraction (OEF) increases and probably does not become critical until it reaches levels that exceed 70–75% [40].

These protective mechanisms may not be as effective in TBI patients. Unlike healthy volunteers in carefully controlled studies, trauma patients often do not have normal cardiopulmonary function. Moreover, autoregulatory mechanisms that usually maintain a relatively constant CBF frequently fail [41]. In these circumstances, a direct linear correlation between mean arterial pressure (MAP) and CBF exists, making patients susceptible to ischemia or hyperemia.

The degree to which classical ischemia contributes to secondary brain injury in TBI remains controversial. Global CBF often is markedly reduced, but this may be appropriately matched relative to a decreased $CMRO_2$ [40, 42, 43], which in turn may reflect mitochondrial dysfunction and impairments in O_2 utilization, rather than inadequate O_2 supply [44, 45]. Indeed, studies using fluorine-18—labeled fluoromisonidazole ([18F]FMISO)—a positron emission tomography (PET) tracer that undergoes irreversible selective bioreduction within hypoxic cells, show that hypoxia is not confined to regions with structural abnormalities and may occur without ischemia in TBI patients. In other words, microvascular collapse, perivascular edema, diffusion abnormalities, and microthrombosis all may contribute to cellular damage [46]. On the other hand, most patients with fatal TBI have evidence of cerebral infarction at autopsy [47]. Decrements in jugular venous O_2 saturation (that reflect the balance between O_2 supply and demand) and brain tissue oxygen tension (pB_tO_2) have been reported to be common, especially in the first 24 h after TBI, and to be associated with worse long-term outcomes [6, 48, 49]. Furthermore, there is considerable heterogeneity in CBF, $CMRO_2$, and OEF; even though *global* levels may be normal, *regional* values can be substantially deranged. In fact, the proportion of brain that maximally extracts O_2 has averaged more than 10% in some studies and may be considerably higher in individual patients [50, 51]. Given that the risk of infarction depends on the degree and duration of ischemia, this raises concerns about the ability of vulnerable brain regions to tolerate even moderate reductions in Hgb concentration for extended periods of time.

The Effects of Anemia on the Brain

The effects of an Hgb decrease on the brain are listed in Table 3. In the brain, mild anemia may increase cerebral vascular tone because of the viscosity decrease, but as the Hgb decreases, <10 g/dL, compensatory vasodilation mediated by nitric oxide occurs, so DO_2 remains constant as anemia initially develops. Since anemia induces cerebral vasodilatation, this Hgb reduction may contribute to or exacerbate cerebral edema and so increase ICP [52]. Brain hypoxia and dysfunction usually manifest when Hgb is <6–7 g/dL. Consistent with this, studies of acute isovolemic anemia in healthy human volunteers demonstrate slower reaction times and impaired memory when Hgb is <7 g/dL [36]. The reduction in Hgb alone is not the sole reason for this; rather, it is reduced DO_2 since these cognitive changes can be reversed by oxygen [37].

Normal cerebral autoregulation compensates for the reduced oxygen carrying capacity caused by anemia by increasing CBF to maintain cerebral oxygenation [53, 54]. Dysfunction of

Table 3 What happens in the brain when Hgb decreases?

- Mild anemia causes vasoconstriction in response to ↓ viscosity
- As Hgb decreases <10 g/dL compensatory vasodilation, mediated by nitric oxide, occurs, to initially keep DO_2 constant
- Cerebral vasodilatation may contribute to or exacerbate cerebral edema and so increase ICP
- Brain hypoxia and dysfunction usually manifest when Hgb is <6–7 g/dL
  - In healthy human volunteers cognitive impairment occurs during acute isovolemic anemia when Hgb is <7 g/dL
  - These cognitive changes can be reversed by increasing Hgb levels or with supplemental oxygen

cerebrovascular autoregulation caused by the trauma, however, could prevent an adequate CBF increase. Alternatively, CBF could be increased sufficiently, but the resulting cerebral vasodilatation needed to achieve the increase in CBF may result in an increased ICP [52]. In addition, impaired cerebral autoregulation can result in regional areas of hypoperfusion [55]. Therefore, patients with TBI may have impaired DO_2 in the setting of anemia that is typically well tolerated in normal subjects.

The mechanisms that compensate for decreased DO_2 are disrupted in acute brain injury, so tissue hypoxia and cell injury may develop at a higher Hgb level. In addition, the injured brain is vulnerable to even small DO_2 decrements. Furthermore, the Hgb threshold at which anemia becomes severe enough for energy failure or hypoxia in the brain to develop varies somewhat, based on the characteristics of individual patients and the nature of their cerebral injuries. Using mathematical modeling based on animal experiments in the setting of cerebral ischemia, this critical threshold is estimated to be as high as 10–12 g/dL in the vulnerable brain tissue surrounding the core of the infarct, commonly referred to as the "ischemic penumbra" [56]. Similarly, experimental evidence suggests that brain injury (contusion or infarct) may be exacerbated when Hgb is <10 g/dL, whereas maximal DO_2 is observed with a Hct of 31% following global brain ischemia [38, 57, 58].

The implications of anemia have been explored in a fluid percussion TBI model, in which animals underwent isovolemic hemodilution to Hgb concentrations of 5–7 g/dL. Compared with brain-injured animals with normal Hgb levels, those with anemia developed more profound and sustained reductions in pB_tO_2, despite (as expected) a significant CBF increase, i.e., impaired oxygen extraction. Exposure to hemodilution also produced substantially larger contusion volumes and increased histological evidence of apoptosis [57]. Similar findings have been reported in another experiment where hemorrhage was used to induce hypotension [58]. It is likely that multiple causes of secondary injury that occur simultaneously (e.g., hypotension, hypoxemia, and anemia), as commonly occurs in the setting of polytrauma, create a "multiple hit" scenario and are particularly deleterious. Since anemia induces cerebral vasodilatation, Hgb reductions could contribute to cerebral edema and raised ICP, especially when intracranial compliance is limited. Indeed, although modest in magnitude, such a relationship has been observed in animal experiments, even when the degree of hemodilution is relatively mild (hematocrit 27–30%) [52, 59, 60].

In patients with high-grade aneurysmal SAH, which has some pathophysiological similarities with TBI, an Hgb concentration of <9–10 g/dL is an independent factor associated with brain tissue hypoxia and cellular energy dysfunction [61, 62]. For example, Oddo et al. [61], using cerebral microdialysis in poor-grade SAH patients, observed that Hgb <9 g/dL was an independent

factor associated with lower pB_tO_2 values and a greater chance of metabolic distress, defined by a microdialysate lactate/pyruvate ratio (LPR) >40. In a similar study, Kurtz et al. [62], who excluded patients who required an $FiO_2 > 60\%$, also found that Hgb <10 g/dL was associated with cellular energy dysfunction. More recently, Oddo and colleagues [9] observed that an Hgb concentration of <9 g/dL is associated with lower pB_tO_2, and more frequent episodes of brain hypoxia (defined as $pB_tO_2 < 15$ mmHg) in severe TBI patients. In addition, the combination of anemia and brain hypoxia, but not anemia alone, was associated with worse outcomes (Fig. 1). Taken together, these studies suggest that cellular injury (or at least biochemical evidence for cellular dysfunction) may begin when Hgb is <9 g/dL in patients with acute brain injury.

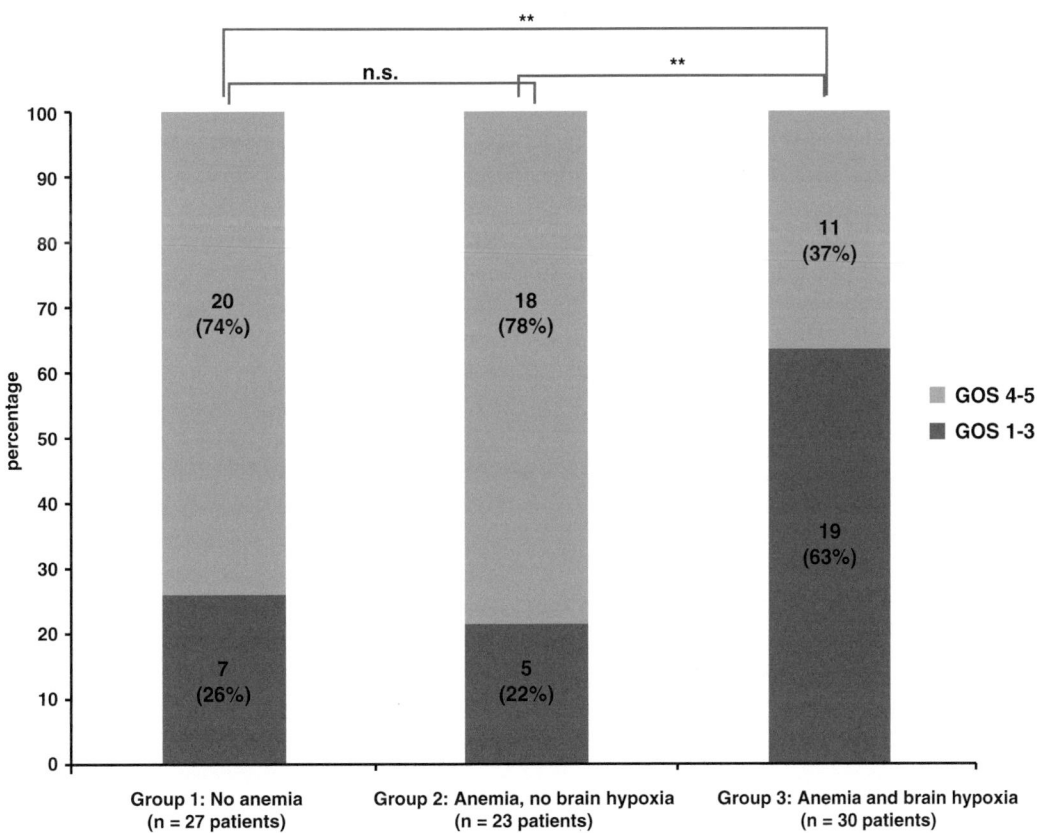

Fig. 1 Anemia and brain hypoxia, but not anemia alone, is associated with worse 30-day outcome [9]

Anemia and Outcome

Anemia in the Surgical Population

There is limited data on the effect of anemia or RBCT in neurosurgical procedures [63–65] although elective neurosurgical procedures are safe and feasible in those patients who refuse allogenic transfusion for religious reasons [66]. What about in other surgical procedures? Preoperative anemia is independently associated with adverse outcomes, including adverse cerebrovascular outcomes after surgery particularly after cardiac operations [67–72]. However, not all studies find an association between preoperative anemia and adverse outcome [73].

Perioperative anemia also is associated with an increased risk for mortality among patients undergoing non-cardiac surgery [74]. In patients with a history of cardiovascular disease, the risk for mortality with perioperative anemia is amplified [75]. The influence of anemia on outcome, however, may depend on change over time rather than absolute values [76]. For example, Spolverato et al. [77] examined 4669 patients who underwent major gastrointestinal surgery. A Δ(Delta)Hgb level of 50% or greater following gastrointestinal surgery was associated with complications, especially ischemic adverse events, even if the nadir Hgb level was 7 g/dL or greater. Larger changes in Hgb were seen in patients with multiple comorbidities and coexisting medical conditions; i.e., "sicker patients" were more vulnerable to anemia.

Anemia in Clinical Traumatic Brain Injury Studies

Several observational studies, summarized, in part, in recent review articles [17, 18, 35] have explored the association between anemia and TBI outcome [3, 24–31, 78]. These studies show a variable relationship between outcome and anemia; i.e., some [27, 78, 79], but not all [24, 80, 81], studies reported that reduced Hgb concentrations are associated with worse outcomes. This variability may be explained by study design since the methodology of these studies varied considerably with respect to the definition of anemia [25, 82, 83], severity and heterogeneity of TBI patients included, timing of Hgb assessments, number of Hgb assessments, outcome measures, and reporting of other confounding factors that are known to be associated with both transfusion and outcome.

One of the largest studies to examine anemia and TBI outcome was the International Mission for Prognosis and Analysis of Clinical Trials in TBI (IMPACT) study, which used prospectively collected data from several thousand patients, most of whom were enrolled in various randomized controlled trials (RCTs) [3]. A clear linear relationship between a lower admission Hgb level and poor 6-month neurological outcome (Glasgow Outcome Scale [GOS] score 1–3) was observed. In addition, an analysis of the MRC CRASH trial, which included more than 10,000 patients, found that an Hgb concentration <9 g/dL at the time of hospital admission was an independent predictor of poor outcome. Along with platelets and pH, Hgb had an inverse linear relation with outcome (i.e., low values are associated with poorer outcome) [79, 84]. Interestingly, this Hgb concentration is similar to that found to be related with metabolic distress in microdialysis and pB_tO_2 studies [61, 62]. On the other hand, not all studies describe an association between reduced Hgb concentrations and worse outcomes. For example, Yang et al. [31], in a review of 234 patients with severe TBI, observed that initial anemia (Hgb < 10 mg/dL) was not a mortality risk factor for patients with isolated severe blunt TBI.

Perhaps more relevant to clinical practice in TBI care are studies where repeated Hgb concentrations, rather than only admission values, are reported [24, 26–28, 30, 31, 78]. The largest of these, a retrospective review of 1150 patients, found the development of anemia (defined as Hgb < 9 g/dL) to be independently associated with mortality [27]. Other smaller retrospective studies also have found that an average Hgb level below 9 g/dL over a period of 7 days was associated, in a multivariate analysis, with increased hospital mortality [78] or that the burden of anemia is associated with poor outcome [85]. Consistent with this, Litofsky et al. [33] in a retrospective review of 939 patients with TBI and a head Abbreviated Injury Scale (AIS) > 3 found that for each 1 g/dL higher Hgb value, the likelihood of a good outcome increased by 33%. However, it remains unclear from these studies whether the association between anemia and poor outcome is causative. Indeed, anemia repeatedly has been demonstrated to be a marker of "severity of illness" in non-neurological critical care populations, and anemia is a variable that is incorporated into commonly used prognostic scales [86, 87].

Thus, although an association between Hgb reductions and poor outcomes provides a strong argument to rigorously avoid anemia in TBI patients as best as possible using blood conservation strategies, it should not necessarily be used as justification for a liberal transfusion approach. Instead, other factors, such as the physiological impact of anemia or patients' cerebrovascular reserve or compensatory response may need to be considered [61].

Red Blood Cell Transfusions : Cerebral Physiologic Effects

The prevention and management of secondary brain injury is the foundation of neurocritical care. In TBI (and other acute brain injuries) the principal concern with anemia is how it affects DO_2. Several factors, including CBF, Hgb concentration, the degree to which Hgb is saturated with oxygen, and the relatively small amount of O_2 dissolved in blood, influence DO_2. Oxygen delivery can be improved by several methods, and because Hgb concentration is important, transfusion is one such technique. However, it is conceivable that avoiding hypoxia, rather than anemia alone, may prevent neuron damage. Consistent with this, clinical studies in SAH show that induced hypertension, rather than hemodilution (viscosity change) or hypervolemia, can improve pB_tO_2 [88]. In addition, studies using PET show that increased FiO_2 allows the metabolic rate of at-risk brain tissue in TBI patients to increase [51], whereas cerebral

microdialysis studies demonstrate that normobaric hyperoxia [89] and hyperbaric oxygen [90, 91] improve biochemical markers in the brain and, in some patients, control ICP. Consequently, pB_tO_2-based therapy combined with control of ICP and CPP is used in some patients, and appears to be associated with improved outcome after TBI [92] and SAH [93]. The implication of these studies is that RBCT should improve DO_2 in the brain to be effective. Recent data from a phase II trial suggests that improved pB_tO_2 is associated with improved outcome after severe TBI [94].

Anemia, which is noted in as many as 50% of patients with TBI, can impair oxygen delivery and further contribute to cerebral ischemia. There also is disruption of cerebral autoregulation and increased ICP that can further contribute to cerebral hypoperfusion. The impact of RBCT on cerebral physiology has been assessed in several clinical studies of brain-injured patients: RBCT appears to provide variable changes in pB_tO_2 [95–100] and markers of cerebral aerobic metabolism, principally the lactate/pyruvate ratio [97]. In general, pB_tO_2 appears to slightly increase with transfusion. However, a reduction also may be observed with about one-third of transfusions [95–100]. Some of this variability may be associated with the age of transfused RBCs, with an increase in pB_tO_2 primarily observed with fresher blood that has been stored for less than 2 weeks, although this finding is not consistent [98]. In addition, a recent study suggested that there is a greater pB_tO_2 increment following transfusion in women and younger patients [100]. Despite the potential increase in pB_tO_2, transfusion does not necessarily influence cerebral metabolism, as demonstrated in another recent study using microdialysate lactate/pyruvate ratios [97]. In a recent randomized clinical trial [101], post hoc analysis showed that, overall, the incidence of brain tissue hypoxia was similar in the two transfusion threshold groups (Hgb 7 or 10 g/dL). When the pB_tO_2 catheter was placed in normal brain, however, tissue hypoxia occurred in 25% of patients in the 7 g/dL threshold group, whereas it was observed in 10.2% of patients in the 10 g/dL threshold group [102]. This may be important since it is well known that the position of a monitor can influence the robustness of the results. Another potential benefit of maintaining a higher Hgb concentration is to avoid increased ICP induced by anemia [52]; however, further post hoc analysis of the same trial [101] did not observe an ICP effect. When ICP has been reported before and after transfusion, RBCs did not appear to modify it significantly [95–98].

The physiologic effects of RBCT also have been assessed using ^{15}O-PET in anemic (Hgb < 10 g/dL) SAH patients [103, 104]. While global CBF remains stable, RBCT increases global DO_2 (18%), associated with a decrease in the oxygen extraction fraction (OEF) but no clear change in $CMRO_2$. The DO_2 increase is greater (28%) in oligemic brain regions (low DO_2 and oxygen extraction fraction >0.5) at baseline, suggesting that RBCT may be protective in these susceptible regions [103]. In a subsequent study of 38 individuals with SAH at risk for delayed cerebral ischemia (DCI), PET imaging was used to measure global and regional CBF and DO_2 before and after (1) a fluid bolus, (2) a 25% increase in mean arterial pressure, or (3) a transfusion of 1 unit of RBC [104]. An increase in global CBF or DO_2 was only observed after RBCT in patients whose Hgb was <9 g/dL but not after other treatments. When DO_2 was impaired at baseline, all treatments improved CBF and DO_2, with the greatest improvement after RBCT. In SAH patients, pB_tO_2 also can be increased by induced hypertension; however, hemodilution appears to have the opposite effect [88]. Together these data suggest that RBCT can be used to augment DO_2 in the brain. Whether this is protective or associated with better outcome is still to be fully elucidated. At the basis of this is whether anemia is an independent factor associated with poor outcome in TBI. Other important unanswered questions include:

1. Is there a ceiling effect to this beneficial response; i.e., what is the optimal Hgb to maximize DO_2?
2. Could fresh blood provide greater improvements in oxygen transport and oxidative metabolism?

3. How do these physiologic findings translate into ability to minimize DCI or brain injury; i.e., does lowering OEF prevent further brain injury or infarction?

Red Blood Cell Transfusion

Surgical Procedures: The Balance of Anemia and Transfusion

Preoperative and perioperative anemia is independently associated with adverse outcomes after surgery [67–72]. Herein lies a paradox, since large surgical datasets continue to suggest an association between RBCT and perioperative morbidity, mortality, stroke, and delirium [68, 105–108]. These effects have been best described in cardiac surgery where a dose-dependent effect is observed [109–111]. For example, in a randomized, non-inferiority clinical trial of 502 patients who underwent cardiac surgery and were transfused to maintain Hct ≥ 30% or ≥24%, 30-day all-cause mortality and severe morbidity was similar in the two groups. The number of transfused red blood cell units was an independent risk factor for clinical complications or death [110]. In another trial of patients undergoing cardiac surgery, there was no significant difference in a composite outcome of infection or ischemic events using an Hgb transfusion trigger of 7.5 vs. 9 g/dL; however, analysis of secondary end points suggested higher rates of 90-day mortality with the lower Hgb trigger [112]. In other surgical procedures—e.g., hip surgery, carotid endarterectomy, and spine surgery—RBCT also adversely affected outcome [11, 113]. For example, the FOCUS trial, a randomized trial of RBCT, using an Hgb transfusion trigger of 8 vs. 10 g/dL in hip surgery, showed that a more restrictive RBCT threshold in the absence of symptoms of anemia may be reasonable, including in elderly patients at risk for cardiovascular events [11]. On the other hand patients with high blood loss (more than 2 L) during spine surgery who are under-resuscitated (Hgb < 8 g/dL) have a significantly increased risk of surgical infections [114]. Importantly, these studies did not address differences with transfusions in patients who developed myocardial infarction (MI) in the postoperative period and in patients presenting with acute coronary syndrome there still is no clear consensus about the appropriate transfusion trigger. Consistent with this there is variation in hospital transfusion thresholds in patients with unstable coronary artery disease (CAD), whereas practice surveys indicate that there remain deficits in the use of recommended patient blood management (PBM) strategies that often vary between geographic region [115].

Red Blood Cell Transfusions in General Critical Care

Allogeneic RBCT has been a lifesaving procedure for decades. Early and aggressive use of blood products continues to be an important component in the resuscitation of bleeding patients, especially in the setting of trauma [8, 116]. However, even after initial resuscitation, critically ill patients were, historically, often transfused when the Hgb concentration was <10 g/dL, to augment global oxygen delivery. As a result, more than half of ICU patients, particularly those who remained in ICU for more than a week, typically received at least 1 unit of RBCs.

Such a "liberal" approach to transfusion has been challenged by accumulating evidence from the past 10–15 years suggesting that RBCTs are associated with the development of various complications in critically ill patients, most importantly immunosuppression with an increased risk of nosocomial infections, and a higher prevalence of non-cardiogenic pulmonary edema and acute respiratory distress syndrome (ARDS) [117, 118]. Transfusion also has been linked to the development of the systemic inflammatory response syndrome (SIRS) and multiple organ dysfunction syndrome (MODS) [119, 120]. In addition, a large body of observational studies has raised the concern that RBCTs may exacerbate outcome in some ICU patients [121]. Consequently, a more restrictive transfusion policy (Hb < 7 g/dL) is now preferred for many patients.

Several randomized trials in adults and in the pediatric population have addressed RBCT in critical care [10, 12, 122]. The Transfusion Requirements in Critical Care (TRICC) trial compared a "liberal" (goal Hgb > 9–10 g/dL) vs. "restricted" (goal Hgb > 7 g/dL) RBCT trigger in 838 ICU patients [10]. There was no advantage to a liberal transfusion strategy, and overall 30-day mortality was similar. Mortality in the restrictive RBCT group was less than the liberal group among younger (<55 years) and less ill (acute physiology and chronic health evaluation [APACHE] II <20) patients [10]. As may often happen in RCTs, practice misalignment was evident: While outcome was similar for all patients, subgroup analysis showed the sicker patient (older, worse APACHE) seemed to do better with a more liberal RBCT strategy. We have observed the same in a retrospective analysis of 421 patients with SAH who underwent surgery. In patients who survived ≥2 days, RBCT was associated with unfavorable outcome particularly if transfused ≥3 units of blood. However, propensity analysis, to control for the probability of exposure to RBCT conditional on observed covariates measured before RBCT, indicates that RBCT is associated with unfavorable outcome in the absence of DCI but not when DCI is present, suggesting that RBCT may be useful in sicker patients with reduced cerebrovascular reserve [123].

A recent Cochrane review pooled data from 31 RCTs, involving 12,587 participants, across a range of clinical specialities (e.g., surgery, critical care) and different thresholds for RBCT to examine the outcome effect [13]. Restrictive RBCT strategies reduced the risk for an RBC transfusion by 43%. Overall, restrictive and more liberal transfusion strategies had similar 30-day mortality (moderate-quality evidence). Other outcomes assessed—i.e., cardiac events (low-quality evidence), myocardial infarction, stroke, thromboembolism (high-quality evidence), and risk of infection (pneumonia, wound, or bacteremia)—also showed no difference. The findings provide good evidence that transfusions with allogeneic RBCs can be avoided in most patients with Hgb thresholds >7–8 g/dL. However, the data do not prove that one strategy is preferable or beneficial. Furthermore, there is insufficient data to inform the safety of RBCT policies in several clinical subgroups, including acute coronary syndrome, myocardial infarction, TBI, other acute neurological disorders such as stroke or SAH, thrombocytopenia, cancer, hematological malignancies, and bone marrow failure [13].

Transfusion in Traumatic Brain Injury

RBCT is frequent in hospitalized TBI patients. Boutin et al. [124] pooled data from 23 studies (7524 patients); approximately 36% (95% confidence interval [CI], [28–44]) of patients received RBC transfusion at some point during their hospital stay. Transfusion was rare in mild TBI and was more likely the lower the GCS, suggesting that perhaps RBCT was a marker of injury severity. However, Hgb thresholds for transfusion were rarely available (reported in only nine studies) and varied from 6 to 10 g/dL [124]. This meta-analysis also showed that mortality was similar among transfused and non-transfused patients in univariate and multivariate analyses. However, there was high heterogeneity, and mortality often is considered a crude and perhaps not relevant marker for TBI outcome. The impact on outcome may in part depend on injury severity or Hgb threshold. For example, Elterman et al. [125] observed an association between mortality and RBCT but only if the initial Hgb was >10 g/dL or there was no evidence for shock in comatose patients.

Despite the findings in general critical care, concern remains that restrictive transfusion practices may not always be appropriate for patients with acute brain injury and that Hgb concentrations as low as 7 g/dL may not be well tolerated given the unique characteristics of neurocritical care patients. The results describing the role of RBCT in TBI are inconsistent: Some find an association with worse outcome while others do not or find an association with complications but not outcome [24, 26, 27, 30, 32, 80, 119, 126–128]. In part, this variation may depend on study methodology or RBCT thresholds or again may simply mean that RBCT is a marker of injury

severity. Several observational studies, largely retrospective, have examined the association between transfusion and clinical outcome after TBI and reported that RBCT can be associated with mortality [26, 27], functional outcome scores at discharge [24], or 6-month outcome assessed by the Glasgow Outcome Score [30]. For example, Salim et al. [27], in a retrospective study on 1150 TBI patients in which 46% of patients received RBCT when Hgb levels were <9 g/dL, found that RBCT was associated with an increased hospital mortality in a logistic regression model, while anemia was not. Leal-Noval et al. [129] examined 1-year neurocognitive and disability levels in 309 TBI patients, 53% of whom received ≥1 unit of blood during their ICU stay. At 1 year, transfused patients were more likely to have a worse functional outcome. Transfused patients, however, were more severely ill upon admission—although propensity analysis suggested that there was an independent relationship between RBCT and unfavorable long-term functional outcomes. It is unclear whether there is a dose effect, although Duane et al. [28] have observed that the number of units of all blood products (RBCs, plasma, platelets, and cryoprecipitate) administered to TBI patients is independently associated with mortality after adjustment for nadir Hgb.

The effect of RBCT on outcome may depend on injury severity and other variables. For example, Litofsky et al. [33], in a retrospective review of 939 patients with TBI and AIS >3, observed that RBCT was associated with poorer outcome at Hgb levels <9 and <10 g/dL but not at lower Hgb thresholds; i.e., sicker patients may benefit from RBCT, or, alternatively, measures other than Hgb alone may be necessary to trigger transfusion. There may be other potential benefits. For example, Carr et al. [130], in a clinical series of 89 severe TBI patients who required an ICP monitor, observed a positive association with decreased length of hospitalization when RBCT occurred at a Hgb threshold >8 mg/dL, and length of ICU stay was shorter for patients transfused at thresholds >9 mg/dL. However, no outcome effect was observed. Surveys of clinicians who care for TBI patients or those with other acute neurological disorders (e.g., stroke or SAH) demonstrate substantial practice variability. Indeed, many clinicians have not adopted a restrictive approach in these settings. Moreover, there is a tendency to individualize anemia management based on the specific characteristics of patients and the perceived risk of ischemia; i.e., use triggers other than Hgb alone [15–17]. Because of such practice individualization, some researchers have criticized the approach of a clinical trial with fixed treatment protocols (e.g., Hgb threshold of 7 vs. 10 g/dL) for therapies that are more commonly "titrated" in clinical practice, because practice misalignment may occur [131].

There is limited rigorous level I evidence to inform RBCT practice in TBI. A subgroup analysis of 67 TBI patients included in the Transfusion Requirements in Critical Care (TRICC) trial, with average daily Hgb concentrations of 10.5 vs. 8.5 g/dL, was performed. Mortality was 13% in the liberal transfusion group and 17% in the restrictive group [80]. Given the small number of patients with TBI or other types of acute brain injury included in the TRICC trial, it is unclear whether the results can be applied to TBI patients. Naidech et al. [132] performed a feasibility RCT of 44 SAH patients and compared goal Hgb concentrations of ≥10 vs. 11.5 g/dL. The sample size was too small to reach definitive conclusions other than a tendency to fewer infarcts on magnetic resonance imaging (MRI) in the higher Hgb threshold group. Robertson et al. [101] prospectively enrolled 200 severe TBI patients within 6 h of injury and randomized them to administration of erythropoietin (EPO) or placebo and to Hgb transfusion thresholds of 7 or 10 g/dL using a 2×2 factorial design to maintain assigned Hgb levels with transfusion of leukocyte-reduced packed red blood cells until ICP monitoring and ventilator support were discontinued. Clinical outcome was similar when maintaining an Hgb of 10 or 7 g/dL [101]. Subsequent analyses showed that delayed mortality rates, after adjusting for injury severity, were greater for patients with a transfusion threshold of 10 g/dL [102].

Several recent reviews have addressed the role of anemia and transfusion in acute neurological disorders including TBI [17, 18, 64, 133, 134].

The information summarized in these reviews indicates that:

1. There is clinical equipoise about optimal transfusion practices in neurocritical care patients.
2. There is considerable variation in transfusion preferences in TBI [15].
3. Recommendations for general critical care patients may not apply to all patients with brain injury.
4. Measures other than Hgb may be needed to trigger transfusion.

It remains to be elucidated whether anemia and transfusion are simply markers of disease severity or are independent factors associated with outcome. There is general consensus that anemia should be avoided using blood conservation strategies, but cogent arguments can be made for liberal and restrictive RBCT strategies. However, other factors, such as the physiological impact of anemia or patients' cerebrovascular reserve or compensatory response may need to be considered; i.e., rather than an Hgb trigger for transfusion, it is conceivable that this trigger varies in individual patients and in the same patient over time and may depend on other measures—specifically how anemia affects the brain, e.g., how anemia and Hgb levels influence oxygenation. Consistent with this, in a retrospective analysis of a prospective cohort of 80 severe TBI patients whose pB_tO_2 was monitored, Oddo et al. [9] observed that anemia (Hgb $\leq$ 9 g/dL) with simultaneous compromised pB_tO_2 (<20 mmHg), but not anemia alone, was a risk factor for unfavorable outcome, irrespective of injury severity.

Complications Associated with Red Blood Cell Transfusions

There are several potential complications from blood or blood product transfusion, including common complications such as acute, delayed, or nonimmune hemolytic reactions and allergic reactions and rare complications such as transfusion-transmitted infections and graft versus host disease. However, in TBI patients, the more common reasons for morbidity and mortality with transfusion are transfusion-related acute lung injury (TRALI) and transfusion-associated circulatory overload (TACO) [135]. Both of these syndromes result in increased pulmonary edema.

TRALI is characterized by pulmonary edema, usually within 6 h of initial transfusion, although more delayed presentations can occur [136]. Patients usually are hypoxic and hypotensive, and TRALI may be difficult to clinically distinguish from acute respiratory distress syndrome. However TRALI usually is transient and reversible. It is caused by immune complex-mediated damage to the pulmonary vasculature that increases its permeability and so contributes to edema. The risk of TRALI increases when a greater number of blood products are transfused, particularly plasma transfusions. Management includes supportive care with oxygen and mechanical ventilation. Diuretics and steroids have limited benefit [137, 138].

In TACO, increased hydrostatic pressure leads to increased edema; hence, the likelihood of developing TACO is associated with the volume transfused [139]. Like TRALI, it is more frequently observed with plasma transfusion [140]. However, unlike TRALI, there are clinical features of fluid overload in addition to hypoxia and respiratory distress. B-type natriuretic peptide can help differentiate TACO and TRALI since it is elevated in TACO and not in TRALI [141, 142]. Treatment of TACO involves prompt diuresis along with supplemental oxygen or mechanical ventilation.

In TBI or other patients with acute brain injury, an increased risk of thromboembolic events has been described after RBCT [101, 143]. Vedantam et al. [144] in post hoc analysis of a recent RCT in TBI suggest that transfusion at a higher Hgb threshold (10 g/dL) may be associated with a greater risk of intracranial hemorrhage progression; the risk was 55% greater for patients transfused at a threshold of 10 g/dL than those in the 7 g/dL threshold group. However, the effect was not significantly different, and patients with hemorrhagic progression also were older, had a higher initial ICP, had mass lesions on CT,

and were more likely to undergo surgery at admission. There were also missing data on coagulation parameters and platelet counts. It is therefore difficult to conclude that transfusion had any causative effect.

How May Transfusion Aggravate Outcome?

The precise mechanism of how transfusion aggravates outcome is still under investigation. The deleterious effects of blood transfusion may be associated with several factors and is likely a result of interactions of these factors. The deleterious effects may be related to immunomodulation and immune system suppression through allogenic red blood cells or leucocytes. Animal studies support the idea that RBCT induces neuroinflammation and impairment of learning and memory [145]. In particular, some of the adverse effects of RBCTs could be attributable to concomitant administration of leukocytes, which then "contaminate" RBC units during blood donation. The burden of leukocytes can be reduced with filters either pre- or post-storage. Whether leukoreduction reduces the occurrence of complications in critically ill patients remains controversial, with conflicting results from RCTs [146, 147]. Consequently, not all blood banks have adopted this practice. However, regions that have transitioned to universal leukoreduction report favorable results [148]. Furthermore, the quality of transfused blood has changed since 1999 when the TRICC trial was published, and this likely will alter outcomes. For example, findings in the Anemia and Blood Transfusion in Critically Ill Patients' (ABC) study were consistent with TRICC [20]. However, in the Sepsis Occurrence in Acutely Ill Patients' (SOAP) study that used the same methodology as ABC, but was performed several years later, RBCT was not associated with worse outcomes [149]. In the last several years leuko-depletion, which may be associated with fewer adverse transfusion effects, has been widely adopted, and, in general, transfusion has become safer.

Large observational studies have suggested a possible association between longer RBC storage duration and mortality in critically ill patients [150]. In trauma studies, age of RBCs has been associated with increased mortality, multi-organ failure including respiratory failure, increased risk of infections, and increased thromboembolic events [151, 152]. However this may depend on the number of units transfused with increased complications only occurring if >3 units are transfused in the first 24 h [153]. The effect of the age of stored blood in TBI has had limited investigation. Leal-Noval et al. [129] observed that the length of RBC storage did not influence the rate of mid- or long-term unfavorable outcomes. A number of potentially important biochemical changes occur in RBCs (and the supernatant) while they are stored in the blood bank before transfusion, referred to as the "storage lesion" [154]. There is a gradual reduction in ATP concentration, loss of membrane phospholipids, and oxidative damage to proteins. The resulting morphological changes and impaired membrane function may reduce the deformability of RBCs and interfere with microcirculatory flow through capillaries and cause endothelial activation and stimulation of inflammatory cascades [155]. Gradual depletion of 2,3-diphosphoglycerate occurs during storage, which in turn interferes with the ability of Hgb to offload O_2 [156]. Thus, even though RBCTs may increase arterial O_2 content, this does not necessarily produce an increment in tissue delivery, let alone an increment in O_2 utilization [157, 158]. It therefore is conceivable that RBCs stored for less time could be more effective at delivering O_2 [158]. However Yamal et al. [102] in post hoc analysis of an RCT in TBI patients showed that RBC age was not associated with $SjvO_2$ or pB_tO_2.

Whether or not transfusions with fresh RBCs are associated with improved outcomes has remained inconclusive in large part because it is difficult to study; i.e., different units have different ages [154]. In addition most RBCT transfusions are now leukoreduced and in many studies the role of other transfusion often is not accounted for; this may be significant since fresh frozen plasma or platelets each may be transfused in about 20% of patients. The impact of RBC storage duration was assessed in the Age of Blood Evaluation (ABLE) trial, where 1211 critically ill patients were randomized to receive either "standard or care" RBCs (stored in the blood bank for 2–42 days) or "fresh" RBCs (stored for less than 8 days). The primary outcome (90-day mortality) was similar in the fresh-blood and standard-blood group. There also were no significant between-group differences in any of the secondary outcomes (major illnesses; duration of respiratory, hemodynamic, or renal support; length of stay in the hospital; and transfusion reactions) [159]. In the 2016 AABB clinical practice guidelines, 13 RCTs that included 5515 participants randomly allocated to receive fresher blood or standard-issue blood were analyzed to examine for RBC storage duration. These RCTs demonstrated that fresher blood did not improve clinical outcomes [12].

The effect of RBCT in TBI may depend on brain metabolism. For example, Sekhon et al. [160] examined 28 severe TBI patients in a single-center observational study and found that pressure reactivity index (PRx) increased after transfusion, indicating worsening cerebrovascular pressure reactivity. This effect, however, depended in part on pB_tO_2; in patients with mean $pB_tO_2 > 20$ mmHg pre-transfusion, the PRx increased significantly, but it did not change in patients with $pB_tO_2 < 20$ mmHg. In other words, the underlying state of ongoing cerebral ischemia and brain hypoxia in individual patients may lead to differential effects of blood. These results suggest that patients with cerebral hypoxia are better candidates for RBC transfusion, as their autoregulation does not deteriorate any further. Hence, while the risks of transfusion are well understood, there also are patients who benefit from RBCT; furthermore, the potential benefit that RBCT may have in patients with cerebral ischemia and prevention of secondary brain injury may far exceed the increased risks. Identification of which patients will benefit optimal transfusion strategies and resuscitation end points remains tantamount.

Hematopoiesis-Stimulating Agents

An intuitive potential approach to avoid both the deleterious effects of anemia and transfusion is the use of hematopoiesis-stimulating drugs, such as erythropoietin or darbepoietin. Erythropoietin also has multiple biological properties that may be neuroprotective [161]. Putative mechanisms of benefit include increased expression of anti-apoptotic genes, antioxidant properties, reduced inflammation, less cerebral edema, and promotion of neural and endothelial progenitor cells [162–164]. In animal models, erythropoietin and its analogues appear to improve outcomes with various types of neurological injury, including TBI [165–171]. This includes improvements in brain oxygen saturation and the microcirculation, raising the question of whether it may alter DO_2 [172].

In 2002, a large multicenter RCT found that weekly administration of 40,000 IU of recombinant erythropoietin reduced the transfusion requirements of critically ill patients [173]. This effect was considerably more modest in a subsequent trial, probably because clinicians had by then adopted more restrictive transfusion practices [174]. However, erythropoietin does not appear to significantly improve survival when administered to critically ill patients in general [173, 174]. Subgroup analyses of these trials suggested that mortality was reduced when erythropoietin was administered to trauma patients. However, the degree to which this potential benefit may be attributable to erythropoietin use in TBI patients was uncertain since no clear interaction between GCS score and erythropoietin was observed [173–175]. Promising phase II trials have been published in patients undergoing cardiac surgery [176] and with SAH [177]. However in acute ischemic stroke patients, mortality is increased in patients who receive erythropoietin [178].

In TBI, retrospective matched cohort studies of erythropoietin suggest a therapeutic benefit [82], but this effect is absent in RCTs. A large multicenter RCT, EPO-TBI, which included 606 patients was recently concluded; 308 patients received erythropoietin in a dose of 40,000 units subcutaneously once a week for a maximum of 3 weeks [179]. The primary outcome, neurologic status at 6 months, was similar in the treatment and placebo groups. There also was no overall effect on survival, although when adjusted for injury severity according to IMPACT prognostic factors, mortality appeared less in the erythropoietin group. By contrast, Li et al. in a smaller RCT that included 159 patients observed better outcomes at 3 months post injury [180]. Interestingly there was no effect on Hgb levels. Similarly, Robertson et al. [101], in a 2 × 2 factorial design RCT of 200 patients that also included RBCT at 2 Hgb thresholds, found that there was no interaction between erythropoietin and Hgb transfusion threshold and no outcome benefit. Meta-analysis of erythropoietin trials in TBI that include 915 patients [181] or of eligible RCTs that include 2607 critically ill patients after trauma [182] shows no benefit of erythropoietin on functional outcome, although mortality and hospital stay were lower in erythropoietin patients. The Operation Brain Trauma Therapy (OBTT), a multicenter, preclinical drug and circulating biomarker screening consortium for TBI, also has found that erythropoietin, among other therapies examined, appears to have limited, if any, clinical benefit [183, 184].

There are concerns that chronic erythropoietin administration has several adverse effects including hypertension, hypertensive encephalopathy, seizures, venous thromboembolism (VTE), and other vascular events. An analogue of erythropoietin (carbamylated erythropoietin) has been produced, which has the same biological effects without promoting hematopoiesis. It is hoped that the use of such analogues will reduce the risk of thromboembolism. However there appears to be limited interaction between VTE and outcome in the various erythropoietin trials including in TBI [185]. The various data taken together, while promising in preclinical studies, do not support widespread use of erythropoietin in TBI patients or in anemia management. There remain several unanswered questions including dosage, timing (initiation, frequency, and duration), patient selection, and interaction with other therapies, specifically RBCT.

Hemoglobin-Based Oxygen Carriers

Hemoglobin (Hgb)-based oxygen carriers (HBOCs) or Hgb-based blood substitutes (HBBSs) are resuscitative fluid preparations that contain free Hgb, not surrounded by an RBC membrane. The theoretical appeal of these products is that they rapidly increase arterial oxygen content and could help circumvent the need for allogeneic RBCs, especially among patients with hemorrhagic shock in the pre-hospital setting. However, free Hgb also appears to have deleterious effects; probably largely mediated by the scavenging of endogenous nitric oxide with consequent vasoconstriction, pro-inflammatory and pro-thrombotic effects, and the generation of reactive oxygen species [186]. Results from RCTs in a variety of settings (perioperative, trauma, stroke) have been universally disappointing, with cumulative data that indicate an increased risk of myocardial infarction and death [187, 188], although HBOC use may decrease the need for allogenic transfusion [189]. HBOCs are volume expanders, and circulatory volume must be carefully monitored. In addition, these agents often are not as effective as RBCs for restoring Hgb content and concentration. More recently, efforts have been made to develop products that avoid the deleterious effects of older generation HBBSs. It remains unclear whether modifications of existing HBSSs will result in products where the potential benefits outweigh the risks.

Animal studies that use HBBSs in TBI models have reported a variety of benefits, including improved pB_tO_2, reductions in cerebral edema, improved cerebrovascular reactivity, and less neuronal death [190–194]. However, in animal models of hemorrhage with TBI, there is no benefit of HBOC-based fluid resuscitation over lactated Ringer's solution [195]. The proportion of TBI patients in previously published RCTs involving trauma patients has been relatively small. However, no interaction between baseline GCS score and the efficacy of the HBBS could be detected in the most recent, large multicenter RCT [196]. At this stage, HBBSs should be regarded as theoretically interesting as supportive treatment in TBI patients. However, their routine use is not justified and is potentially dangerous. Indeed, no HBOC has gained the US Food and Drug Administration (FDA) approval for human use.

Transfusion Guidelines

In the last several years, a variety of organizations have published transfusion guidelines, e.g., Guidelines for Transfusion [8], recommendations of the American Society of Anesthesiologists Task Force [197, 198], the American College of Physicians [199], the Society of Thoracic Surgeons [200], the Canadian Guidelines [201], the American Association of Blood Banks [12, 202], the Association of Anaesthetists of Great Britain and Ireland [203], the National Clinical Guideline Center in the United Kingdom [204, 205], the British Committee for Standards in Haematology [206], the American College of Surgeons [207], and the Neurocritical Care Society [208]. In addition, several Cochrane reviews are available [13, 14, 209]. In large part these guidelines focus on hospitalized, anemic adult patients who are hemodynamically stable, and in general the recommendations apply more to general critical care than patients with acute brain injury. There are several common themes:

1. A restrictive transfusion strategy (7–8 g/dL) is safe and recommended in stable patients.
2. Transfusion requirements may need to be titrated to parameters of illness severity rather than arbitrarily defined Hgb levels; i.e., transfusion decisions should be made based on symptoms as well as Hgb concentration, and the overall clinical context, patient preferences, and alternative therapies each should be considered.
3. All recognize the paucity of high-quality data and trials in high-risk groups, e.g., acute coronary syndrome, TBI, or other types of acute brain injury.

There often are important differences in national and international societies' recommendations for transfusion and patient blood management (PBM). There is also often significant heterogeneity in clinical protocols across centers and specialties. Indeed, transfusions in the ICU often occur outside evidence-based guidelines or agency recommendations [210–212]. However, education programs, transfusion care bundles, peer-to-peer physician feedback, or institutional benchmarking with similar types of hospitals in such benchmarking systems as the National Surgical Quality Improvement Program (NSQIP) database can help to improve compliance with transfusion guidelines in daily practice [213, 214].

Recent reviews, opinions, and consensus statements have addressed the role of anemia and transfusion in acute neurological disorders including TBI [18, 35], SAH [208], and neurocritical care [17]. The information summarized in these reviews indicates that there is clinical equipoise about optimal transfusion practices in neurocritical care patients. These reviews also suggest that the data from general critical care may not apply to patients with acute brain injury. However, it remains to be elucidated whether anemia and RBCT are simply markers of disease severity or are independent factors associated with outcome. Further RCTs comparing transfusion strategies in TBI or SAH patients are required. This is especially important, as extrapolating data from one disease to another is often ill-advised. Consistent with this, evidence from cardiac surgery RCTs refutes evidence from observational studies and non-cardiac surgery trials [215]. In healthy patients without cardiac disease, a restrictive transfusion trigger of Hgb 7–8 g/dL is safe and appropriate, whereas in select cardiac patients, an Hgb trigger of 8–10 g/dL may be preferable [216]. Similarly there is evidence that a more liberal RBCT strategy may be beneficial in perioperative patients, whereas there is no difference in mortality in liberal or restrictive strategies in general critical care [217]. Data from the Department of Veterans Affairs Surgical Quality Improvement Program database that included 424,015 major non-cardiac operations among elderly patients (≥65 years) in 117 veterans' hospitals observed that hospitals with higher transfusion rates in patients with an indication for transfusion had lower risk-adjusted 30-day postoperative mortality rates [218].

The conclusion from the various guidelines and consensus statements indicates that restrictive RBC transfusion practices are cost-effective, reduce the risk of adverse events specific to transfusion, introduce no harm, and are no worse than liberal strategies in stable anemic patients. However, this same strategy may not apply to anemic patients with ongoing hemorrhage, with risk of significant bleeding, or with concurrent ischemic brain, spinal cord, or myocardium, or patients with acute brain injury. In these patients the optimal Hgb transfusion trigger is still being elucidated. It is in these patients that broad-based adherence to guideline recommendations may not apply. Instead, other measures may be important, and decisions about transfusion must respect the individual patient and his or her pathology [9, 34, 35, 219].

Which Is the Optimal Tranfusion Strategy for Patients with Traumatic Brain Injury?

Studies in TBI patients and other forms or acute brain injury (such as SAH) have shown worse outcomes and evidence for metabolic distress and secondary injury in the brain in anemic patients (Hgb < 9.0 g/dL). However, transfusion of red blood cells may not be associated with improved outcome and in some patients may aggravate outcome. This creates a clinical dilemma or paradox: overtransfusion vs. undertransfusion. In TBI there is a paucity of rigorous clinical evidence, and hence there is no consensus on appropriate transfusion thresholds in neurocritically ill patients [101, 124]. Once again, practice surveys and meta-analytic studies in TBI show that there is considerable practice variation and this varies by clinical specialty [15, 124]. In addition, indicators of poor anemia tolerance—e.g., increased lactate, low mixed venous saturation, or pB_tO_2—to decide about RBCT are used heterogeneously, although many agree that these markers can be useful [15,

17]. In SAH, it appears that RBCT decisions often are made based on the perceived cerebrovascular reserve or the severity of the brain injury although these decisions do show geographic variation [16].

How can anemia and RBCT be best managed in TBI? A "restrictive" transfusion practice can be considered safe for TBI patients who are awake and can undergo repeated clinical examination. In these patients, RBCT should be administered to maintain Hgb levels >7.0 g/dL. When there is neurological deterioration or in poor-grade or comatose patients, a target Hgb > 9 g/dL may be a more optimal target. However, this one-size-fits-all approach is far from ideal, and in these patients the decision to initiate RBCT should be individualized to triggers that suggest poor tolerance to anemia; i.e., the transfusion should occur when there is evidence for cerebral ischemia, cell energy dysfunction in the brain, or brain hypoxia [8, 9, 18, 34, 35, 134, 206]. This suggested approach is illustrated in Fig. 2.

Specific "brain" triggers include the invasive or noninvasive assessment of brain oxygen (venous saturation in the jugular vein [$SvjO_2$], pB_tO_2, or skeletal muscle oxygenation [StO_2]), cerebral metabolism (microdialysis measures of lactate and pyruvate), or CBF that can be used to individualize transfusion requirements. In this approach, only patients with anemia (e.g., Hgb < 9–10 g/dL) and coexistent brain hypoxia (pB_tO_2 <15–20 mmHg, $SvjO_2$ < 55%) or cerebral metabolic distress (lactate/pyruvate ratio [LPR] >40) should be considered as potential candidates for RBCT. Whether this approach will make a difference is unclear, although accumulating data from several sources suggest it may. For example, Oddo et al. [9], in a retrospective review of 90 TBI patients, observed that the combination of anemia and brain hypoxia, but not anemia alone, was associated with worse outcome. Secondly, Hollis et al. [220], in a retrospective cohort study involving Veterans Affairs facilities and 7361 patients with coronary artery disease who underwent inpatient non-cardiac surgery and had a nadir postoperative hematocrit between 20 and 30% observed that patients with a lower Hgb and a myocardial infarct had better outcomes with RBCT. On the other hand, transfusion in septic shock to optimize oxygen delivery to reach a mixed $SvjO_2$ or superior vena cava ($ScvO_2$) oxygen saturation >70% does not always alter outcome [221]. The key issue then appears to be maintaining a lower Hgb transfusion threshold, without compromising cerebral perfusion or oxygenation. Hence, there are potential detrimental effects of simply targeting a

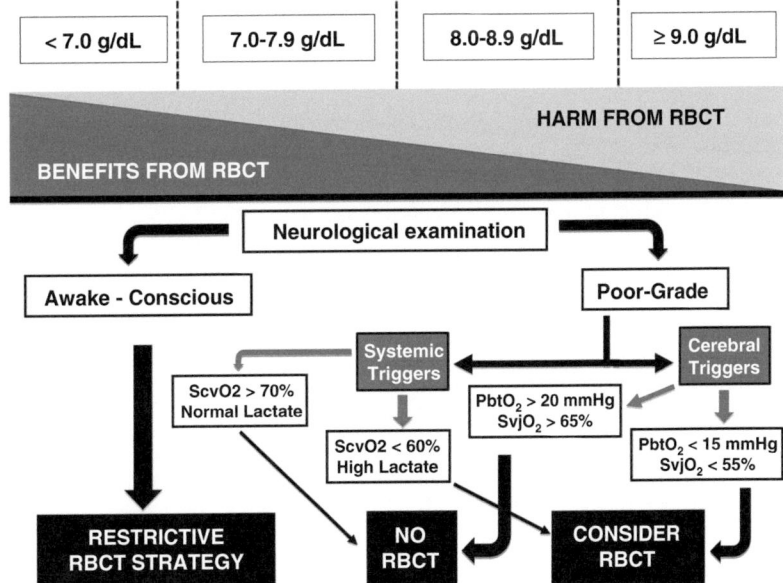

Fig. 2 An approach to transfusion in TBI. Reprinted under Creative Commons license from Lelubre C, Bouzat P, Crippa IA, Taccone FS. Anemia management after acute brain injury. Critical Care. 2016;20:152. http://creativecommons.org/licenses/by/4.0/

particular Hgb value after severe TBI. Instead, a combination of physiological parameters to measure cerebral and systemic perfusion and brain oxygenation is likely more useful to determine when severe TBI patients require transfusion. This strategy is similar to newer approaches to ICP management, i.e., using other parameters of brain health to decide the optimal threshold at which to treat a patient [222–224]. In many respects this recognition of phenotypic differences and the need to individualize care based on several rather than single parameters are the conceptual bases of large studies such as Collaborative European NeuroTrauma Effectiveness Research in Traumatic Brain Injury (CENTER-TBI). The reason that so many RCTs that simply dichotomize management have failed in TBI likely reflects this heterogeneity [225, 226].

Conclusions

In summary, anemia is very common among patients with moderate and severe TBI, such that clinicians often are faced with the question at which Hgb threshold to transfuse. However, there is limited high-quality, prospective data to help make decisions. Randomized trials have involved far too few TBI patients to reach definitive conclusions. Thus, it is not surprising that there is widespread practice variation. The brain also has a strict O_2 requirement that makes it vulnerable to hypoperfusion and hypoxia. In addition, anemia is a risk factor for secondary cerebral injury, and evidence for cellular energy dysfunction can occur when Hgb is <9–10 g/dL. In our opinion, an Hgb transfusion threshold of 7 g/dL may not be safe in TBI patients, as it is in other critically ill patients. Instead a higher Hgb threshold (~Hgb 9 g/dL) may be suitable in select TBI patients.

RBC transfusions frequently have immediate, seemingly beneficial effects on cerebral physiology. The magnitude of this effect may depend in part upon the duration that RBCs have been stored before administration. In light of existing physiological data, we generally aim to keep Hgb concentrations >9 g/dL during the initial several days after TBI. An increasing number of centers use multimodal neurological monitoring, which may help individualize transfusion goals based on the degree of cerebral hypoxia or metabolic distress. When available, pB_tO_2 values less than 15–20 mmHg or a lactate/pyruvate ratio >30–40 would influence us to use more aggressive Hgb correction (e.g., transfusion threshold of 10 g/dL).

Clinicians can attempt to reduce transfusion requirements by limiting phlebotomy, minimizing hemodilution, and providing appropriate prophylaxis against gastrointestinal hemorrhage. Administration of exogenous erythropoietin may have a small impact to further reduce the need for transfusion, but also may increase complications, most notably deep venous thrombosis. Erythropoietin is currently of great interest as a potential neuroprotective agent. However, it should not be used routinely for this purpose. HBBSs are also of interest, but existing preparations have not been shown to be beneficial, let alone safe, in the context of TBI.

The risks of transfusion are well known. Use of transfusion needs to be considered not only in terms of risk but also in terms of potential benefit. Herein is the dilemma for the physician: over-transfuse or under-transfuse. To make this decision requires an understanding of patient physiology. In the ICU, clinicians routinely adjust treatment dose and care based on multiple factors and an individual assessment of patients' signs, symptoms, and comorbidity. It is conceivable that more physiological transfusion triggers using direct signals coming from the brain or other measures of "brain health" will progressively replace arbitrary Hgb-based transfusion triggers.

References

1. Maas AIR, Stocchetti N, Bullock R. Moderate and severe traumatic brain injury in adults. Lancet Neurol. 2008;7:728–41.
2. Langlois JA, Rutland-Brown W, Thomas KE. Traumatic brain injury in the United States: emergency department visits, hospitalizations, and deaths. Georgia: Centers for Disease Control and Prevention, National Center for Injury Prevention and Control; 2004.

3. McHugh GS, Engel DC, Butcher I, Steyerberg EW, Lu J, Mushkudiani N, et al. Prognostic value of secondary insults in traumatic brain injury: results from the IMPACT study. J Neurotrauma. 2007;24:287–93.

4. Chesnut RM, Marshall LF, Klauber MR, Blunt BA, Baldwin N, Eisenberg HM, et al. The role of secondary brain injury in determining outcome from severe head injury. J Trauma. 1993;34:216–22.

5. Manley G, Knudson MM, Morabito D, Damron S, Erickson V, Pitts L. Hypotension, hypoxia, and head injury: frequency, duration, and consequences. Arch Surg. 2001;136:1118–23.

6. Maloney-Wilensky E, Gracias V, Itkin A, Hoffman K, Bloom S, Yang W, et al. Brain tissue oxygen and outcome after severe traumatic brain injury: a systematic review. Crit Care Med. 2009;37:2057–63.

7. Brain Trauma Foundation; American Association of Neurological Surgeons; Congress of Neurological Surgeons; Joint Section on Neurotrauma and Critical Care, AANS/CNS, Bratton SL, Chestnut RM, Ghajar J, McConnell Hammond FF, Harris OA, Hartl R, et al. Guidelines for the management of severe traumatic brain injury. I. Blood pressure and oxygenation. J Neurotrauma. 2007;24(1):S7–13.

8. Napolitano LM, Kurek S, Luchette FA, Corwin HL, Barie PS, Tisherman SA, et al.; American College of Critical Care Medicine of the Society of Critical Care Medicine; Eastern Association for the Surgery of Trauma Practice Management Workgroup. Clinical practice guideline: red blood cell transfusion in adult trauma and critical care. Crit Care Med. 2009;37:3124–57.

9. Oddo M, Levine JM, Kumar M, Iglesias K, Frangos S, Maloney-Wilensky E, Le Roux P. Anemia and brain oxygen after severe traumatic brain injury. Intensive Care Med. 2012;38(9):1497–504.

10. Hébert PC, Wells G, Blajchman MA, Marshall J, Martin C, Pagliarello G, et al. A multicenter randomized, controlled clinical trial of transfusion requirements in critical care. Transfusion Requirements in Critical Care Investigators, Canadian Critical Care Trials Group. N Engl J Med. 1999;340(6):409–17.

11. Carson JL, Terrin ML, Noveck H, Sanders DW, Chaitman BR, Rhoads GG, et al.; FOCUS Investigators. Liberal or restrictive transfusion in high-risk patients after hip surgery. N Engl J Med. 2011;365(26):2453–62.

12. Carson JL, Guyatt G, Heddle NM, Grossman BJ, Cohn CS, Fung MK, et al. Clinical practice guidelines from the AABB: Red Blood Cell Transfusion Thresholds and Storage. JAMA. 2016;316(19):2025–35.

13. Carson JL, Stanworth SJ, Roubinian N, Fergusson DA, Triulzi D, Doree C, Hebert PC. Transfusion thresholds and other strategies for guiding allogeneic red blood cell transfusion. Cochrane Database Syst Rev. 2016;(10):CD002042.

14. Carless PA, Henry DA, Carson JL, Hebert PP, McClelland B, Ker K. Transfusion thresholds and other strategies for guiding allogeneic red blood cell transfusion. Cochrane Database Syst Rev. 2010;(10):CD002042.

15. Sena MJ, Rivers RM, Muizelaar JP, Battistella FD, Utter GH. Transfusion practices for acute traumatic brain injury: a survey of physicians at US trauma centers. Intensive Care Med. 2009;35:480–8.

16. Kramer AH, Diringer MN, Suarez JI, Naidech AM, Macdonald LR, Le Roux PD. Red blood cell transfusion in patients with subarachnoid hemorrhage: a multidisciplinary North American survey. Crit Care. 2011;15:R30.

17. Kramer AH, Zygun DA. Anemia and red blood cell transfusion in neurocritical care. Crit Care. 2009;13(3):R89.

18. Utter GH, Shahlaie K, Zwienenberg-Lee M, Muizelaar JP. Anemia in the setting of traumatic brain injury: the arguments for and against liberal transfusion. J Neurotrauma. 2011;28:155–65.

19. WHO. Haemoglobin concentrations for the diagnosis of anaemia and assessment of severity. Vitamin and Mineral Nutrition Information System. Geneva: World Health Organization, (WHO/NHD/MnM/11.1). 2011. Available at: http://www.who.int/vmnis/indicators/haemoglobin.pdf. Accessed 11 June 2017.

20. Vincent JL, Baron JF, Reinhart K, Gattinoni L, Thijs L, Webb A, et al.; ABC (Anemia and Blood Transfusion in Critical Care) Investigators. Anemia and blood transfusion in critically ill patients. JAMA. 2002;288:1499–507.

21. Corwin HL, Getinger A, Pearl RG. The CRIT Study: anemia and blood transfusion in the critically ill – current practice in the United States. Crit Care Med. 2004;32:39–52.

22. Rodriguez RM, Corwin HL, Gettinger A, Corwin MJ, Gubler D, Pearl RG. Nutritional deficiencies and blunted erythropoietin response as causes of anemia of critical illness. J Crit Care. 2001;16:36–41.

23. Walsh TS, Saleh EE. Anemia during critical illness. Br J Anesth. 2006;97:278–91.

24. Carlson AP, Schermer CR, Lu SW. Retrospective evaluation of anemia and transfusion in traumatic brain injury. J Trauma. 2006;61:567–71.

25. Schirmer-Makalsen K, Vik A, Gisvold SE, Skandsen T, Hynne H, Klepstad P. Severe head injury: control of physiological variables, organ failure and complications in the intensive care unit. Acta Anaesthesiol Scand. 2007;51:1194–201.

26. George ME, Skarda DE, Watts CR, Pham HD, Beilman GJ. Aggressive red blood cell transfusion: no association with improved outcome for victims of isolated traumatic brain injury. Neurocrit Care. 2008;8:337–43.

27. Salim A, Hadjizacharia P, DuBose J, Brown C, Inaba K, Chan L, et al. Role of anemia in traumatic brain injury. J Am Coll Surg. 2008;207:398–406.

28. Duane TM, Mayglothling J, Grandhi R, Warrier N, Aboutanos MB, Wolfe LG, et al. The effect of anemia and blood transfusions on mortality in closed head injury patients. J Surg Res. 2008;147:163–7.

29. Flückiger C, Béchir M, Brenni M, Ludwig S, Sommerfeld J, Cottini SR, et al. Increasing hematocrit above 28% during early resuscitative phase is not associated with decreased mortality following severe traumatic brain injury. Acta Neurochir. 2010;152:627–36.

30. Warner MA, O'Keeffe T, Bhavsar P, Shringer R, Moore C, Harper C, et al. Transfusions and long-term functional outcome in traumatic brain injury. J Neurosurg. 2010;133:539–46.

31. Yang CJ, Hsiao KY, Su IC, Chen IC. The association between anemia and the mortality of severe traumatic brain injury in emergency department. J Trauma. 2011;71(6):E132–5.

32. Al-Dorzi HM, Al-Humaid W, Tamim HM, Haddad S, Aljabbary A, Arifi A, et al. Anemia and blood transfusion in patients with isolated traumatic brain injury. Crit Care Res Pract. 2015;2015:672639.

33. Litofsky NS, Martin S, Diaz J, Ge B, Petroski G, Miller DC, Barnes SL. The negative impact of anemia in outcome from traumatic brain injury. World Neurosurg. 2016;90:82–90.

34. Le Roux P. Hemoglobin management in acute brain injury. Curr Opin Crit Care. 2013;19(2):83–91.

35. Kramer A, Le Roux P. Red blood cell transfusion and transfusion alternatives in traumatic brain injury. Curr Treat Options Neurol. 2012;14:150–63.

36. Weiskopf RB, Kramer JH, Viele M, Neumann M, Feiner JR, Watson JJ, et al. Acute severe isovolemic anemia impairs cognitive function and memory in humans. Anesthesiology. 2000;92:1646–52.

37. Weiskopf RB, Feiner J, Hopf HW, Viele MK, Watson JJ, Kramer JH, et al. Oxygen reverses deficits of cognitive function and memory and increased heart rate induced by acute severe isovolemic anemia. Anesthesiology. 2002;96:871–7.

38. Weiskopf RB, Viele MK, Feiner J, Kelley S, Lieberman J, Noorani M, et al. Human cardiovascular and metabolic response to acute, severe isovolemic anemia. JAMA. 1998;279:217–21.

39. Hare GMT, Tsui AKY, McLaren AT, Ragoonanan TE, Yu J, Mazer CD. Anemia and cerebral outcomes: many questions, fewer answers. Anesth Analg. 2008;107:1356–70.

40. Coles JP, Fryer TD, Smielewski P, Rice K, Clark JC, Pickard JD, et al. Defining ischemic burden after traumatic brain injury using ^{15}O PET imaging of cerebral physiology. J Cereb Blood Flow Metab. 2004;24:191–201.

41. Todd MM, Wu B, Warner DS. The hemispheric cerebrovascular response to hemodilution is attenuated by a focal cryogenic brain injury. J Neurotrauma. 1994;11:149–60.

42. Bouma GJ, Muizelaar JP, Stringer WA, Choi SC, Fatouros P, Young HF. Ultra-early evaluation of regional cerebral blood flow in severely head-injured patients using xenon-enhanced computerized tomography. J Neurosurg. 1992;77:360–8.

43. Vespa PM. The implications of cerebral ischemia and metabolic dysfunction for treatment strategies in neurointensive care. Curr Opin Crit Care. 2006;12:119–23.

44. Verweij BH, Muizelaar JP, Vinas FC, Peterson PL, Xiong Y, Lee CP. Impaired cerebral mitochondrial function after traumatic brain injury in humans. J Neurosurg. 2000;93:815–20.

45. Menon DK, Coles JP, Gupta AK, Fryer TD, Smielewski P, Chatfield DA, et al. Diffusion limited oxygen delivery following head injury. Crit Care Med. 2004;32:1384–90.

46. Veenith TV, Carter EL, Geeraerts T, Grossac J, Newcombe VF, Outtrim J, et al. Pathophysiologic mechanisms of cerebral ischemia and diffusion hypoxia in traumatic brain injury. JAMA Neurol. 2016;73(5):542–50.

47. Graham DI, Ford I, Adams JH, Doyle D, Teasdale GM, Lawrence AE, et al. Ischemic brain damage is still common in fatal non-missile head injury. J Neurol Neurosurg Psychiatry. 1989;52:346–50.

48. Gopinath SP, Robertson CS, Contant CF, Hayes C, Feldman Z, Narayan RK, et al. Jugular venous desaturation and outcome after head injury. J Neurol Neurosurg Psychiatry. 1994;57:717–23.

49. Van Santbrink H, Maas AI, Avezaat CJ. Continuous monitoring of parital pressure of brain tissue oxygen in patients with severe head injury. Neurosurgery. 1996;38:21–31.

50. Abate MG, Trivedi M, Fryer TD, Smielewski P, Chatfield DA, Williams GB, et al. Early derangements in oxygen and glucose metabolism following head injury: the ischemic penumbra and pathophysiological heterogeneity. Neurocrit Care. 2008;9:319–25.

51. Nortje J, Coles JP, Timofeev I, Fryer TD, Aigbirhio FI, Smielewski P, et al. Effect of hyperoxia on regional oxygenation and metabolism after severe traumatic brain injury: preliminary findings. Crit Care Med. 2008;36:273–81.

52. Tango HK, Schmidt AP, Mizumoto N, Lacava M, Cruz RJ Jr, Auler JO Jr. Low hematocrit levels increase intracranial pressure in an animal model of cryogenic brain injury. J Trauma. 2009;66(3):720–6.

53. Brown MM, Marshall J. Regulation of cerebral blood flow in response to changes in blood viscosity. Lancet. 1985;1:604–9.

54. Brown MM, Wade JP, Marshall J. Fundamental importance of arterial oxygen content in the regulation of cerebral blood flow in man. Brain. 1985;108:81–93.

55. Engelborghs K, Haseldonckx M, Van Reempts J, Van Rossem K, Wouters L, Borgers M, Verlooy J. Impaired autoregulation of cerebral blood flow in an experimental model of traumatic brain injury. J Neurotrauma. 2000;17:667–77.

56. Dexter F, Hindman BJ. Effect of haemoglobin concentration on brain oxygenation in focal stroke: a mathematical modeling study. Br J Anaesth. 1997;79:346–51.

57. Hare GM, Mazer CD, Hutchison JS, McLaren AT, Liu E, Rassouli A, et al. Severe hemodilutional ane-

mia increases cerebral tissue injury following acute neurotrauma. J Appl Physiol. 2007;103:1021–9.

58. Matsushita Y, Bramlett HM, Kuluz JW, Alonso O, Dietrich WD. Delayed hemorrhagic hypotension exacerbates the hemodynamic and histopathologic consequences of traumatic brain injury in rats. J Cereb Blood Flow Metab. 2001;21:847–56.

59. Hariri RJ, Firlick AD, Shepard SR, Cohen DS, Barie PS, Emery JM III, et al. Traumatic brain injury, hemorrhagic shock, and fluid resuscitation: effects on intracranial pressure and brain compliance. J Neurosurg. 1993;79(3):421–7.

60. Chappell JE, Shackford SR, McBride WJ. Effect of hemodilution with diaspirin cross-linked hemoglobin on intracranial pressure, cerebral perfusion pressure, and fluid requirements after head injury and shock. J Neurosurg. 1997;86:131–8.

61. Oddo M, Milby A, Chen I, Frangos S, MacMurtrie E, Maloney-Wilensky E, et al. Hemoglobin concentration and cerebral metabolism in patients with aneurysmal subarachnoid hemorrhage. Stroke. 2009;40:1275–81.

62. Kurtz P, Schmidt JM, Claasssen J, Carrera E, Fernandez L, Helbok R, et al. Anemia is associated with metabolic distress and brain tissue hypoxia after subarachnoid hemorrhage. Neurocrit Care. 2010;13(1):10–6.

63. Couture DE, Ellegala DB, Dumont AS, Mintz PD, Kassell NF. Blood use in cerebrovascular neurosurgery. [erratum appears in Stroke 2002 May;33(5):1442]. Stroke. 2002;33(4):994–7.

64. Le Roux P, Elliott JP, Winn HR. Blood transfusion during aneurysm surgery. Neurosurgery. 2001;49:1068–75.

65. de Gray LC, Matta BF. The health economics of blood use in cerebrovascular aneurysm surgery: the experience of a UK centre. Eur J Anaesthesiol. 2005;22(12):925–8.

66. Hardesty DA, Doerfler S, Sandhu S, Whitmore RG, Ford P, Rushton S, Le Roux P. Neurosurgery among Jehovah's Witnesses: a comparison with matched concurrent controls. World Neurosurg. 2017;97:132–9.

67. Karkouti K, Djaiani G, Borger MA, Beattie WS, Fedorko L, Wijeysundera D, et al. Low hematocrit during cardiopulmonary bypass is associated with increased risk of perioperative stroke in cardiac surgery. Ann Thorac Surg. 2005;80:1381–7.

68. Bahrainwala ZS, Grega MA, Hogue CW, Baumgartner WA, Selnes OA, McKhann GM, Gottesman RF. Intraoperative hemoglobin levels and transfusion independently predict stroke after cardiac operations. Ann Thorac Surg. 2011;91(4):1113–8.

69. Park HW, Song JM, Choo SJ, Chung CH, Lee JW, Kim DH, Kang DH, Song JK. Effect of preoperative ejection fraction, left ventricular systolic dimension and hemoglobin level on survival after aortic valve surgery in patients with severe chronic aortic regurgitation. Am J Cardiol. 2012;109(12):1782–6.

70. Ranucci M, Di Dedda U, Castelvecchio S, Menicanti L, Frigiola A, Pelissero G, Surgical and Clinical Outcome Research (SCORE) Group. Impact of preoperative anemia on outcome in adult cardiac surgery: a propensity-matched analysis. Ann Thorac Surg. 2012;94(4):1134–41.

71. Dündar C, Oduncu V, Erkol A, Tanalp AC, Sırma D, Karagöz A, et al. In-hospital prognostic value of hemoglobin levels on admission in patients with acute ST segment elevation myocardial infarction undergoing primary angioplasty. Clin Res Cardiol. 2012;101(1):37–44. Epub 2011 Sep 20.

72. Leichtle SW, Mouawad NJ, Lampman R, Singal B, Cleary RK. Does preoperative anemia adversely affect colon and rectal surgery outcomes? J Am Coll Surg. 2011;212(2):187–94.

73. Zhang L, Hiebert B, Zarychanski R, Arora RC, Cardiovascular Health Research in Manitoba (CHaRM) Investigator Group. Preoperative anemia does not increase the risks of early surgical revascularization after myocardial infarction. Ann Thorac Surg. 2013;95(2):542–7.

74. Musallam KM, Tamim HM, Richards T, Spahn DR, Rosendaal FR, Habbal A, et al. Preoperative anaemia and postoperative outcomes in non-cardiac surgery: a retrospective cohort study. Lancet. 2011;378(9800):1396–407.

75. Carson JL, Duff A, Poses RM, Berlin JA, Spence RK, Trout R, et al. Effect of anaemia and cardiovascular disease on surgical mortality and morbidity. Lancet. 1996;348(9034):1055–60.

76. Calderaro D, Gualandro SM, Gualandro DM, Yu PC, Carmo GLA, Marques AC, et al. Acute anemia and cardiovascular events after vascular surgery. Eur Heart J. 2013;34(Suppl 1):P358.

77. Spolverato G, Kim Y, Ejaz A, Frank SM, Pawlik TM. Effect of relative decrease in blood hemoglobin concentrations on postoperative morbidity in patients who undergo major gastrointestinal surgery. JAMA Surg. 2015;150(10):949–56.

78. Sekhon MS, McLean N, Henderson WR, Chittock DR, Griesdale DE. Association of hemoglobin concentration and mortality in critically ill patients with severe traumatic brain injury. Crit Care. 2012;16(4):R128.

79. Steyerberg EW, Van Beek JG, Mushkudiani NA, Steyerberg EW, Butcher I, McHugh GS, et al. Prognostic value of admission laboratory parameters in traumatic brain injury: results from the IMPACT study. J Neurotrauma. 2007;24(2):315–28.

80. McIntyre LA, Fergusson DA, Hutchison JS, Pagliarello G, Marshall JC, Yetisir E, et al. Effect of a liberal versus restrictive transfusion strategy on mortality in patients with moderate to severe head injury. Neurocrit Care. 2006;5:4–9.

81. Sanchez-Olmedo JI, Flores-Cordero JM, Rincon-Ferrari MD, Perez-Ale M, Munoz-Sanchez MA, Dominguez-Roldan JM, et al. Brain death after severe traumatic brain injury: the role of systemic secondary brain insults. Transplant Proc. 2005;37(5):1990–2.

82. Talving P, Lustenberger T, Kobayashi L, Inaba K, Barmparas G, Schnüriger B, et al. Erythropoiesis stimulating agent administration improves survival after severe traumatic brain injury. Ann Surg. 2010;251:1–4.

83. Ariza M, Mataró M, Poca MA, Junqué C, Garnacho A, Amorós S, et al. Influence of extraneurological insults on ventricular enlargement and neuropsychological functioning after moderate and severe traumatic brain injury. J Neurotrauma. 2004;21:864–76.

84. Steyerberg EW, Mushkudiani N, Perel P, Butcher I, Lu J, McHugh GS, et al. Predicting outcome after traumatic brain injury: development and international validation of prognostic scores based on admission characteristics. PLoS Med. 2008;5:e165.

85. Griesdale DE, Sekhon MS, Menon DK, Lavinio A, Donnelly J, Robba C, et al. Hemoglobin area and time index above 90 g/L are associated with improved 6-month functional outcomes in patients with severe traumatic brain injury. Neurocrit Care. 2015;23(1):78–84.

86. Knaus WA, Draper EA, Wagner DP, Zimmerman JE. APACHE II: a severity of disease classification system. Crit Care Med. 1985;13:818–29.

87. Harrison DA, Parry GJ, Carpenter JR, Short A, Rowan K. A new risk prediction model for critical care: The Intensive Care National Audit and Research Centre (ICNARC) model. Crit Care Med. 2007;35:1091–8.

88. Muench E, Horn P, Bauhuf C, Roth H, Philipps M, Hermann P, et al. Effects of hypervolemia and hypertension on regional cerebral blood flow, intracranial pressure, and brain tissue oxygenation after subarachnoid hemorrhage. Crit Care Med. 2007;35:1844–51.

89. Tolias CM, Reinert M, Seiler R, Gilman C, Scharf A, Bullock MR. Normobaric hyperoxia–induced improvement in cerebral metabolism and reduction in intracranial pressure in patients with severe head injury: a prospective historical cohort-matched study. J Neurosurg. 2004;101(3):435–44.

90. Rockswold SB, Rockswold GL, Zaun DA, Zhang X, Cerra CE, Bergman TA, Liu J. A prospective, randomized clinical trial to compare the effect of hyperbaric to normobaric hyperoxia on cerebral metabolism, intracranial pressure, and oxygen toxicity in severe traumatic brain injury. J Neurosurg. 2010;112(5):1080–94.

91. Rockswold SB, Rockswold GL, Vargo JM, Erickson CA, Sutton RL, Bergman TA, Biros MH. Effects of hyperbaric oxygenation therapy on cerebral metabolism and intracranial pressure in severely brain injured patients. J Neurosurg. 2001;94(3):403–11.

92. Nangunoori R, Maloney-Wilensky E, Stiefel MDM, Park S, Kofke WA, Levine J, Yang W, Le Roux P. Brain tissue oxygen based therapy and outcome after severe traumatic brain injury: a systematic literature review. Neurocrit Care. 2012;17(1):131–8.

93. Bohman LE, Sanborn M, Pisapia J, Levine J, Frangos S, Stiefel M, Le Roux P. Long term outcome of patients with aneurysmal subarachnoid hemorrhage treated with brain oxygen-directed therapy. In: Neurocritical Care Society Meeting, Denver; 2012.

94. Okonkwo D, Shutter L, Moore C, Temkin N, Puccio A, Madden C, Andaluz N, Chesnut R, Bullock MR, Grant G, McGregor J, Weaver M, Jallo J, Le Roux P, Moberg R, Barber J, Lazaridis C, Diaz-Arristia R. Brain Tissue Oxygen Monitoring and Management in Severe Traumatic Brain Injury (BOOST-II): a Phase II randomised trial. Crit Care Med. 2017;45(11):1907–14.

95. Smith MJ, Stiefel MF, Magge S, Frangos S, Bloom S, Gracias V, et al. Packed red blood cell transfusion increases local cerebral oxygenation. Crit Care Med. 2005;33:1104–8.

96. Leal-Noval SR, Rincón-Ferrari MD, Marin-Niebla A, Cayuela A, Arellano-Orden V, Marín-Caballos A, et al. Transfusion of erythrocyte concentrates produces a variable increment on cerebral oxygenation in patients with severe traumatic brain injury: a preliminary study. Intensive Care Med. 2006;32:1733–40.

97. Zygun D, Nortje J, Hutchinson PJ, Timofeev I, Menon DK, Gupta AK. The effect of red blood cell transfusion on cerebral oxygenation and metabolism following severe traumatic brain injury. Crit Care Med. 2009;37:1074–8.

98. Leal-Noval SR, Muñoz-Gómez M, Arellano-Orden V, Marín-Caballos A, Amaya-Villar R, Marín A, et al. Impact of age of transfused blood on cerebral oxygenation in male patients with severe traumatic brain injury. Crit Care Med. 2008;36:1290–6.

99. Figaji AA, Zwane E, Kogels M, Fieggen AG, Argent AC, Le Roux PD, et al. The effect of blood transfusion on brain oxygenation in children with severe traumatic brain injury. Pediatr Crit Care Med. 2010;11:325–31.

100. Arellano-Orden V, Leal-Noval SR, Cayuela A, Muñoz-Gómez M, Ferrándiz-Millón C, García-Alfaro C, et al. Gender influences cerebral oxygenation after red blood cell transfusion in patients with severe traumatic brain injury. Neurocrit Care. 2011;14:18–23.

101. Robertson CS, Hannay HJ, Yamal JM, Gopinath S, Goodman JC, Tilley BC, Epo Severe TBI Trial Investigators, et al. Effect of erythropoietin and transfusion threshold on neurological recovery after traumatic brain injury: a randomized clinical trial. JAMA. 2014;312(1):36–47.

102. Yamal JM, Rubin ML, Benoit JS, Tilley BC, Gopinath S, Hannay HJ, et al. Effect of hemoglobin transfusion threshold on cerebral hemodynamics and oxygenation. J Neurotrauma. 2015;32(16):1239–45.

103. Dhar R, Zazulia AR, Videen TO, Zipfel GJ, Derdeyn CP, Diringer MN. Red blood cell transfusion increases cerebral oxygen delivery in anemic patients with subarachnoid hemorrhage. Stroke. 2009;40:3039–44.

104. Dhar R, Scalfani MT, Zazulia AR, TO V, Derdeyn CP, Diringer MN. Comparison of induced hyperten-

sion, fluid bolus, and blood transfusion to augment cerebral oxygen delivery after subarachnoid hemorrhage. J Neurosurg. 2012;116(3):648–56.

105. Thiele RH, Huffmyer JL, Raphael J. Perioperative morbidity: lessons from recent clinical trials. Curr Opin Crit Care. 2012;18(4):358–65.

106. Sabaté S, Mases A, Guilera N, Canet J, Castillo J, Orrego C, et al.; ANESCARDIOCAT Group. Incidence and predictors of major perioperative adverse cardiac and cerebrovascular events in noncardiac surgery. Br J Anaesth 2011;107(6):879–90.

107. Koster S, Hensens AG, Schuurmans MJ, van der Palen J. Risk factors of delirium after cardiac surgery: a systematic review. Eur J Cardiovasc Nurs. 2011;10(4):197–204.

108. Reeves BC, Murphy GJ. Increased mortality, morbidity, and cost associated with red blood cell transfusion after cardiac surgery. Curr Opin Cardiol. 2008;23(6):607–12.

109. Mikkola R, Gunn J, Heikkinen J, Wistbacka JO, Teittinen K, Kuttila K, Lahtinen J, Juvonen T, Airaksinen JK, Biancari F. Use of blood products and risk of stroke after coronary artery bypass surgery. Blood Transfus. 2012;10(4):490–501.

110. Hajjar LA, Vincent JL, Galas FR, Nakamura RE, Silva CM, Santos MH, et al. Transfusion requirements after cardiac surgery: the TRACS randomized controlled trial. JAMA. 2010;304:1559–67.

111. Whitson BA, Huddleston SJ, Savik K, Shumway SJ. Risk of adverse outcomes associated with blood transfusion after cardiac surgery depends on the amount of transfusion. J Surg Res. 2010;158(1):20–7.

112. Murphy GJ, Pike K, Rogers CA, Wordsworth S, Stokes EA, Angelini GD, et al.; TITRe2 Investigators. Liberal or restrictive transfusion after cardiac surgery. N Engl J Med. 2015;372(11):997–1008

113. Kang JL, Chung TK, Lancaster RT, Lamuraglia GM, Conrad MF, Cambria RP. Outcomes after carotid endarterectomy: is there a high-risk population? A National Surgical Quality Improvement Program report. J Vasc Surg. 2009;49(2):331–8, 339.e1; discussion 338–9.

114. Pull ter Gunne AF, Skolasky RL, Ross H, van Laarhoven CJ, Cohen DB. Influence of perioperative resuscitation status on postoperative spine surgery complications. Spine J. 2010;10(2):129–35.

115. Baron DM, Metnitz PG, Fellinger T, Metnitz B, Rhodes A, Kozek-Langenecker SA. Evaluation of clinical practice in perioperative patient blood management. Br J Anaesth. 2016;117(5):610–6.

116. Spahn DR, Cerny V, Coats TJ, Duranteau J, Fernández-Mondéjar E, Gordini G, et al. Management of bleeding following major trauma: a European guideline. Crit Care. 2007;11(1):R17.

117. Gunst MA, Minei JP. Transfusion of blood products and nosocomial infection in surgical patients. Curr Opin Crit Care. 2007;13:428–32.

118. Silverboard H, Aisiku I, Martin GS, Adams M, Rozycki G, Moss M. The role of acute blood transfusion in the development of acute respiratory distress syndrome in patients with severe trauma. J Trauma. 2005;59:717–23.

119. Moore FA, Moore EE, Sauaia A. Blood transfusion. An independent risk factor for postinjury multiple organ failure. Arch Srug. 1997;132:620–4.

120. Schorr AF, Duh MS, Kelly KM, Kollef MH, CRIT Study Group. Red blood cell transfusion and ventilator-associated pneumonia: a potential link? Crit Care Med. 2004;32:666–74.

121. Marik PE, Corwin HL. Efficacy of red blood cell transfusion in the critically ill: a systematic review of the literature. Crit Care Med. 2008;36:2667–74.

122. Lacroix J, Hébert PC, Hutchison JS, Hume HA, Tucci M, Ducruet T, et al. Transfusion strategies for patients in pediatric intensive care units. N Engl J Med. 2007;356:1609–19.

123. Kumar M, Levine J, Faerber J, Elliott JP, Winn HR, Doerfler S, Le Roux P. The effects of red blood cell transfusion on functional outcome after aneurysmal subarachnoid hemorrhage. World Neurosurg. 2017;108:807–16.

124. Boutin A, Chassé M, Shemilt M, Lauzier F, Moore L, Zarychanski R, Griesdale D, Desjardins P, Lacroix J, Fergusson D, Turgeon AF. Red blood cell transfusion in patients with traumatic brain injury: a systematic review and meta-analysis. Transfus Med Rev. 2016;30(1):15–24.

125. Elterman J, Brasel K, Brown S, Bulger E, Christenson J, Kerby JD, et al. Transfusion of red blood cells in patients with a prehospital Glasgow Coma Scale score of 8 or less and no evidence of shock is associated with worse outcomes. J Trauma Acute Care Surg. 2013;75:8–14.

126. Malone DL, Dunne J, Tracy JK, Putnam AT, Scalea TM, Napolitano LM. Blood transfusion, independent of shock severity, is associated with worse outcome in trauma. J Trauma. 2003;54:898–905; discussion 905–7.

127. Takeuchi S, Nagatani K, Otani N, Nawashiro H. The association between anemia and traumatic brain injury. J Trauma. 2011;71:784.

128. Shapiro MJ, Gettinger A, Corwin HL, Napolitano L, Levy M, Abraham E, et al. Anemia and blood transfusion in trauma patients admitted to the intensive care unit. J Trauma. 2003;55:269–73.

129. Leal-Noval SR, Muñoz-Serrano Á, Arellano-Orden V, Cayuela A, Muñoz-Gómez M, Recio A, Alcántara A, Amaya-Villar R, Casado-Méndez M, Murillo-Cabezas F. Effects of red blood cell transfusion on long-term disability of patients with traumatic brain injury. Neurocrit Care. 2016;24(3):371–80.

130. Carr KR, Rodriguez M, Ottesen A, Michalek J, Son C, Patel V, Jimenez D, Seifi A. Association between relative anemia and early functional recovery after severe traumatic brain injury (TBI). Neurocrit Care. 2016;25(2):185–92.

131. Deans KJ, Minneci PC, Suffredini AF, Danner RL, Hoffman WD, Ciu X, et al. Randomization in clinical trials of titrated therapies: unintended conse-

quences of using fixed treatment protocols. Crit Care Med. 2007;35:1509–16.

132. Naidech AM, Shaibani A, Garg RK, Duran IM, Liebling SM, Bassin SL, et al. Prospective, randomized trial of higher goal hemoglobin after subarachnoid hemorrhage. Neurocrit Care. 2010;13:313–20.

133. Travers S, Martin S, Litofsky NS. The effects of anaemia and transfusion on patients with traumatic brain injury: a review. Brain Inj. 2016;30(13–14):1525–32.

134. Lelubre C, Bouzat P, Crippa IA, Taccone FS. Anemia management after acute brain injury. Crit Care. 2016;20(1):152.

135. Vlaar AP, Juffermans NP. Transfusion-related acute lung injury: a clinical review. Lancet. 2013;382(9896):984–94.

136. El Kenz H, Van der Linden P. Transfusion-related acute lung injury. Eur J Anaesthesiol. 2014;31(7):345–50.

137. Sayah DM, Looney MR, Toy P. Transfusion reactions: newer concepts on the pathophysiology, incidence, treatment, and prevention of transfusion-related acute lung injury. Crit Care Clin. 2012;28(3):363–72.

138. Goldberg AD, Kor DJ. State of the art management of transfusion-related acute lung injury (TRALI). Curr Pharm Des. 2012;18(22):3273–84.

139. Clifford L, Jia Q, Yadav H, Subramanian A, Wilson GA, Murphy SP, Pathak J, Schroeder DR, Ereth MH, Kor DJ. Characterizing the epidemiology of perioperative transfusion-associated circulatory overload. Anesthesiology. 2015;122(1):21–8.

140. Alam A, Lin Y, Lima A, Hansen M, Callum JL. The prevention of transfusion-associated circulatory overload. Transfus Med Rev. 2013;27(2):105–12.

141. Skeate RC, Eastlund T. Distinguishing between transfusion related acute lung injury and transfusion associated circulatory overload. Curr Opin Hematol. 2007;14(6):682–7.

142. Gajic O, Gropper MA, Hubmayr RD. Pulmonary edema after transfusion: how to differentiate transfusion-associated circulatory overload from transfusion-related acute lung injury. Crit Care Med. 2006;34(5 Suppl):S109–13.

143. Kumar MA, Boland TA, Baiou M, Moussouttas M, Herman JH, Bell RD, Rosenwasser RH, Kasner SE, Dechant VE. Red blood cell transfusion increases the risk of thrombotic events in patients with subarachnoid hemorrhage. Neurocrit Care. 2014;20(1):84–90.

144. Vedantam A, Yamal JM, Rubin ML, Robertson CS, Gopinath SP. Progressive hemorrhagic injury after severe traumatic brain injury: effect of hemoglobin transfusion thresholds. J Neurosurg. 2016;125(5):1229–34.

145. Tan H, Bi J, Wang Y, Zhang J, Zuo Z. Transfusion of old RBCs induces neuroinflammation and cognitive impairment. Crit Care Med. 2015;43:e276–86.

146. Ferguson D, Khanna MP, Tinmouth A, Hebert PC. Transfusion of leukoreduced red blood cells may decrease postoperative infections: two meta-analyses of randomized controlled tirals. Can J Anaesth. 2004;51:417–24.

147. Dzik WH, Anderson JK, O'Neill EM, Assmann SF, Kalish LA, Stowell CP. A prospective, randomized clinical trial of universal WBC reduction. Transfusion. 2002;42:1114–22.

148. Hébert PC, Fergusson D, Blajchman MA, Wells GA, Kmetic A, Coyle D, et al.; Leukoreduction Study Investigators. Clinical outcomes following institution of the Canadian universal leukoreduction program for red blood cell transfusions. JAMA. 2003;289:1941–9.

149. Vincent JL, Sakr Y, Sprung C, Harboe S, Damas P, Sepsis Occurrence in Acutely Ill Patients (SOAP) Investigators. Are blood transfusions associated with greater mortality rates? Results of the sepsis occurrence in acutely ill patients study. Anesthesiology. 2008;108(1):31–9.

150. Pettilä V, Westbrook AJ, Nichol AD, Bailey MJ, Wood EM, Syres G, et al. Age of red blood cells and mortality in the critically ill. Crit Care. 2011;15:R116.

151. Gauvin F, Spinella PC, Lacroix J, Choker G, Ducruet T, Karam O, et al.; Canadian Critical Care Trials Group and the Pediatric Acute Lung Injury and Sepsis Investigators (PALISI) Network. Association between length of storage of transfused red blood cells and multiple organ dysfunction syndrome in pediatric intensive care patients. Transfusion. 2010;50(9):1902–13.

152. Pettilä V, Westbrook AJ, Nichol AD, Bailey MJ, Wood EM, Syres G, et al.; Blood Observational Study Investigators for ANZICS Clinical Trials Group. Age of red blood cells and mortality in the critically ill. Crit Care. 2011;15(2):R116.

153. Weinberg JA, McGwin G Jr, Vandromme MJ, Marques MB, Melton SM, Reiff DA, Kerby JD, Rue LW III. Duration of red cell storage influences mortality after trauma. J Trauma. 2010;69(6):1427–31; discussion 1431–2.

154. Lelubre C, Vincent JL. Relationship between red cell storage duration and outcomes in adults receiving red cell transfusions: a systematic review. Crit Care. 2013;17(2):R66.

155. Zallen G, Offner PJ, Moore EE, Blackwell J, Ciesla DJ, Gabriel J, et al. Age of transfused blood is an independent risk factor for postinjury multiple organ failure. Am J Surg. 1999;178:570–2.

156. Tinmouth A, Fergusson D, Yee IC, Hébert PC, ABLE Investigators; Canadian Critical Care Trials Group. Clinical consequences of red cell storage in the critically ill. Transfusion. 2006;46:2014–27.

157. Walsh TS, McArdle F, McLellan SA, Maciver C, Maginnis M, Prescott RJ, et al. Does the storage time of transfused red blood cells influence regional or global indexes of tissue oxygenation in anemic critically ill patients? Crit Care Med. 2004;32:364–71.

158. Marik PE, Sibbald WJ. Effect of stored-blood transfusion on oxygen delivery in patients with sepsis. JAMA. 1993;269:3024–9.

159. Lacroix J, Hébert PC, Fergusson DA, Tinmouth A, Cook DJ, Marshall JC, Clayton L, McIntyre L, Callum J, Turgeon AF, Blajchman MA, Walsh TS, Stanworth SJ, Campbell H, Capellier G, Tiberghien P, Bardiaux L, van de Watering L, van der Meer NJ, Sabri E, Vo D, ABLE Investigators; Canadian Critical Care Trials Group. Age of transfused blood in critically ill adults. N Engl J Med. 2015;372(15):1410–8.

160. Sekhon MS, Griesdale DE, Czosnyka M, Donnelly J, Liu X, Aries MJ, et al. The effect of red blood cell transfusion on cerebral autoregulation in patients with severe brain injury. Neurocrit Care. 2015;23:210–6.

161. Kabadi SV, Faden AI. Neuroprotective strategies for traumatic brain injury: improving clinical translation. Int J Mol Sci. 2014;15(1):1216–36.

162. Gatto R, Chauhan M, Chauhan N. Anti-edema effects of rhEpo in experimental traumatic brain injury. Restor Neurol Neurosci. 2015;33(6):927–41.

163. Mammis A, McIntosh TK, Maniker AH. Erythropoietin as a neuroprotective agent in traumatic brain injury. Surg Neurol. 2009;71:527–31.

164. Wang L, Wang X, Su H, Han Z, Yu H, Wang D, Jiang R, Liu Z, Zhang J. Recombinant human erythropoietin improves the neurofunctional recovery of rats following traumatic brain injury via an increase in circulating endothelial progenitor cells. Transl Stroke Res. 2015;6(1):50–9.

165. Lu D, Mahmood A, Qu C, Goussev A, Schallert T, Chopp M. Erythropoietin enhances neurogenesis and restores spatial memory in rats after traumatic brain injury. J Neurotrauma. 2005;22:1011–7.

166. Cherian L, Goodman JC, Robertson C. Neuroprotection with erythropoietin administration following controlled cortical impact injury in rats. J Pharmacol Exp Ther. 2007;322:789–94.

167. Grasso G, Sfacteria A, Meli F, Fodale V, Buemi M, Iacopino DG. Neuroprotection by erythropoietin administration after experimental traumatic brain injury. Brain Res. 2007;1182:99–105.

168. Bouzat P, Fracony G, Thomas S, Valable S, Mauconduit F, Fevre MC, et al. Reduced brain edema and functional deficits after treatment of diffuse traumatic brain injury by carbamylated erythropoietin derivative. Crit Care Med. 2011;39(9):2099–105.

169. Ning R, Xiong Y, Mahmood A, Zhang Y, Meng Y, Qu C, et al. Erythropoietin promotes neurovascular remodeling and long-term functional recovery in rats following traumatic brain injury. Brain Res. 2011;1384:140–50.

170. Schober ME, Requena DF, Block B, Davis LJ, Rodesch C, Casper TC, Juul SE, Kesner RP, Lane RH. Erythropoietin improved cognitive function and decreased hippocampal caspase activity in rat pups after traumatic brain injury. J Neurotrauma. 2014;31(4):358–69.

171. Wang B, Kang M, Marchese M, Rodriguez E, Lu W, Li X, Maeda Y, Dowling P. Beneficial effect of erythropoietin short peptide on acute traumatic brain injury. Neurotherapeutics. 2016;13(2):418–27.

172. Bouzat P, Millet A, Boue Y, Pernet-Gallay K, Trouve-Buisson T, Gaide-Chevronnay L, Barbier EL, Payen JF. Changes in brain tissue oxygenation after treatment of diffuse traumatic brain injury by erythropoietin. Crit Care Med. 2013;41(5):1316–24.

173. Corwin HL, Gettinger A, Pearl RG, Fink MP, Levy MM, Shapiro MJ, et al.; EPO Critical Care Trials Group. Efficacy of recombinant human erythropoietin in critically ill patients: a randomized controlled trial. JAMA. 2002;288:2827–35.

174. Corwin HL, Gettinger A, Fabian TC, May A, Pearl RG, Heard S, et al.; EPO Critical Care Trials Group. Efficacy and safety of epoetin alfa in critically ill patients. N Engl J Med. 2007;357:965–76.

175. Napolitano LM, Fabian TC, Kelly KM, Bailey JA, Block EF, Langholff W, et al. Improved survival of critically ill trauma patients treated with recombinant human erythropoietin. J Trauma. 2008;65:285–97.

176. Haljan G, Maitland A, Buchan A, Arora RC, King M, Haigh J, et al. The erythropoietin neuroprotective effect: assessment in CABG surgery (TENPEAKS): a randomized, double-blind, placebo controlled, proof-of-concept clinical trial. Stroke. 2009;40:2769–75.

177. Tseng MY, Hutchinson PJ, Richards HK, Czosnyka M, Pickard JD, Erber WN, et al. Acute systemic erythropoietin therapy to reduce delayed ischemic deficits following aneurismal subarachnoid hemorrage: a phase II randomized, double-blind, placebo-controlled trial. J Neurosurg. 2009;111: 171–80.

178. Ehrenreich H, Weissenborn K, Prange H, Schneider D, Weimar C, Wartenberg K, et al.; EPO Stroke Trial Group. Recombinant human erythropoietin in the treatment of acute ischemic stroke. Stroke. 2009;40:647–56.

179. Nichol A, French C, Little L, Haddad S, Presneill J, Arabi Y, Bailey M, Cooper DJ, Duranteau J, Huet O, Mak A, McArthur C, Pettilä V, Skrifvars M, Vallance S, Varma D, Wills J, Bellomo R, EPO-TBI Investigators; ANZICS Clinical Trials Group. Erythropoietin in traumatic brain injury (EPO-TBI): a double-blind randomised controlled trial. Lancet. 2015;386(10012):2499–506.

180. Li ZM, Xiao YL, Zhu JX, Geng FY, Guo CJ, Chong ZL, Wang LX. Recombinant human erythropoietin improves functional recovery in patients with severe traumatic brain injury: a randomized, double blind and controlled clinical trial. Clin Neurol Neurosurg. 2016;150:80–3.

181. Liu WC, Wen L, Xie T, Wang H, Gong JB, Yang XF. Therapeutic effect of erythropoietin in patients with traumatic brain injury: a meta-analysis of randomized controlled trials. J Neurosurg. 2016;1:1–8.

182. French CJ, Glassford NJ, Gantner D, Higgins AM, Cooper DJ, Nichol A, Skrifvars MB, Imberger G, Presneill J, Bailey M, Bellomo R. Erythropoiesis-stimulating agents in critically ill trauma patients: a systematic review and meta-analysis. Ann Surg. 2017;265(1):54–62.

183. Kochanek PM, Bramlett HM, Shear DA, Dixon CE, Mondello S, Dietrich WD, Hayes RL, Wang KK, Poloyac SM, Empey PE, Povlishock JT, Mountney A, Browning M, Deng-Bryant Y, Yan HQ, Jackson TC, Catania M, Glushakova O, Richieri SP, Tortella FC. Synthesis of findings, current investigations, and future directions: operation brain trauma therapy. J Neurotrauma. 2016;33(6):606–14.

184. Bramlett HM, Dietrich WD, Dixon CE, Shear DA, Schmid KE, Mondello S, Wang KK, Hayes RL, Povlishock JT, Tortella FC, Kochanek PM. Erythropoietin treatment in traumatic brain injury: operation brain trauma therapy. J Neurotrauma. 2016;33(6):538–52.

185. Skrifvars MB, Bailey M, Presneill J, French C, Nichol A, Little L, Duranteau J, Huet O, Haddad S, Arabi Y, McArthur C, Cooper DJ, Bellomo R, EPO-TBI investigators and the ANZICS Clinical Trials Group. Venous thromboembolic events in critically ill traumatic brain injury patients. Intensive Care Med. 2017;43(3):419–28.

186. Rother RP, Bell L, Hillmen P, Gladwin MT. The clinical sequelae of intravascular hemolysis and extracellular plasma hemoglobin: a novel mechanism of human disease. JAMA. 2005;293:1653–62.

187. Natanson C, Kern SJ, Lurie P, Banks SM, Wolfe SM. Cell-free haemoglobin-based blood substitutes and risk of myocardial infarction and death: a meta-analysis. JAMA. 2008;299:2304–12.

188. Wigginton JG, Roppolo L, Pepe PE. Advances in resuscitative trauma care. Minerva Anestesiol. 2011;77(10):993–1002.

189. Van Hemelrijck J, Levien LJ, Veeckman L, Pitman A, Zafirelis Z, Standl T. A safety and efficacy evaluation of hemoglobin-based oxygen carrier HBOC-201 in a randomized, multicenter red blood cell controlled trial in noncardiac surgery patients. Anesth Analg. 2014;119(4):766–76.

190. Regan RF, Rogers B. Delayed treatment of hemoglobin neurotoxicity. J Neurotrauma. 2003;20:111–20.

191. Shellington DK, Du L, Wu X, Exo J, Vagni V, Ma L, et al. Polynitroxylated pegylated hemoglobin: a novel neuroprotective hemoglobin for acute volume-limited fluid resuscitation after combined traumatic brain injury and hemorrhagic hypotension in mice. Crit Care Med. 2011;39:494–505.

192. Rosenthal G, Morabito D, Cohen M, Roeytenberg A, Derugin N, Panter SS, et al. Use of hemoglobin-based oxygen-carrying solution-201 to improve resuscitation parameters and prevent secondary brain injury in a swine model of traumatic brain injury and hemorrhage. J Neurosurg. 2008;108:575–87.

193. King DR, Cohn SM, Proctor KG. Resuscitation with a hemoglobin-based oxygen carrier after traumatic brain injury. J Trauma. 2005;59:553–62.

194. Stern S, Rice J, Philbin N, McGwin G, Arnaud F, Johnson T, et al. Resuscitation with the hemoglobin-based oxygen carrier HBOC-201, in a swine model of severe uncontrolled hemorrhage and traumatic brain injury. Shock. 2009;31:64–79.

195. White NJ, Wang X, Bradbury N, Moon-Massat PF, Freilich D, Auker C, McCarron R, Scultetus A, Stern SA. Fluid resuscitation of uncontrolled hemorrhage using a hemoglobin-based oxygen carrier: effect of traumatic brain injury. Shock. 2013;39(2):210–9.

196. Moore EE, Moore FA, Fabian TC, Bernard AC, Fulda GJ, Hoyt DB, et al.; PolyHeme Study Group. Human polymerized hemoglobin for the treatment of hemorrhagic shock when blood is unavailable: the USA multicenter trial. J Am Coll Surg. 2009;208:1–13.

197. Practice guidelines for perioperative blood transfusion and adjuvant therapies. An updated report by the American Society of Anesthesiologists Task Force on perioperative blood transfusion and adjuvant therapies. Anesthesiology. 2008;105:198–208.

198. [no authors listed]. American Society of Anesthesiologists Task Force on Perioperative Blood Management. Practice guidelines for perioperative blood management: an updated report by the American Society of Anesthesiologists Task Force on Perioperative Blood Management. Anesthesiology. 2015;122(2):241–75.

199. Qaseem A, Humphrey LL, Fitterman N, Starkey M, Shekelle P, Clinical Guidelines Committee of the American College of Physicians. Treatment of anemia in patients with heart disease: a clinical practice guideline from the American College of Physicians. Ann Intern Med. 2013;159:770–9.

200. Society of Thoracic Surgeons Blood Conservation Guideline Task Force, Ferraris VA, Brown JR, Despotis GJ, Hammon JW, Reece TB, Saha SP, et al. 2011 update to the Society of Thoracic Surgeons and the Society of Cardiovascular Anesthesiologists blood conservation clinical practice guidelines. Ann Thorac Surg. 2011;91:944–82.

201. [no authors listed] Expert Working Group. Guidelines for red blood cell and plasma transfusion for adults and children. Can Med Assoc J. 2008;156(Suppl 11):1–24.

202. Carson JL, Grossman BJ, Kleinman S, Tinmouth AT, Marques MB, Fung MK, Holcomb JB, Illoh O, Kaplan LJ, Katz LM, Rao SV, Roback JD, Shander A, Tobian AA, Weinstein R, Swinton McLaughlin LG, Djulbegovic B, Clinical Transfusion Medicine Committee of the AABB. Red blood cell transfusion: a clinical practice guideline from the AABB*. Ann Intern Med. 2012;157(1):49–58.

203. Klein AA, Arnold P, Bingham RM, Brohi K, Clark R, Collis R, Gill R, McSporran W, Moor P, Rao Baikady R, Richards T, Shinde S, Stanworth S, Walsh TS. AAGBI guidelines: the use of blood components and their alternatives 2016. Anaesthesia. 2016;71(7):829–42.

204. Padhi S, Kemmis-Betty S, Rajesh S, Hill J, Murphy MF. Guideline Development Group Blood transfusion: summary of NICE guidance. BMJ. 2015;351:h5832.

205. [no authors listed] National Clinical Guideline Centre (UK). Blood transfusion. London: National Institute for Health and Care Excellence (UK); 2015.

206. Retter A, Wyncoll D, Pearse R, Carson D, McKechnie S, Stanworth S, Allard S, Thomas D, Walsh T, British Committee for Standards in Haematology. Guidelines on the management of anaemia and red cell transfusion in adult critically ill patients. Br J Haematol. 2013 Feb;160(4):445–64.

207. [no authors listed] American College of Surgeons. ACS TQIP Best practices in the management of traumatic brain injury. Chicago: American College of Surgeons; 2015. https://www.east.org/content/documents/45_podcast_acstqip_tbi_guidelines_2.pdf

208. Le Roux PD, Participants in the International Multidisciplinary Consensus Conference on the Critical Care Management of Subarachnoid Hemorrhage. Anemia and transfusion after subarachnoid hemorrhage. Neurocrit Care. 2011;15(2):342–53.

209. Carson JL, Carless PA, Hebert PC. Transfusion thresholds and other strategies for guiding allogeneic red blood cell transfusion. Cochrane Database Syst Rev. 2012;(4):CD002042.

210. Chen JH, Fang DZ, Tim Goodnough L, Evans KH, Lee Porter M, Shieh L. Why providers transfuse blood products outside recommended guidelines in spite of integrated electronic best practice alerts. J Hosp Med. 2015;10(1):1–7.

211. Norgaard A, De Lichtenberg TH, Nielsen J, Johansson PI. Monitoring compliance with transfusion guidelines in hospital departments by electronic data capture. Blood Transfus. 2014;12(4):509–19.

212. Seitz KP, Sevransky JE, Martin GS, Roback JD, Murphy DJ. Evaluation of RBC transfusion practice in adult ICUs and the effect of restrictive transfusion protocols on routine care. Crit Care Med. 2017;45(2):271–81.

213. Yeh DD, Naraghi L, Larentzakis A, Nielsen N, Dzik W, Bittner EA, Chang Y, Kaafarani HM, Fagenholz P, Lee J, DeMoya M, King DR, Velmahos G. Peer-to-peer physician feedback improves adherence to blood transfusion guidelines in the surgical intensive care unit. J Trauma Acute Care Surg. 2015;79(1):65–70.

214. Borgert M, Binnekade J, Paulus F, Vroom M, Vlaar A, Goossens A, Dongelmans D. Implementation of a transfusion bundle reduces inappropriate red blood cell transfusions in intensive care - a before and after study. Transfus Med. 2016;26(6):432–9.

215. Patel NN, Avlonitis VS, Jones HE, Reeves BC, Sterne JA, Murphy GJ. Indications for red blood cell transfusion in cardiac surgery: a systematic review and meta-analysis. Lancet Haematol. 2015;2(12):e543–53.

216. Chan AW, de Gara CJ. An evidence-based approach to red blood cell transfusions in asymptomatically anaemic patients. Ann R Coll Surg Engl. 2015;97(8):556–62.

217. Fominskiy E, Putzu A, Monaco F, Scandroglio AM, Karaskov A, Galas FR, Hajjar LA, Zangrillo A, Landoni G. Liberal transfusion strategy improves survival in perioperative but not in critically ill patients. A meta-analysis of randomised trials. Br J Anaesth. 2015;115(4):511–9.

218. Chen A, Trivedi AN, Jiang L, Vezeridis M, Henderson WG, Wu WC. Hospital blood transfusion patterns during major noncardiac surgery and surgical mortality. Medicine (Baltimore). 2015;94(32):e1342.

219. Mirski MA, Frank SM, Kor DJ, Vincent JL, Holmes DR Jr. Restrictive and liberal red cell transfusion strategies in adult patients: reconciling clinical data with best practice. Crit Care. 2015;19:202.

220. Hollis RH, Singletary BA, McMurtrie JT, Graham LA, Richman JS, Holcomb CN, Itani KM, Maddox TM, Hawn MT. Blood transfusion and 30-day mortality in patients with coronary artery disease and anemia following noncardiac surgery. JAMA Surg. 2016;151(2):139–45.

221. Sadaka F, Trottier S, Tannehill D, Donnelly PL, Griffin MT, Bunaye Z, O'Brien J, Korobey M, Lakshmanan R. Transfusion of red blood cells is associated with improved central venous oxygen saturation but not mortality in septic shock patients. J Clin Med Res. 2014;6(6):422–8.

222. Chesnut RM. A conceptual approach to managing severe traumatic brain injury in a time of uncertainty. Ann N Y Acad Sci. 2015;1345:99–107.

223. Lazaridis C, DeSantis SM, Smielewski P, Menon DK, Hutchinson P, Pickard JD, Czosnyka M. Patient-specific thresholds of intracranial pressure in severe traumatic brain injury. J Neurosurg. 2014;120(4):893–900.

224. Le Roux P. Intracranial pressure monitoring and management. In: Laskowitz D, Grant G, editors. Translational research in traumatic brain. Boca Raton: CRC Press/Taylor and Francis Group; 2016.

225. Maas AI, Menon DK, Steyerberg EW, Citerio G, Lecky F, Manley GT, Hill S, Legrand V, Sorgner A, CENTER-TBI Participants and Investigators. Collaborative European NeuroTrauma Effectiveness Research in Traumatic Brain Injury (CENTER-TBI): a prospective longitudinal observational study. Neurosurgery. 2015;76(1):67–80.

226. Maas AI, Menon DK, Lingsma HF, Pineda JA, Sandel ME, Manley GT. Re-orientation of clinical research in traumatic brain injury: report of an international workshop on comparative effectiveness research. J Neurotrauma. 2012;29(1):32–46.

Timing of Extracerebral Operations in Severe Traumatic Brain Injury Patients

P. B. Raksin

Introduction

An anecdote sets the stage: A young male patient presents to an urban trauma center after being struck by a passing vehicle as he crossed the street. His arrival Glasgow Coma Scale (GCS) score is documented as 10. Initially, he is mildly tachycardic and hypertensive. He has obvious deformity of his distal right lower extremity. He is transferred to the radiology suite for imaging studies. CT (computed tomography) of the head reveals a 12 mm right acute subdural hematoma with an associated 7 mm of midline shift and obliteration of cisterns. The patient's neurologic status declines to a GCS of 7 while in the scanner. Additional imaging is deferred, and he is promptly intubated for airway protection. He is taken emergently to the operating room for a right decompressive craniectomy and evacuation of subdural hematoma. The trauma team follows him to the operating room to perform chest tube placement for a hemopneumothorax and a FAST (*f*ocused *a*ssessment with *s*onography in *t*rauma) scan that is negative.

P. B. Raksin, MD
Department of Neurosurgery, Rush University
Medical Center, Chicago, IL, USA

Division of Neurosurgery, John H. Stroger Jr.
Hospital of Cook County (formerly Cook
County Hospital), Chicago, IL, USA
e-mail: patricia_raksin@rush.edu

The orthopedics team indicates their intention to follow the craniectomy immediately thereafter with open reduction and internal fixation for a tibia-fibula fracture. The orthopedics resident repeatedly comes to the threshold of the operating room—near the foot of the bed—inquiring as to when the case would be finished. Meanwhile, the neurosurgical team is struggling with malignant edema and the manifestations of presumed coagulopathy. The patient becomes hypotensive. The immediate priority becomes "getting off the table" and over to the intensive care unit (ICU) for further resuscitation. Just then, the orthopedics resident reappears in the doorway. This time, when asking for an update, he is invited to come around to the *head* of the table to observe the hemorrhagic hemisphere swelling out of the cranium to help him understand the gravity of the situation.

Determining the order of operations—figuratively and, in some cases, quite literally—may pose considerable challenges in the care of the polytrauma patient. The presence of traumatic brain injury (TBI) in this setting compounds the complexity of the decision-making process. An awareness of the epidemiology of multiple system trauma allows the clinician to anticipate likely combinations of injury and their relative severity. An appreciation of basic principles of trauma resuscitation and an understanding of their interplay with evolving secondary brain injury are essential to direct care that is both neuroprotective and neuroproactive. A familiarity with the considerations being weighed by the subspecialists consulted for comorbid injuries is helpful in prioritizing interventions. A systematic, multidisciplinary approach that is geared toward optimizing outcomes, while minimizing potential harms, is the (sometimes unattainable) goal.

Epidemiology

Unintentional injury remains the leading cause of death for individuals under the age of 45 [1]. TBI is a contributing factor in approximately 30% of all injury deaths [2]. For the year 2010, approximately 2.5 million emergency department visits, hospitalizations, or deaths were associated with TBI—alone or in combination with additional injuries. The majority (75%) of these cases are classified as concussion or other types of mild traumatic brain injury (mTBI). TBI was a diagnosis in more than 280,000 hospitalizations. More than 50,000 individuals ultimately die from TBI-associated injuries each year.

Trauma-related mortality occurs in three waves: (1) "immediate" death, in the field, due to lethal primary injury; (2) "early" death, within minutes to hours, due to airway compromise, hemorrhagic shock, and/or catastrophic intracranial injury; and (3) "late" death, in the days to weeks after injury, due to multisystem organ failure, malignant systemic inflammation, overwhelming sepsis, and/or refractory increased intracranial pressure (ICP) [3]. Primary injury prevention and efficient prehospital transport may help offset the first peak. Rapid assessment and prompt intervention help mitigate the second. Comprehensive, multidisciplinary ICU care provides the best defense against the third. It is notable that neurologic injury is a factor at each of these outcome intervals.

Outcomes

The terms "polytrauma," "multiple system trauma," and "major" trauma often are used interchangeably. However, the term "polytrauma" lacks a validated definition. "Polytrauma" was initially used to denote two or more comorbid injuries [4]. Tscherne et al. adopted a definition of greater than or equal to two severe injuries, where one—or the sum total of all—of the injuries was considered life-threatening [5]. Others have tried to define polytrauma in terms of Injury Severity Score (ISS) or Abbreviated Injury Score (AIS), although there is no consensus regarding threshold values [6, 7].

Any discussion of outcomes among patients with polytrauma, therefore, is limited by heterogeneity of injury classification. Still, a few generalizations can be made. The primary determinant of mortality in the polytrauma patient is often the severity of the head injury [8]. The presence of head injury may confer an up to threefold increase in mortality. Even moderate traumatic brain injury (TBI) doubles predicted mortality when associated with extracranial injury [9, 10]. Regel et al. analyzed their experience in the management of 3406 polytrauma patients over a 20-year period in Germany [11]. Sixty-nine percent of patients presented with TBI. The most frequent combination was head and extremity injury (63%). Increasing total injury severity correlated with increased head injury severity. Prognosis was worse with injuries involving the brain, thorax, and extremities. Mortality was significantly higher in the presence of head injury (30.5% with TBI versus 24.4% without).

In a cohort study examining functional outcome and quality of life at least 2 years following major trauma, Gross et al. reported that significantly fewer survivors with TBI were living independently; head injury patients also demonstrated a more profound decrease in their capacity to work [12]. Polytrauma patients—with or without TBI—demonstrated significantly reduced long-term outcomes as compared with pre-injury level in all domains of the short form (SF)-36. The mental sum component of the SF-36 and cognitive subdomains of other investigated functional outcome scores best discriminated between survivors with and without TBI. Even at 10 years post-injury, there is evidence to suggest significantly worse functional outcomes for polytrauma patients with TBI as compared those without [13].

A large European registry cataloguing 26,541 trauma cases offers some perspective on the impact of polytrauma in general and, more specifically, the impact of TBI in this setting [14]. Fifty percent of registry cases included a diagnosis of head or thoracic trauma. Thoracic trauma was seen principally in conjunction with polytrauma, whereas two-thirds of head injury patients presented with significant TBI alone. Polytrauma with abdominal injury was associated with the highest rate of mortality across all age groups (33.1% ages 16–65, 64.1% age > 65); comorbid head injury demonstrated the next highest mortality rate (29.3% ages 16–65; 56.2% age > 65). Isolated head injury accounted for 12.9% of deaths among patients 16–65 years of age and 35.4% of those older than 65 years. The authors noted that mortality was greater for *polytrauma* than for the sum of the individual injury components. Though only 16% of patients in the registry met criteria for polytrauma, this subgroup accounted for nearly half of the recorded deaths (43%). The remainder were due primarily to a combination of isolated TBI and limb fractures in elderly patients. While the incidence of polytrauma among elderly patients was lower, such patients demonstrated mortality rates twice that of younger adults.

The patient presenting with multiple system trauma should be managed in accordance with Advanced Trauma Life Support (ATLS®) guidelines [15]. A methodical, organized team approach is essential in this setting. Establishment of an adequate airway ("A")—whether by endotracheal or nasotracheal intubation or by surgical cricothyroidotomy—is the initial priority. Intubation for airway protection should be considered for those with decreased level of consciousness (GCS ≤ 8), with severe maxillofacial fractures, with risk for aspiration, or with risk for obstruction. Cervical spine precautions should be observed. Supplemental oxygen should be provided. Breathing ("B") and ventilation comprise the second priority. This includes recognition and treatment of tension pneumothorax, hemothorax, flail chest, and subcutaneous emphysema, if present.

Assessment of circulation ("C") and control of hemorrhage follows. It is crucial to recognize the signs and symptoms of shock, remembering that hypotension *is* hypovolemia in trauma patients until proven otherwise. Blood loss of greater than 750 ml—representing approximately 15% of blood volume—results in tachycardia (class II shock). Hypotension develops in adults with blood loss approaching 1500–2000 ml, or approximately 30–40% of circulating blood volume (class III shock). Hemodynamic status may be impaired by uncontrolled external hemorrhage, massive hemoperitoneum, unstable pelvic fracture, hemothorax, and/or cardiac tamponade. Basic chest and pelvic X-rays, as well as a FAST scan, may be performed at that time. Fluid resuscitation and transfusion of blood products, if indicated, are initiated. External bleeding should be identified and controlled. Internal bleeding may require emergent operative intervention. In short, the patient's hemodynamic status dictates the imaging and management priorities from that point forward.

Once the "ABCs" have been addressed, the trauma team arrives at "D" for "disability." It is during this portion of the initial assessment that the patient's neurologic exam comes into sharper focus. Pupillary symmetry, size, and reactivity are documented. The GCS score is calculated. A patient with a GCS less than or equal to 8 should be intubated promptly for airway protection. An observed decreased level of consciousness may reflect decreased cerebral oxygenation ("A"), decreased cerebral perfusion ("C"), direct cerebral injury ("D"), intoxication with alcohol or drugs, metabolic derangement, or seizure. Hypoxemia and hypovolemia should be excluded first. Mannitol may be considered if a lateralizing exam and/or signs of herniation are present. A CT head is requested for the hemodynamically stable patient. The hemodynamically unstable patient may require so-called "damage control" lifesaving surgery, followed by ongoing resuscitation in the ICU setting [16]. The secondary survey, including a thorough history and complete neurologic exam, follows completion of the primary survey (the aforementioned elements, supplemented by "E" for "exposure and environment"). The resuscitative effort should be well-established, ideally with normalization of physiologic parameters. Indicated diagnostic radiographic studies and special procedures may be undertaken.

Coincident with the initial resuscitation effort, the clinician must consider that polytrauma patients—who might present in hemorrhagic shock and/or with comorbid lung injury—are particularly susceptible to secondary injury in the setting of TBI. Secondary injury unfolds over the minutes, hours, and days after the primary insult. While radiographic hyperdensity is certain to generate a request for neurosurgical consultation, secondary injury is not visible on the initial CT head and, therefore, may not be foremost in the minds of the frontline trauma team resuscitating the patient. The primary brain injury—with disruption of the blood-brain barrier—exposes neuronal cells to circulating immune cells and inflammatory mediators, setting into motion a series of inflammatory cascades. The release of cytokines, chemokines, and complement anaphylatoxins may drive leukocytes across the abnormally permeable blood-brain barrier, leading to further inflammation and injury of neural tissue [17, 18]. Additional insults—hypoxemia, hypotension, ischemia, cerebral edema, raised ICP—all threaten to exacerbate this inflammatory response. Furthermore, there is evidence to suggest that polytrauma patients presenting with concomitant musculoskeletal injury are subject to the activation of multiple inflammatory cascades in parallel [19, 20].

Secondary injury is insidious and can be lethal. The Trauma Coma Data Bank study demonstrated that a single episode of hypotension between injury and arrival to the trauma center *doubled* mortality, increased morbidity, and was associated with poorer outcomes [21, 22]. Similarly, hypoxia, which may be present at the scene in up to 60% of cases, has been associated with higher mortality and worse neurologic outcomes [23, 24]. Stocchetti et al. observed hypotension in nearly one-quarter (24%) and hypoxemia in greater than half (57%) of patients with TBI (mean GCS 7) in the field. While 80% of those with preserved blood pressure and saturation in the field went on to favorable outcomes, the prognosis for those with compromise of both was uniformly poor [23]. Chi et al. reported that nearly 40% of isolated TBI patients sustain a secondary insult (hypotension, hypoxia, or both) in the field and that the presence of hypoxia resulted in a significant increase in the odds of mortality (OR 2.66, $p < 0.05$) [25]. Therefore, care must be taken to avoid hypotension and hypoxia.

Jeremitsky et al. examined physiologic factors that might impact outcomes over the first 24 h after injury, finding that hypotension, hyperglycemia, and hypothermia were associated with increased mortality, while hypocapnia, acidosis, and hypoxemia were associated with significantly longer ICU length of stay [26]. Cerebral blood flow (CBF) has been shown to be at its nadir in the first 24 h after TBI, and low CBF at any point post-injury has been associated with worse neurologic outcomes, underscoring the critical need to support blood pressure and oxygenation [27]. Using xenon CT, Marion et al. demonstrated that low CBF in patients without mass lesions in the first few hours after injury was followed by a 24-h period of hyperemia [28]. Low CBF in the first 24 h was associated with (but not statistically significant for) poor outcome. Data derived from the Trauma Coma Data Bank patients suggested that avoidance of the shock state would have provided an estimated 9.3% reduction in unfavorable outcomes, prompting Piek et al. to recommend vigilance for the recognition of hypotension through the period of triage and transition to the ICU setting, coupled with prompt and aggressive treatment to restore normal perfusion [21].

A facility with the language of trauma and a fundamental understanding of the considerations relevant to providers in different specialty areas are invaluable in navigating the optimal management of the polytrauma patient. This chapter will address the timing of interventions for comorbid abdominal, craniofacial, and orthopedic injuries in the setting of traumatic brain injury—with particular attention to the interplay of pathophysiology and coordination of care.

Abdominal Trauma

The patient presenting with comorbid abdominal and intracranial trauma poses potential competing concerns: (1) life-threatening hemorrhage that compromises hemodynamic stability and (2) intracranial mass lesion that threatens herniation. Most central nervous system (CNS) deaths in this setting result from delays in craniotomy to evacuate mass lesions, while most non-CNS deaths result from inadequate resuscitation for intra-abdominal injuries [29–31]. Determining management priorities in this setting sometimes involves a delicate balancing act. On rare occasion, simultaneous interventions are indicated.

It bears repeating that the patient's hemodynamic status is a primary driver of clinical decision-making—particularly in the polytrauma patient who might present with multiple potential etiologies for physiologic instability (Fig. 1a). In the hypotensive trauma patient, hypovolemia due to ongoing hemorrhage is the presumption. Initial therapy is directed toward resuscitation, a search for the source, and elimination of life-threatening hemorrhage. If the patient is too unstable to permit transport to the CT scanner, a FAST scan may be performed at bedside. ATLS® guidelines rec-

ommend emergent laparotomy for control of bleeding in the setting of a positive FAST scan with hemorrhagic shock [15]. In this case, CT head may be deferred at the discretion of the trauma team.

However, if a patient with a depressed level of consciousness demonstrates lateralizing findings on initial neurologic exam, a space-occupying intracranial process—with the likelihood of raised intracranial pressure—should be presumed. The neurosurgeon should be apprised of the patient promptly and given the opportunity to determine whether intervention—medical or surgical—is reasonable and feasible. If the patient is hemodynamically unstable, attention to resuscitation, with a goal of restoring and maintaining sufficient mean arterial pressure (MAP) to achieve an adequate cerebral perfusion pressure

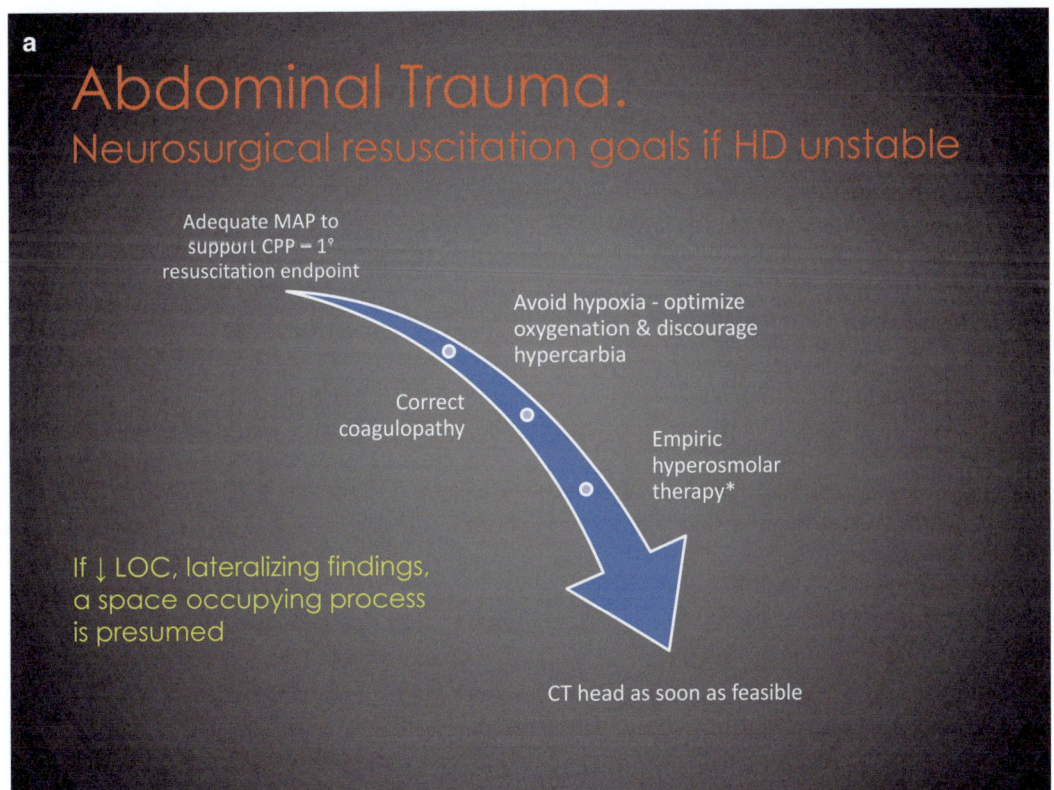

Fig. 1 Abdominal trauma. (**a**) Hemodynamically (HD) unstable. (**b**) HD stable. Abbreviations: *MAP* mean arterial pressure, *CPP* cerebral perfusion pressure, *LOC* loss of consciousness, *CT* computed tomography, *GCS* Glasgow Coma Scale, *ICP* intracranial pressure

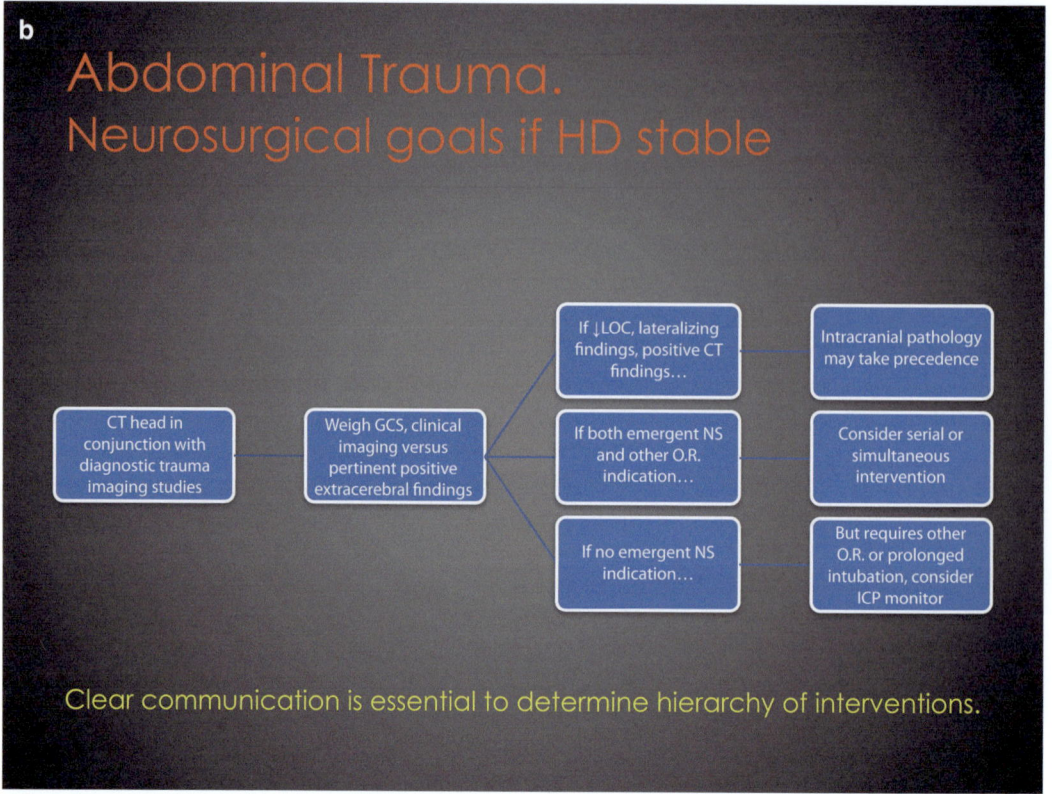

Fig. 1 (continued)

(CPP), becomes the immediate endpoint. Hypoxia, likewise, should be avoided; ventilation strategies should optimize oxygenation and discourage hypercarbia. The presence of coagulopathy may limit invasive intracranial procedures such as placement of an intracranial pressure (ICP) monitor and/or exploratory burr hole coincident with the trauma team intervention. While hyperosmolar therapy might be considered in the absence of ICP monitoring for patients with acute neurologic decline and/or signs of herniation, the introduction of bolus-dose mannitol may exacerbate hypotension and potentially contribute to expansion of an extra-axial hematoma, if present [32]. Hypertonic saline may be an option for osmolar therapy and mini-resuscitation of cerebral blood flow (CBF). Diagnostic CT imaging of the brain should be performed as soon as clinical stability permits to guide further therapy.

If the patient is sufficiently stable (Fig. 1b) to allow for formal diagnostic imaging, CT head should be performed in conjunction with imaging of the cervical spine, chest, abdomen, and pelvis. CT head findings and GCS must be weighed against pertinent positive extracerebral findings. If a patient presents with obvious depressed level of consciousness and/or focal neurologic findings and without evidence of hemodynamic compromise, intracranial pathology may take precedence over other considerations. If, on the other hand, imaging reveals intracranial pathology that does not require emergent craniotomy and it is anticipated that the patient will require surgical intervention by the trauma team and/or a prolonged course of mechanical ventilation, consideration should be given to placement of an ICP monitor. The presence of an invasive monitor allows the anesthesiologist to track and treat ICP, tailor anesthetic to maintain adequate CPP, and, ideally, mitigate the risk of contributing to secondary injury. A sudden and/or precipitous change in measured values may also provide an indication of the patient's evolving intracranial condition. In this setting, clear communication between the neurosurgical and trauma teams is essential to determine the hierarchy for necessary interventions.

Indeed, multiple algorithmic approaches have been proposed for the triage of patients with comorbid intracranial and abdominal injury. Wisner et al. retrospectively reviewed 800 patients presenting with comorbid intracranial and abdominal injuries, noting that the number of cases of therapeutic laparotomy delayed to obtain (what turned out to be) negative imaging of the head exceeded the number of craniotomies delayed by negative laparotomy [33]. Diagnostic peritoneal lavage was advocated for patients with likely cranial and abdominal injuries who were deemed "stable." If nondiagnostic, CT head should follow. If gross blood were present, clinical neurologic status should dictate the order of operations. In the presence of lateralizing signs, CT head should precede operative intervention for abdominal pathology. In the absence of lateralizing signs, Wisner et al. advocated immediate laparotomy if abdominal hemorrhage were suggested by diagnostic studies [33].

In 1995, Huang et al. reported their experience with a system to triage competing intracranial and intra-abdominal pathology [34]. A score of zero to 8 was assigned on the basis of an ultrasound assessment of the presence and relative amount of hemoperitoneum. Patients with a score of greater than or equal to 3 (at least 1000 ml blood present) were taken for urgent laparotomy, with the caveat that pupillary size and light reflex were monitored frequently during the procedure and immediate burr hole exploration performed if indicated. CT imaging was performed prior to consideration of laparotomy if the score was less than 3 (less than 1000 ml blood present). The neurosurgical procedure took precedence if CT head findings provided an indication for emergent intervention, and, in such cases, intra-abdominal pathology was followed with serial ultrasound. Laparotomy was considered simultaneously or immediately post-craniotomy if CT abdomen suggested surgical pathology, the amount of hemoperitoneum increased, the patient developed peritoneal signs, and/or intestinal perforation was documented (by diagnostic peritoneal lavage or gastrografin study).

The concept of simultaneous operative interventions by multiple different surgical teams is perhaps more developed in the military theater; however, there is a small body of literature to suggest a role in the civilian sphere. Moore et al. presented two such cases, accompanied by a review of existing literature [35]. They emphasized the importance of multidisciplinary planning to permit efficient transfer and coordinated care, noting that integration must occur not only across surgical service lines but at other levels of hospital infrastructure as well. They suggested the implementation of protocols to account for the complexity of coordinating multiple surgical setups and the movement of personnel, as well as the incorporation of simulation exercises to train staff in their (sometimes multiple) roles. Hernandez et al. described a hybrid position—with an ipsilateral shoulder roll to permit head turn and extension of the arms at a 90° angle to permit unfettered abdominal access—that would optimize access of multiple teams to permit simultaneous operative interventions at the head and abdomen [36]. The potential benefits of simultaneous interventions include more prompt and efficient care for emergent conditions, resulting in control of life-threatening bleeding and minimization of secondary injury, and the possibility of decreased overall operative and anesthesia time.

Craniofacial Trauma

Given anatomic proximity to the intracranial compartment, one would expect that craniofacial trauma would occur quite frequently in association with TBI. Several published investigations have endeavored to quantify this relationship, not only from the standpoint of simple co-occurrence but also with respect to associations between certain fracture patterns and intracranial injury [37]. The reported incidence of comorbid TBI and facial trauma has been reported variously as 5.4–85% [38–41].

Using a large data set—comprising more than 1.3 million injured individuals—derived from the National Trauma Data Bank (NTDB), Mulligan et al. sought to correlate the incidence of TBI, facial fractures, and cervical spine injury [42]. The incidence of facial fracture was 21.7% in patients with a head injury, 13.5% in patients with cervical spine injury, and 24% in patients presenting with combined TBI and cervical spine injury. Head injury was present in 67.9% of patients with facial fracture, 40.2% of those with cervical spine injury, and 71.5% of those with combined facial fracture and cervical spine injury. The authors note that using NTDB data does potentially skew the data toward a younger, more severely injured population presenting to larger trauma centers.

In a further investigation, the same authors attempted to establish the prevalence of head and/or cervical injuries in conjunction with certain types of facial fractures [43]. The overall prevalence of head injury ranged from 28.7% to 79.9% in the setting of isolated facial bone fracture; with two or more facial fractures, the prevalence of head injury was 65.5–88.7%. Head injuries were identified in 60.2%, 66.7%, and 69% of patients presenting with nasal, orbital floor, and malar area fractures, respectively. While the authors included concussion with loss of consciousness in the category of head injury—potentially overestimating the prevalence—the link between facial fractures and TBI was unambiguous. Lee et al. further defined the relationship between specific facial bone fractures and the likelihood of head injury; their data indicated the greatest association between upper-level facial fractures and TBI [44]. Isolated mandibular fractures and midface fractures associated with mandibular fracture, conversely, were associated with a low incidence of comorbid intracranial injury, suggesting a possible protective effect for such fractures with respect to the brain due to location of the impact.

Alvi and colleagues described the types of co-occurring injuries observed in patients presenting with maxillofacial trauma [45]. Cerebral hematoma was identified in 43.7% of patients in their series; subdural hematoma was the most frequent subtype of hemorrhage (accounting for 41.3% of identified cerebral hematomas). Twenty-four percent required invasive neurosurgical intervention for ICP monitoring and/or evacuation of hematoma. Orbital fracture was the most common associated fracture type (though nasal fracture was seen most commonly in isolation). Pulmonary injury was the next most common injury associated with facial trauma (31.1%). Cervical spine injury occurred in 7.3%. Eleven of 13 recorded deaths were attributed to "neurologic cause."

In a retrospective analysis of 2195 patients with facial fracture, Holrieder et al. identified factors predictive of potential intracranial hemorrhage and/or need for surgical evacuation of hemorrhage [46]. Orbital fracture again was the most common facial fracture present. Extra-facial injuries were present in nearly one-third of patients reviewed; closed head injury (defined as transient loss of consciousness and/or post-traumatic amnesia) was most common, followed by intracranial hemorrhage. The presence of nausea/vomiting (OR 20.2) or seizure (OR 22.1) emerged as the strongest predictive factors for the presence of comorbid intracranial hemorrhage. Only 1.2% of patients without these findings were diagnosed with intracranial hemorrhage. Closed head injury (OR 9.75) and cranial vault fracture (OR 5) were associated with hematoma requiring surgical evacuation.

While the literature suggests that early operative intervention for repair of facial fractures might result in improved functional and aesthetic outcomes, the patient presenting with comorbid severe TBI poses challenges to achieving these goals [47, 48]. Intraoperative factors such as supine positioning, fluid shifts due to blood loss and/or fluid replacement, and vasodilatory anesthetic agents may negatively impact management of the intracranial injury. It remains that the vast majority of facial fractures are not life-threatening and do not require emergent intervention. The incidence of life-threatening hemorrhage in association with facial fractures is fairly low [49–51]. Respiratory distress, however, is more common—whether attributable to anxiety, associated TBI, airway obstruction (from soft tissue swelling or direct trauma to airway), concomitant pulmonary injury, hemorrhagic shock, or any combination of these conditions. The overall rate of endotracheal intubation among patients with facial trauma is commonly cited as 2–6% [37, 52]. However, in the Alvi et al. study, 42% of included patients required intubation, and nearly 15% went on to require tracheostomy.

Tung and colleagues reviewed 1025 cases of facial fracture admitted to their trauma center over a 4-year period to establish the prevalence of comorbid life-threatening injuries [53]. The most common facial bone fractured was the maxilla. Sixty-four patients (6.2%) presented with conditions requiring emergent intervention: 21 requiring craniotomy for intracranial hematoma, 19 with hemorrhagic shock requiring transfusion of greater than 1500 mL, 17 with airway compromise requiring intubation or tracheostomy, and 7 requiring chest tube placement for management of hemopneumothorax. Five patients died: three secondary to intracranial injury and two related to hemorrhagic shock. The authors cautioned that the "grotesque" appearance of certain facial injuries may detract from investigation for additional, potentially life-threatening conditions.

Luce et al. argued that the occurrence of associated life-threatening injuries was predictable on the basis of mechanism of injury and facial fracture pattern [40]. The authors classified the mechanism of injury as high or low velocity, further dividing high-velocity injuries by the nature of the impact: either low (affecting facial bones with low resistance to impact) or high G (affecting facial bones with high resistance to impact). In their series of 1020 patients, only 4% who sustained facial fracture in a low-velocity circumstance had an associated life-threatening injury, while 32% of those involved in high-velocity events so presented. Twenty-one percent in the low-G group and 50% in the high-G group had "major" associated injuries. Fracture of the supraorbital ridge—the area of highest impact tolerance—was associated with "major" injury in 70% of cases (though TBI was not specified). Central nervous system injury was present in 12% of low-G versus 36% of high-G injuries.

Derdyn et al. reviewed 49 patients (from a pool of 4000 TBI patients over 7 years) presenting with co-occurring displaced facial fractures and TBI to determine whether certain clinical and radiographic features might predict poor prognosis, as well as whether these factors might influence the time of surgical repair [54]. Patients requiring—at a minimum—invasive ICP monitor placement were included. Multisystem trauma, low presentation GCS, intracranial hemorrhage, displacement of normally midline cerebral structures, and upper-level facial fractures (i.e., supraorbital rim or frontal sinus) were associated with a statistically significant poorer prognosis. Patients with additional body system trauma, likewise, demonstrated significantly worse outcomes. Such patients should be considered for delayed surgical repair (or no intervention if assessed to have no reasonable functional outcome).

For patients with ICP < 15 mmHg at the time of intervention, the time interval from injury to surgical repair—whether early (0–3 days), middle (4–7 days), or late (>7 days)—did not affect survival. There was, in fact, a trend toward improved survival in the setting of early repair; however, this observation must be tempered by the knowledge that patients selected for early repair were more likely to have presented with more mild TBI. The authors concluded that there appeared to be no contraindication to early surgical repair of facial fractures in this subgroup, but cautioned that the presence of a dural tear and/or cerebrospinal fluid (CSF) leak might mask the patient's true pressure status. The authors suggested ICP monitoring for patients undergoing early facial fracture repair to assist in detection of increased ICP that might occur in the setting of delayed hematoma.

Shibuya et al. reported a perioperative complication rate of 11% in a retrospective cohort of 99 TBI patients (out of 600) with facial fractures requiring surgical repair [55]. The majority of patients presented with injuries involving the middle third of the face. Initial GCS and injury involving the upper one-third of the face correlated with a higher complication rate. ICU monitoring, immediate intubation, ICP monitoring, mannitol use, and phenytoin use were also associated with increased complication rates. The interval between injury and surgical repair of facial fractures was significantly different among groups (longest in the group with major complications). The length of procedure approached statistical significance ($p = 0.07$). In multivariate analysis, the odds of complication increased by 1.3 for each additional hour of surgery and by 1.2 for each additional day to repair. Patients in the major complication (defined as loss of vision, major neurologic injury, death, or severe infection) group, not surprisingly, presented with lower initial GCS, required more intensive ICU therapy for TBI, were not medically stable to proceed with facial fracture repair for longer periods, and required longer operative times to manage more complex craniofacial trauma. These findings are consistent with the data presented by Derdyn et al. suggesting an association between similar factors and worse neurologic outcomes, providing an argument for deferred surgical repair of facial fractures in patients with significant intracranial injury [54].

The development of CSF leak in the setting of facial trauma with comorbid severe TBI adds an additional layer of complexity to the decision-making process regarding the timing of interventions. The onset of clinically evident CSF leak often is delayed in this setting. Cerebral edema or hematoma related to the intracranial injury may effectively tamponade the egress of fluid; rhinorrhea or otorrhea may not become manifest until the period of peak swelling has passed. Likewise, the use of temporary CSF diversion for management of raised ICP also may mask the problem until the drain is "challenged" for removal. Delayed development of a CSF fistula also may occur as a complication of surgical intervention for other traumatic pathology. Certain fracture patterns, coupled with the presence of pneumocephalus, may alert the clinician to anticipate the likelihood of an eventual issue. CSF fistula is estimated to occur in 10–30% of patients presenting with skull base fracture [56–58]. Clinical monitoring for signs and symptoms of a CSF leak is indicated for patients deemed to be at risk. A patient with facial fractures and substantial radiographic pneumocephalus—but no clinically evident leak—might be managed conservatively with lowering of the head of bed (if not at odds with management of the head injury) and the use of supplemental oxygen (100% nonrebreather face mask) to promote dissipation of intracranial air.

Initial conservative management of clinically evident CSF leak may be a reasonable option. Elevation of the head of bed and rhinorrhea precautions (avoidance of nose-blowing, Valsalva maneuvers, use of straws, use of incentive spirometry, coughing with the mouth closed, etc.) alone may prove effective. Investigators have reported spontaneous cessation of CSF rhinorrhea in up to 85% of patients managed nonsurgically over 1 week (and according to one study by Mincy et al., up to 68% within 48 h) [59, 60]. For cases of persistent leakage, consideration may be given to temporary CSF diversion, bearing in mind that the presence of significant intracranial traumatic pathology may provide a contraindication to the use of lumbar cisternal drainage. In such cases, an external ventricular drain may be necessary and provides not only the opportunity for therapeutic drainage of CSF but also for continuous monitoring of ICP. There remains some controversy with respect to what constitutes a reasonable duration of drainage prior to declaring failure.

The incidence of meningitis has been estimated at 7–30% in patients with post-traumatic CSF leak [61]. Two large meta-analyses published in close order (though nearly 20 years ago) offer a window onto the controversy regarding the efficacy of antimicrobial prophylaxis [62, 63]. The first study, published in the infectious diseases literature, suggested no benefit to the use of antibiotics for the prevention of meningitis. The second study, published in the otolaryngology literature, conceded that there was no clear evidence that prophylactic antibiotics were effective; however, the authors continued to advocate for prophylaxis based on the observation that while two of five patients not treated developed meningitis, no patient receiving antibiotics did. A recent Cochrane review on this topic concluded that current evidence does not support the use of prophylaxis and suggests that prophylaxis may alter the normal mucosal flora [64]. The implication is that antibiotic use would simply select out for more resistant organisms if the patient were to develop meningitis at a future time. Source control—with temporary CSF diversion if necessary prior to definitive management—is the preferred management strategy to minimize the risk of infection.

The timing of surgical management is influenced by the goals of intervention in this setting: (1) identification and repair of the dural breach to minimize the risk of ongoing CSF leak and meningitis, (2) elimination of large bony defects that might contribute to brain sag and potential neurologic deficit, (3) reestablishment of normal bony anatomy to minimize the risk of mucocele, and (4) optimization of cosmesis. While early intervention may be desirable to minimize the risk of infection, the management of intracranial injury—including treatment for raised ICP—should take precedence; from a functional standpoint, definitive repair is often deferred for the first 5–7 days post-injury. In their series of 43 patients, Archer and colleagues documented an average time from admission to repair of 5 days [65]. Twelve percent of patients required hematoma evacuation, 12% required external ventricular drainage, and 7% ultimately required ventriculoperitoneal (VP) shunt placement. If a patient requires emergent neurosurgical intervention for decompression and/or evacuation of hematoma, it may be reasonable to consider primary repair of a CSF fistula at that time [66]; however, some have advocated deferral of definitive repair pending restoration of normal physiologic parameters, subsidence of cerebral edema, and better assessment of the patient's neurologic and functional status [56, 67]. A discussion of surgical techniques for skull base reconstruction is beyond the scope of this chapter.

Orthopedic Trauma

More than 60% of traumatic injuries involve the musculoskeletal system, and more than 50% of trauma patients have at least one musculoskeletal injury that, if not life-threatening, might be limb-threatening and/or result in functional impairment. In the European registry cited earlier, the incidence of at least one limb and/or pelvic fracture was 71.3% [14]. Most of these fractures, however, occurred in isolation. Another large European (German) registry cataloguing 24,885 patients recorded the presence of significant extremity injury (defined as AIS ≥ 2) in 56% of polytrauma patients [68]. The average number of fractures was 2.1 per patient. Significant extremity injury was associated with comorbid thoracic trauma, an increased likelihood of transfusion, more operative interventions, and longer ICU, as well as hospital, length of stay. Interestingly, patients who *did not* present with significant extremity injuries were more likely to have a lower GCS score in the field, a more severe brain injury, and higher rates of both in-hospital and 30-day mortality. The authors concluded that the presence of significant extremity injury constituted a distinguishing feature with respect to hospital course and mortality.

The arguments for early definitive fracture fixation are compelling (Fig. 2). Early operative intervention has been linked to reduced inflammation at the fracture site, decreased pain and narcotic use, improved pulmonary mechanics, and earlier mobilization. In the setting of isolated femur injury, early fixation has been associated with decreased morbidity and mortality, as well as lower rates of pulmonary complications such as fat embolization syndrome, venous thromboembolic events (VTE), and acute respiratory distress syndrome (ARDS). Controversy regarding early definitive management weighs these anticipated benefits against the potential for perioperative morbidity related to other injuries, possibly precipitating decompensation in a patient who is incompletely resuscitated or otherwise physiologically compromised.

Indeed, these concerns are paramount in the management of fractures in patients with comorbid severe TBI, where the goal of achieving early surgical fixation may complicate efforts to manage the acute brain injury. Prolonged operative time, blood loss, perioperative fluid requirements, variations in blood pressure under

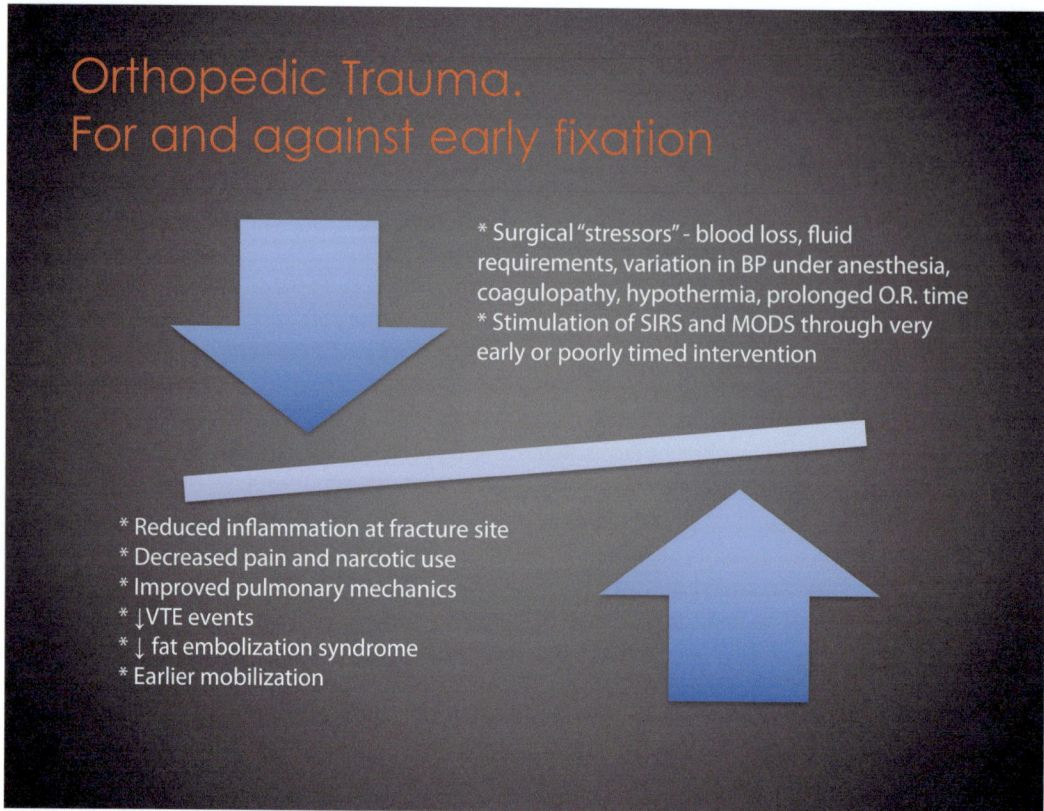

Fig. 2 Pros and cons of early fixation for orthopedic trauma. Abbreviations: *BP* blood pressure, *OR* operating room, *SIRS* systemic inflammatory response syndrome, *MODS* multiple organ dysfunction syndrome, *VTE* venous thromboembolic events

anesthesia, coagulopathy, and hypothermia may threaten a precarious neurologic status, potentially contributing to secondary brain injury. It bears noting that very early, or poorly timed, orthopedics intervention also has been correlated with stimulation of systemic inflammatory response syndrome (SIRS) and multiple organ dysfunction syndrome (MODS)—with potentially lethal consequences [69, 70]. As a result, the goal of early definitive fixation may be accorded lower priority in the multisystem trauma patient.

Practice patterns for the management of orthopedic injuries in the polytrauma patient with severe TBI have evolved over time, influenced by developments within orthopedics as well as advances in general trauma care. The concept of early fracture fixation initially came into favor in the mid-1970s, fueled by an observed reduction

in the rate of fat embolism [71, 72]. A desire to reduce the number of days in traction—associated with considerable medical morbidity—was another driver of this strategy [73]. Other perceived benefits included the ability to mobilize a patient at an earlier time point, decreased stimulation of inflammatory responses (associated with prolonged traction), decreased rates of pulmonary infection, and improved pulmonary hygiene.

Bone et al. investigated complications associated with early (less than 24 h) versus delayed (greater than 48 h) fixation in 178 patients who were subdivided into isolated and multiple injury groups [74]. Not surprisingly, a significantly increased incidence of pulmonary complications, as well as increased ICU and hospital length of stay, was observed when fixation was delayed for patients with multiple injuries. Three patients in the early stabilization group required craniotomy (versus none in the delayed group). On the basis of their data, the authors advocated for early fixation of fractures in multiple trauma patients, suggesting that judicious use of early intubation, ventilator support, and fluid management would limit potential pulmonary complications.

The 1990s was marked by publication of a number of studies offering conflicting conclusions regarding the advisability and safety of early fracture fixation among polytrauma patients with severe TBI. An investigation by Poole et al. found that the risk of pulmonary complications was related more to the severity of comorbid head and chest injuries than to the timing of fracture fixation [75]. The risk of central nervous system complication correlated with the severity of TBI. At the same time, early fracture fixation did not prevent pulmonary morbidity. The group reported higher rates of pneumonia (15.6% versus 3.8%), as well as mortality (4.3% versus 0%), for early versus delayed intervention.

Jaicks and colleagues observed that patients undergoing early fracture fixation both received significantly more fluid at the 24-h and 48-h time points and experienced higher rates of intraoperative hypotension and hypoxia [76]. While the rate of neurologic complication was similar between cohorts, those in the early group demonstrated a lower discharge GCS score. These data raised concerns regarding the "stress" that surgery might place on the injured brain and the potential negative influence on secondary brain injury. Another study reported a mortality rate of 8.9% for patients undergoing early fixation in the setting of TBI—exceeding that for patients with comorbid thoracic injury (4.3%) twofold [77]. The subset of patients with femur fracture and ISS > 15 who underwent fixation in the 2- to 4-day window demonstrated shorter hospital length of stay and lower mortality than those who underwent fixation within the first 24 h after injury.

These findings were challenged a few years later by published data from the R Adams Cowley Shock Trauma Center suggesting no difference in discharge GCS score or central nervous system complications among moderate or severe TBI patients undergoing early fracture fixation for injuries to the pelvis and/or lower extremities [78]. Most patients in this series, in fact, underwent early fixation. No differences were noted with respect to ICU length of stay, the need for ventilator support, or rates of pneumonia and ARDS. Interestingly, the same group also published a retrospective analysis of a series of patients treated preferentially with initial external fixation, comparing them to a cohort of who had undergone early definitive management [79]. The external fixation group, overall, presented with more severe injuries, a significantly higher ISS, a significantly lower GCS, and greater fluid and transfusion requirements. They noted that application of the external fixator device was accomplished with short operative time (mean 35 min) and modest blood loss (90 ml) as compared with intramedullary nailing (mean operating time 135 min with blood loss 400 ml). The average time to definitive stabilization was 4.8 days.

Taking a slightly different approach, Reynolds et al.—in a review of 424 multiple system trauma patients—asserted that delayed fixation was not deleterious with respect to outcome [80]. Observed pulmonary complications correlated more with the severity of thoracic or brain injury than the timing of fixation. The incidence of head injury and, specifically, low GCS was higher in the subgroup undergoing delayed intervention. The authors described two patients who experienced neurologic decline after fracture fixation performed either in the less-than-24-h or 24- to 48-h window, as well as 1 patient with a presentation GCS of 13 who underwent early fixation only to deteriorate neurologically and progress to herniation and death. The latter patient's course underscores the need to weigh the potential risks and benefits of a given procedure for the individual patient.

Brundage et al. took the concept of treatment intervals a step further, stratifying patients with femoral shaft fractures into five groups based on the timing of fracture fixation (less than 24 h to greater than 120 h or no fixation) [81]. Overall, patients undergoing fixation within 24 h experienced the lowest rates of ARDS and pneumonia, as well as the shortest ICU and hospital lengths of stay. Those undergoing interventions in the 2- to 5-day window demonstrated a higher incidence of ARDS, pneumonia, and fat embolism. The subset with comorbid head injury had the highest discharge GCS if fixed within 24 h; however, there was no statistically significant difference in discharge GCS with respect to all other patients who ultimately underwent surgical fixation. This conclusion stands in contrast to the findings of Jaicks et al. [76]. The authors emphasize judicious preoperative resuscitation and stabilization of hemodynamic status as possible factors influencing favorable outcomes.

It follows that a series of management paradigms have emerged from efforts to delineate potential "windows of opportunity" for safe operative intervention in this population (Fig. 3). Pape and colleagues described this evolution in the context of their own practice—transitioning from "early total care" (early, definitive stabilization) to

an "intermediate" model (in which certain *at-risk* patients with multiple injuries underwent early temporary fixation) to "damage control" [79] orthopedics (where early temporary stabilization was followed by conversion to intramedullary nailing)—and discussed the influence of their change in treatment protocols on complications and outcomes [82]. They noted an overall significant decrease in systemic complications over time, regardless of fixation strategy employed. This was attributed to generalized improvement in emergency services over the study period. However, even in the damage control era, intramedullary nailing was associated with a higher rate of ARDS than external fixation. The authors asserted the higher "surgical burden" associated with the procedure as the likely explanation for this observation. They suggested that damage control is a reasonable alternative for patients at high risk for systemic complications. The princi-

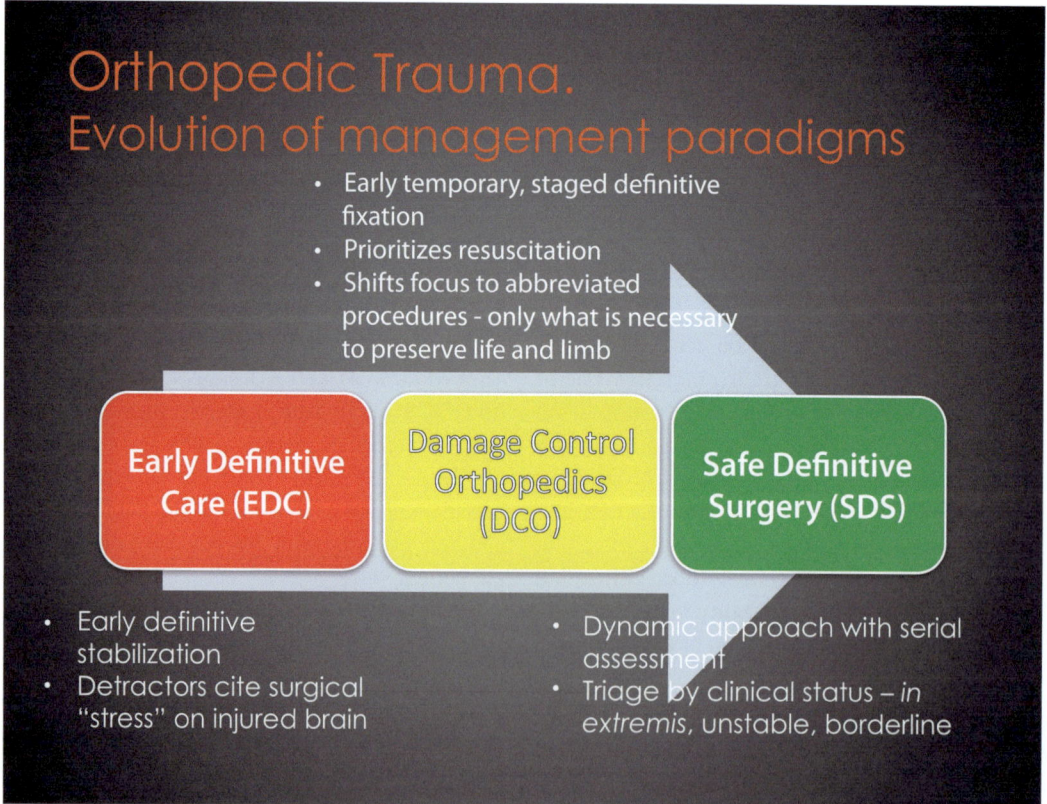

Fig. 3 Evolution of management paradigms for orthopedic trauma

ple underlying damage control is to perform only those interventions required for preservation of life and limb. The article did not specifically address the subset of patients with comorbid TBI, though head injury was cited as the indication for external fixation in 4.2–7.3% of cases over the study period—comparable to shock (3.8–6.3%) and somewhat less frequent than for thoracic or abdominal injury (8.1–17.3%).

Grotz et al. furthered the argument for the damage control paradigm in their 2004 review of the timing and method of fracture stabilization for polytrauma patients with comorbid TBI, suggesting that it is ultimately the severity of the head injury that drives survival and functional outcome [83]. They offered a series of management recommendations for this subpopulation, emphasizing the need to avoid conditions that might exacerbate secondary brain injury and stressing the use of invasive ICP monitoring when clinically appropriate—not only in the ICU but also in the operating room. They advocate an individualized treatment plan for patients deemed physiologically unstable—which may veer toward damage control principles—but also contend that orthopedic injuries should be managed aggressively, with the mind-set that neurologic recovery will occur.

Flierl and colleagues applied principles of immunopathophysiology in an attempt to identify the optimal window for surgical fixation in polytrauma patients with femoral fracture and TBI [84]. The authors tracked and superimposed anticipated inflammatory responses on brain and systemic pathophysiology across time to arrive at a physiologic rationale for damage control orthopedics. Early total care was advocated for patients with a GCS of 14 or 15, unremarkable head CT, and isolated femur fracture. Damage control management was recommended for patients presenting with a GCS of 8 or less and/or CT findings suggestive of significant intracranial injury. Patients presenting with a GCS in the moderate range or GCS in the mild range—with radiographic intracranial pathology—might also benefit from an initial damage control approach. They proposed conversion of damage to definitive intervention for patients

recovering to a GCS of greater than 12 and/or a comatose patient with stable ICP and CPP over a 48-h period.

In short, there is a body of conflicting evidence regarding both the timing and type of intervention for fractures in the setting of multiple system trauma with comorbid fracture and severe TBI. At the same time, multiple studies have demonstrated no significant differences between early and late fixation groups in terms of perioperative morbidity or mortality. The EAST Practice Management Guidelines Work Group (2001) concluded that there was no compelling evidence that early fracture fixation exerted a significant influence on outcome for patients with comorbid TBI of any severity [85]. The work group recommended an individualized approach, taking into consideration elements such as the overall severity of injury (by GCS, radiographic findings, and ICP), the severity of pulmonary dysfunction, hemodynamic status, estimated operative time, and whether the fracture in question is open or closed. A 2014 update to the original document did not specifically address patients with comorbid TBI but did advocate for early (less than 24 h) fracture fixation to reduce mortality, infection, and venous thromboembolic events [86]. This was provided as a "conditional" recommendation, based on a low overall quality of evidence.

Pape and Pfeifer recently have advanced the concept of "safe definitive surgery" (SDS) as a means of reconciling the dichotomy between early total care and damage control surgery [87]. They propose a dynamic approach to the severely injured multiple trauma patient that involves a series of assessments over time. Patients initially are triaged by clinical status: borderline, unstable, or in extremis. Those in the latter group require resuscitation and perhaps surgical hemorrhage control. The likely orthopedic intervention is damage control/traction in this setting, with ongoing reassessment until stable for definitive surgical fixation. Patients in the borderline and unstable groups, likewise, benefit from initial resuscitation but remain potential candidates for operation at secondary and tertiary time points, dependent upon overall clinical stability.

While their model does not specifically reference patients with severe TBI, it provides a reasonable framework to approach decision-making regarding fracture management in this subpopulation. Damage control should be considered as the first stage of intervention when definitive treatment is not feasible or advisable due to critical injury or significant soft tissue injury. Damage control—performing only those procedures required to preserve life or limb—prioritizes resuscitation and correction of coagulopathy, hypothermia, acidosis, and metabolic derangement over early definitive care. This pathway commits the orthopedic surgeon to staged interventions over time and shifts the focus to abbreviated procedures for hemorrhage control, debridement to reduce contamination, and stabilization of bone and soft tissue. External fixation is employed commonly in this setting. The decision regarding the timing of definitive management must be individualized and depends not only on normalization of hemodynamic parameters but also on evidence of improving acidosis, coagulopathy, and hypothermia. Adequate resuscitation also helps ensure that CPP will be maintained in a patient with comorbid TBI. Reasonable clinical benchmarks to consider proceeding with definitive fixation include improvement in neurologic status to a GCS in the mild range (13–15) or, in the persistently comatose patient, stability of ICP (at a level < 20 mmHg) and CPP (at a level > 60 mmHg) for at least 48 h. In either case, serial imaging should demonstrate stability with respect to the size and distribution of hemorrhage. Invasive ICP monitoring, if present, should be maintained during the operative intervention to augment the physiologic information available to anesthesia staff and provide an indication of evolving clinical condition.

Conclusions

Optimal surgical management of extracranial injuries in the polytrauma patient with severe TBI demands a systematic approach to care that emphasizes multidisciplinary involvement and effective communication among team members.

While treating the greatest threat to life initially transcends other considerations, ongoing management requires repeated assessment of relative risks and benefits for a given intervention for the individual patient. Hemodynamic status dictates initial priorities for imaging and management. If hemodynamically stable, the neurologic injury may take precedence. If unstable, the primary focus shifts to resuscitation and damage control. The treating neurosurgeon must take an active role in this process, remaining cognizant of the potential impact of care decisions with respect to the primary (and secondary) brain injury and exercising vigilance about advocating for treatment strategies that are neuroprotective and neuro-proactive. Goals of therapy must be directed toward the dual tasks of preventing multi-organ failure and mitigating secondary brain injury. Where no specific evidence-based recommendations exist to guide treatment decisions, clinical judgment assumes even greater importance. Understanding the interplay between traumatic brain injury and factors relevant to the care of other injured organ systems renders one more adept in navigating discussion of management priorities, as well as risks and benefits of any contemplated interventions.

References

1. Leading causes of death age group 2014 [dataset on the Internet]. National Vital Statistics System, National Center for Health Statistics, CDC; 2016 [cited 2016 Dec 26]. Available from: https://www.cdc.gov/injury/wisqars/leadingcauses.html
2. Faul M, Xu L, Wald MM, Coronado VG. Traumatic brain injury in the United States: emergency department visits, hospitalizations, and deaths: Atlanta, Centers for Disease Control and Prevention, National Center for Injury Prevention and Control; 2010.
3. Sauaia A, Moore FA, Moore EE, Haenel J, Read R, Lezotte D. Early predictors of postinjury multiple organ failure. Arch Surg. 1994;129:39–45.
4. Border JR, LaDuca J, Seibel R. Priorities in the management of the patient with polytrauma. Prog Surg. 1975;14:84–120.
5. Tscherne H, Oestern HJ, Sturm JA. Stress tolerance of patients with multiple injuries and its significance for operative care [in German]. Langenbecks Arch Chir. 1984;364:71–7.

6. Baker SP, O'Neill B, Haddon W, Long WB. The injury severity score: a method for describing patients with multiple injuries and evaluating emergency care. J Trauma. 1974;14:187–96.

7. Butcher N, Enninghorst N, Sisak K, Balogh ZJ. The definition of polytrauma: variable interrater versus intrarater agreement – a prospective international study among trauma surgeons. J Trauma. 2013;74:884–9.

8. Lefering R, Paffrath T, Linker R, Bouillon B, Neugebauer EAM, German Society for Trauma. Head injury and outcome – what influence do concomitant injuries have? J Trauma. 2008;65:1036–44.

9. Sumann G, Kampfl A, Wenzel V, Schobersberger W. Early intensive care unit intervention for trauma care: what alters the outcome? Curr Opin Crit Care. 2002;8:587–92.

10. McMahon C, Yates D, Campbell F, Hollis S, Woodford M. Unexpected contribution of moderate traumatic brain injury to death after major trauma. J Trauma. 1999;47(5):891.

11. Regel G, Lobenhoffer P, Grotz M, Pape H-C, Lehmann U, Tscherne H. Treatment results of patients with multiple trauma: an analysis of 3406 cases treated between 1972 and 1991 at a German level I trauma center. J Trauma. 1995;38:70–8.

12. Gross T, Schüepp M, Attenberger C, Pargger H, Amsler F. Outcomes in polytraumatized patients with and without brain injury. Acta Anaesthesiol Scand. 2012;56:1163–74.

13. Zeckey C, Hildebrand F, Pape H-C, Mommsen P, Panzica M, Zelle BA, et al. Head injury in polytrauma – is there an effect on outcome more than 10 years after the injury? Brain Inj. 2011;25:551–9.

14. Lecky FE, Bouamra O, Woodford M, Alexandrescu R, O'Brien SJ. Epidemiology of polytrauma. In: Pape H-C, Peitzman AB, Schwab CW, Giannoudis PV, editors. Damage control management in the polytrauma patient. Berlin: Springer Science + Business Media, LLC; 2010. p. 13–23. https://doi.org/10.1007/978-0-387-89508-6_2.

15. The ATLS Subcommittee, American College of Surgeons' Committee on Trauma, International ATLS Working Group. Advanced trauma life support (ATLS®): the ninth edition. J Trauma Acute Care Surg. 2013;74:1363–6.

16. Tisherman SA, Barie P, Bokhari F, Bonadies J, Daley B, Diebel L, et al. Resuscitation endpoints. J Trauma. 2004;57:898–912.

17. Ransahoff RM. The chemokine system in neuroinflammation: an update. J Infect Dis. 2002;186(Suppl 2):S152–6.

18. Stahel PF, Mc M-K, Kossmann T. The role of the complement system in traumatic brain injury. Brain Res Rev. 1998;27:243–56.

19. Gebhard F, Huber-Lang M. Polytrauma – pathophysiology and management principles. Langenbeck's Arch Surg. 2008;393:825–31.

20. Stahel PF, Smith WR, Moore EF. Role of biological modifiers regulating the immune response after trauma. Injury. 2007;38:1409–22.

21. Piek J, Chesnut RM, Marshall LF, van Berkum-Clark M, Klauber MR, Blunt BA, et al. Extracranial complications of severe head injury. J Neurosurg. 1992;77:901–7.

22. Chesnut RM, Marshall LF, Klauber MR, Blunt BA, Baldwin N, Eisenberg HM, et al. The role of secondary brain injury in determining outcome from severe head injury. J Trauma. 1993;34:216–22.

23. Stocchetti N, Furlan A, Volta F. Hypoxemia and arterial hypotension at the accident scene in head injury. J Trauma. 1996;40:764–7.

24. Wald SL, Shackford SR, Fenwick J. The effect of secondary insults on mortality and long-term disability after severe head injury in a rural region without a trauma system. J Trauma. 1993;34:377–81.

25. Chi JH, Knudson M, Vassar MJ, McCarthy MC, Shapiro MB, Mallet S, et al. Prehospital hypoxia affects outcome in patients with traumatic brain injury: a prospective multicenter study. J Trauma. 2006;61:1134–41.

26. Jeremitsky E, Omert L, Dunham CM, Protetch J, Rodriguez A. Harbingers of poor outcome the day after severe brain injury: hypothermia, hypoxia, and hypoperfusion. J Trauma. 2003;54:312–9.

27. Bouma GJ, Muizelaar JP. Cerebral blood flow, cerebral blood volume, and cerebrovascular reactivity after severe head injury. J Neurotrauma. 1992;9(Suppl 1):S333–48.

28. Marion D, Darby J, Yonas H. Acute regional cerebral blood flow changes caused by severe head injuries. J Neurosurg. 1991;74:407–13.

29. Rose J, Valtonen S, Jennett B. Avoidable factors contributing to death after head injury. Br Med J. 1977;2:615.

30. Certo TF, Rogers FB, Pilcher DB. Review of care of fatally injured patients in a rural state: five year follow up. J Trauma. 1983;23:559–65.

31. Foley RW, Harris LS, Pilcher DB. Abdominal injuries in automobile injuries. J Trauma. 1977;23:611–5.

32. Carney N, Totten AM, O'Reilly C, Ullman JS, Hawryluk GW, Bell MJ, et al. Guidelines for the management of severe traumatic brain injury, fourth edition. Neurosurgery. 2017;80(1):6–15.

33. Wisner DH, Victor NS, Holcroft JW. Priorities in the management of multiple trauma: intracranial versus intra-abdominal injury. J Trauma. 1993;35:271–8.

34. Huang M-S, Shih H-C, Wu J-K, Ko T-J, Fan V-K, Pan R-G, et al. Urgent laparotomy versus emergency craniotomy for multiple trauma with head injury patients. J Trauma. 1995;38:154–7.

35. Moore JM, Thomas PAW, Gruen RL, Rosenfled CP. Simultaneous multisystem surgery: an important capability for the civilian trauma hospital. Clin Neurol Neurosurg. 2016;148:13–6.

36. Hernandez AM, Roguski M, Qiu RS, Shepard MJ, Riesenburger RI. Surgeons' perspectives on optimal patient positioning during simultaneous cranial procedures and exploratory laparotomy. South Med J. 2013;106:679–83.

37. Gwyn PP, Carraway JH, Horton CE, Adamson JE, Mladick RA. Facial fractures: associated injuries and complications. Plast Reconstr Surg. 1971;47:225–30.

38. Lim LH, Lam LK, Moore MH, Trott JA, David DJ. Associated injuries in facial fractures: review of 839 patients. Br J Plast Surg. 1993;46(8):635.

39. Gautam V, Leonard EM. Bony injuries in association with minor head injury: lessons for improving the diagnosis of facial fractures. Injury. 1994;25:47–9.

40. Luce EA, Tubb TD, Moore AM. Review of 1000 major facial fractures and associated injuries. Plast Reconstr Surg. 1979;63:26–30.

41. Sinclair D, Schwartz M, Gruss JS, McLellan B. A retrospective review of the relationship between facial fractures, head injuries, and cervical spine injuries. J Emerg Med. 1988;6:109–12.

42. Mulligan RP, Friedman JA, Mahabir RC. A nationwide review of the associations among cervical spine injuries, head injuries, and facial fractures. J Trauma. 2010;68:587–92.

43. Mulligan RP, Mahabir RC. The prevalence of cervical spine injury, head injury, or both with isolated and multiple craniomaxillofacial fractures. Plast Reconstr Surg. 2010;126:1647–51.

44. Lee KF, Wagner LK, Lee YE, Suh JH, Lee SR. The impact-absorbing effects of facial fractures in closed head injuries: an analysis of 210 patients. J Neurosurg. 1987;66:542–7.

45. Alvi A, Doherty T, Lewen G. Facial fractures and concomitant injuries in trauma patients. Laryngoscope. 2003;113:102–6.

46. Hohlrieder M, Hinterhoelzl J, Ulmer H, Lang C, Hackl W, Kampfl A, et al. Traumatic intracranial hemorrhages in facial fracture patients: review of 2,195 patients. Intensive Care Med. 2003;29:1095–100.

47. Manson PN, Crawley WA, Yaremchuk MJ, Rochman GM, Hoopes JE, French JH. Midface fractures: advantages of immediate extended open reduction and bone grafting. Plast Reconstr Surg. 1985;76:1–12.

48. Gruss JS, Mackinnon SE. Complex maxillary fractures: role of buttress reconstruction and immediate bone grafts. Plast Reconstr Surg. 1986;78:9–22.

49. Thaller SR, Beal SL. Maxillofacial trauma; a potentially fatal injury. Ann Plast Surg. 1991;27(3):281.

50. Ardekian L, Samet N, Shoshani Y, Taicher S. Life-threatening bleeding following maxillofacial trauma. J Craniomaxillofac Surg. 1993;21(8):336.

51. Murakami WT, Davidson TM, Marshall LF. Fatal epistaxis in craniofacial trauma. J Trauma. 1983;23:57–61.

52. Busuito MJ, Smith DJ, Robinson MC. Mandibular fractures in an urban trauma center. J Trauma. 1986;26(9):826.

53. Tung T-C, Tseng W-S, Chen C-T, Lai J-P, Chen Y-R. Acute life-threatening injuries in facial fracture patients: a review of 1,025 patients. J Trauma. 2000;49:420–4.

54. Derdyn C, Persing JA, Broaddus WC, Delashaw JB, Jane J, Levine PA, et al. Craniofacial trauma: and assessment of risk related to timing of surgery. Plast Reconstr Surg. 1990;86:238–45.

55. Shibuya TY, Karam AM, Doerr T, Stachler RJ, Zormeier M, Mathog RH, et al. Facial fracture repair

56. Yilmazlar S, Arslan E, Kocaeli H, Dogan S, Aksoy K, Korfali E, et al. Cerebrospinal fluid leakage complicating skull base fractures: analysis of 81 cases. Neurosurg Rev. 2006;29:64–71.

57. Brodie H, Thompson TC. Management of complications from 820 temporal bone fractures. Am J Otol. 1997;18:188–97.

58. Lewin W. Cerebrospinal fluid rhinorrhea in nonmissile head injuries. Clin Neurosurg. 1966;12:237–52.

59. Bell RB, Dierks EJ, Homer L, Potter BE. Management of cerebrospinal fluid leak associated with craniomaxillofacial trauma. J Oral Maxillofac Surg. 2004;62:676–84.

60. Mincy JE. Posttraumatic cerebrospinal fluid fistula of the frontal fossa. J Trauma. 1966;6:618–22.

61. Friedman JA, Ebersold MJ, Quast LM. Persistent posttraumatic cerebrospinal fluid leakage. Neurosurg Focus. 2000;9:e1–5.

62. Brodie H. Prophylactic antibiotics for posttraumatic cerebrospinal fluid fistulae. A meta-analysis. Arch Otolaryngol Head Neck Surg. 1997;123:749–52.

63. Villalobos T, Arango C, Kubilis P, Rathore M. Antibiotic prophylaxis after basilar skull fractures: a meta-analysis. Clin Infect Dis. 1998;27:364–9.

64. Ratilal BO, Costa J, Pappamikail L, Sampaio C. Antibiotic prophylaxis for preventing meningitis in patients with basilar skull fractures. Cochrane Database Syst Rev. 2015;(4):CD004884.

65. Archer JB, Sun H, Bonney PA, Zhao YD, Hiebert JC, Sanclement JA, et al. Extensive traumatic anterior skull base fractures with cerebrospinal fluid leak: classification and repair techniques using combined vascularized tissue flaps. J Neurosurg. 2016;124: 647–56.

66. Ziu M, Savage JG, Jimenez DF. Diagnosis and treatment of cerebrospinal fluid rhinorrhea following accidental traumatic anterior skull base fractures. Neurosurg Focus. 2012;32:e3.

67. Rocchi G, Caroli I, Belli E, Salvati M, Cimatti M, Delfini R. Severe craniofacial fractures with frontobasal involvement and cerebrospinal fluid fistula: indications for surgical repair. Surg Neurol. 2005;63:559–64.

68. Banerjee M, Bouillon B, Shafizadeh S, Paffrath T, Lefering R, Wafaisade A, German Trauma Registry Group. Epidemiology of extremity injuries in multiple trauma patients. Injury. 2013;44:1015–21.

69. Giannoudis PV. Surgical priorities in damage control in polytrauma. J Bone Joint Surg. 2003;85-B:478–83.

70. Pape H-C, Giannoudis P, Krettek C. The timing of fracture treatment in polytrauma patients: relevance of damage control orthopedic surgery. Am J Surg. 2002;183:622–9.

71. Riska E, Von Bonsdorf H, Hakkinen S. Prevention of fat embolism by early internal fixation of fractures in patients with multiple injuries. Injury. 1976;8:110–6.

72. Riska E, Nyllynen P. Fat embolism in patients with multiple injuries. J Trauma. 1982;22:891–4.

73. Seibel R, LaDuca J, Hassett JM, Babikian G, Mills B, Border DO, et al. Blunt multiple trauma (ISS 36), femur traction, and the pulmonary failure, septic state. Ann Surg. 1985;202:283–95.

74. Bone LB, Johnson KD, Weigelt J, Schienberg R. Early versus delayed stabilization of femoral fractures. J Bone Joint Surg. 1989;71:336–40.

75. Poole GV, Miller JD, Agnew SG, Griswold JA. Lower extremity fracture fixation in head-injured patients. J Trauma. 1992;32:654–9.

76. Jaicks RR, Cohn SM, Moller BA. Early fracture fixation may be deleterious after head injury. J Trauma. 1997;42:1–5.

77. Fakhry SM, Rutledge R, Dahners LE, Kessler D. Incidence, management, and outcome of femoral shaft fracture: a statewide population-based analysis of 2805 adult patients in a rural state. J Trauma. 1994;37:255–60.

78. Scalea T, Scott JD, Brumback RJ, Burgess AR, Mitchell KA, Kufera JA, et al. Early fracture fixation may be "just fine" after head injury: no difference in central nervous system outcomes. J Trauma. 1999;46:839–46.

79. Scalea TM, Boswell SA, Scott JD, Mitchell KA, Kramer ME, Pollack AN. External fixation as a bridge to intramedullary nailing for patients with multiple injuries and with femur fractures: damage control orthopedics. J Trauma. 2000;48:613–23.

80. Reynolds MA, Richardson JD, Spain DA, et al. Is the timing of fracture fixation important for the patient with multiple trauma? Ann Surg. 1995;222:470–81.

81. Brundage S, McGhan R, Jurkovich GJ, Mack C, Maier RV. Timing of femur fracture fixation: effect on outcome in patients with thoracic and head injuries. J Trauma. 2002;52:299–307.

82. Pape H-C, Hildebrand F, Pertschy S, Zelle B, Garapati R, Grimme K, et al. Changes in management of femoral shaft fractures in polytrauma patients: from early total care to damage control orthopedic surgery. J Trauma. 2002;53:452–62.

83. Grotz MRW, Giannoudis PV, Pape H-C, Allami MK, Dinopoulos H, Kretteck C. Traumatic brain injury and stabilization of long bone fractures: an update. Injury. 2004;35:1077–86.

84. Flierl MA, Stoneback JW, Beauchanp KM, Hak DJ, Morgan SJ, Smith WR, et al. Femur shaft fracture fixation in head-injured patients: when is the right time? J Orthop Trauma. 2010;24:107–14.

85. Dunham CM, Bosse MJ, Clancy TV, Cole FJ, Coles MJM, Knuth T, et al. Practice management guidelines for the optimal timing of long-bone fracture stabilization in trauma patients: the EAST practice management guidelines work group. J Trauma. 2001;50:958–67.

86. Gandhi RR, Overton T, Haut ER, Lau B, Vallier HA, Rohs T, et al. Optimal timing of femur fracture stabilization in polytrauma patients–update. J Trauma. 2014;77:787–95.

87. Pape H-C, Pfeifer R. Safe definitive orthopedic surgery (SDS); repeated assessment for tapered application of early definitive care and damage control? Injury. 2015;46:1–3.

Optimal Treatment of Dysautonomia

Gabriel N. Friedman, Ziev B. Moses, Ian Tafel, and William B. Gormley

Introduction

Summary of the Problem and Context Relative to Traumatic Brain Injury

Dysautonomia following traumatic brain injury (TBI) is a clinical syndrome that has been recognized for decades but has recently begun receiving increased awareness due to the severity of its symptoms and its common prevalence in the post-TBI patient population [1]. This syndrome has been referred to by at least 31 different names in the literature including clinical descriptors such as "autonomic storming," "paroxysmal autonomic instability with dystonia," and "central autonomic instability" in addition to other terminologies such as "acute midbrain syndrome" or "diencephalic seizures" that have reflected putative structural or mechanistic hypotheses [2]. The wide diversity in nomenclature has been considered a crucial obstacle to producing more precise diagnostic and treatment guidelines [3]. In response, a consensus group of experts in the field met in 2014 in order to develop uniform nomenclature and diagnostic guidelines and settled on the term "paroxysmal sympathetic hyperactivity" (PSH) to describe this syndrome (which will be used throughout the remainder of this chapter) [4].

The clinical features of PSH include symptoms related to sympathetic overactivity including tachycardia, hypertension, hyperhidrosis, hyperthermia, and tachypnea, in addition to muscle hypertonia with decerebrate or decorticate posturing, often occurring in short intervals with abrupt onset and offset [5]. These paroxysmal episodes are thought to be sometimes triggered by stimuli such as pain, turning, stretching, constipation, urinary retention, or endotracheal suctioning [6]. There are thought to be three stages to PSH, with patients in the first stage displaying relatively few clinical manifestations. Following the withdrawal of sedation, patients in the second stage have been found to experience dysautonomia for an average

G. N. Friedman, BA
Department of Neurosurgery, Harvard Medical School, Massachusetts General Hospital, Boston, MA, USA
e-mail: Gabriel_Friedman@hms.harvard.edu

Z. B. Moses, MD · I. Tafel, MD
W. B. Gormley, MD, MPH, MBA (✉)
Department of Neurosurgery, Brigham and Women's Hospital, Boston, MA, USA
e-mail: ZMOSES@partners.org; itafel@partners.org; wgormley@bwh.harvard.edu

© Springer International Publishing AG, part of Springer Nature 2018
S. D. Timmons (ed.), *Controversies in Severe Traumatic Brain Injury Management*,
https://doi.org/10.1007/978-3-319-89477-5_14

of 74 days; and in the third stage, dysautonomic symptoms abate, with the exception of spasticity and dystonia, which remain for a longer course [5].

One particular challenge of diagnosing PSH is that many of the symptoms overlap with other conditions often seen in the acute post-TBI setting. For example, intermittent hypertension and tachypnea can be seen with pain, seizures, or elevated intracranial pressure, while fever, diaphoresis, and tachypnea can be seen with infection, pulmonary embolus, or drug reactions [7]. With this wide range of symptoms that are commonly seen in the neurosurgical intensive care unit (ICU), there is a considerable differential diagnosis for PSH that also includes neuroleptic malignant syndrome, malignant hyperthermia, autonomic dysreflexia, central fever, and agitation [8].

There are two major manifestations of PSH that have been categorized in the literature: one is a short-duration syndrome that lasts for around a week and is typically seen in the neurosurgical ICU, and the other is a longer-term condition that can continue for months [2]. These varying time courses are responsible for the widely divergent reported incidences that typically range from around 7 to 33%. While as many as 90% of post-TBI patients in the acute setting can show signs of autonomic arousal [9], it is thought that the most accurate estimate for the incidence of patients who meet the rigorous diagnostic criteria for chronic PSH is around 8–12% [10, 11], while the shorter-duration syndrome may be seen in roughly 24–33% of cases [10, 12]. Given the high incidence of TBI in the general population on an annual basis [13], PSH represents a substantial and often unrecognized disease burden.

While the precise origins of autonomic dysregulation following TBI is unknown, there are several theories that have been put forth to explain its possible etiology. The earliest investigations into this syndrome posited that the occurrence of paroxysmal sympathetic activity could result from an epileptogenic focus [14], consistent with the brief and abrupt nature of seizure activity. However, electroencephalography (EEG) analysis of what were believed to be diencephalic seizures has not revealed epileptiform activity [15],

and treatment with anticonvulsive medication has not been effective, suggesting an alternative mechanistic link [16]. An alternative theory suggests that dysautonomia following TBI is a disconnection syndrome caused by a loss of contact between areas such as the upper brainstem and diencephalon to the anterior hypothalamus, representing a disruption of communication between autonomic centers of the brain in the diencephalon and connections to cortical, subcortical, or brainstem regions that are involved in autonomic regulation [8, 17]. A more recent proposal, which contrasts with this conventional disconnection theory, is the excitatory/inhibitory ratio (EIR) model. This theory advances the notion that with brain injury, diencephalic processes that normally mediate an inhibitory influence on spinal afferents become damaged, producing an "allodynic tendency" that, in essence, overreacts to normally non-nociceptive stimuli and subsequently results in a positive feedback loop that manifests as sympathetic overactivity [1]. One advantage of the EIR model over the conventional disconnection theory is that the latter requires that an excitatory pathway from the upper brainstem to the diencephalon remains undamaged (which may be unlikely given that brainstem damage is often associated with PSH), while the EIR theory does not require any particular pathway to remain intact [1]. Nevertheless, a significant amount of investigation remains in order to fully understand the origins of this clinical syndrome.

Even while the etiology of PSH remains unknown, at a pathophysiological level, it is believed that the mechanism of PSH is related to elevated catecholamine levels, which is a common finding following TBI [18]. For example, one analysis found a strong association between Glasgow Coma Scale (GCS) and norepinephrine elevation, with patients in a coma having norepinephrine levels up to seven times the normal level [18]. In addition to producing dysautonomic symptoms, these elevated levels of circulating catecholamines can also produce harmful extracranial complications including arrhythmias and pulmonary edema [19] in addition to immunosuppression as a result of increases in interleukin pathways that dampen monocyte function and suppress the immune response [20]. Thus, taken together, patients with PSH following TBI are in a particularly precarious state of health with the potential for numerous complications and an impeded path to recovery.

Indeed, several studies have found correlations between severity of injury and the extent of autonomic symptoms experienced following TBI. Patients who suffer from PSH have been found to have the most serious brain injuries as assessed via the GCS and Disability Rating Scale (DRS) at 1 week [10]. Additional studies have shown that patients who met the criteria for dysautonomia had a strong association with other factors that indicated a more complicated recovery including admission with a GCS of 3, spending a longer period of time in a coma, requiring longer periods of mechanical ventilation, and experiencing increased comorbidity such as decubitus ulcers and deep venous thromboses [11]. As a result of these complications, it is unsurprising that patients with PSH have longer hospital stays and increased risk for infection and thus represent an increased utilization of healthcare resources [10].

In addition to these more direct measures of medical complications, there is also a range of other comorbidities that have been found to result from dysautonomia following TBI. Extreme hypermetabolism in the setting of sympathetic storms has been reported [21], which may account for observations of weight loss up to 25% during the acute recovery phase [10]. Malnourishment that arises from this hypermetabolism can place patients at risk of other complications such as critical illness neuropathy [22]. Dystonic posturing, which is a frequent occurrence during paroxysmal episodes, can heighten the risk of pain and contractures [22]. Furthermore, hyperthermia following TBI has been found to predict poor outcomes [23]. It has also been suggested that autonomic instability during rehabilitation may cause disruptions to a physical therapy regimen [24]. In summary, while PSH has been recognized in various forms going back decades, it has only been in the last 10–20 years that its full impact has been elucidated. Given that patients who experi-

ence TBI are already among the most complex patients seen in the acute hospital setting, PSH represents a serious complication that is made even more difficult to manage due to limited diagnostic and treatment guidelines.

Evidence Bases for Diagnosis, Prognosis, and Treatment

Diagnosis

As discussed previously, diagnosis of PSH has remained difficult due to a high initial prevalence of autonomic symptoms, diverse nomenclature, dearth of large case series, and until 2014, the absence of formal diagnostic criteria. Despite precise diagnostic guidelines, there have been several different approaches used to help determine which patients have either developed PSH or are most at risk of developing the syndrome. These approaches have generally relied on assessing patients for a combination of clinical symptoms that together meet a threshold for diagnosis of PSH, while other groups have looked at autonomic parameters themselves to determine whether a rigorous investigation of physiological data can help differentiate those with PSH from those without.

Even with the limited number of large patient studies, several groups have attempted to develop formal diagnostic criteria that can be used to determine which patients should be treated for PSH. Altogether there have been nine different sets of criteria developed for the purpose of diagnosing [25]. These criteria are generally based both on the presence of specific symptoms and the number of total autonomic symptoms present. For example, virtually all sets of criteria proposed use clinical features such as elevated heart rate, blood pressure, respiratory rate, sweating, temperature, and motor activity as inclusion criteria for a diagnosis of PSH. There is general consensus that patients must exhibit at least five of these manifestations in order to be considered undergoing paroxysmal autonomic hyperactivity [5, 26]. Several studies also include other less commonly seen clinical features such as agitation, mydriasis, and flushing as other signs that can be used to classify autonomic dysfunction [8, 26, 27].

In addition to clinical features, other quantitative and qualitative measures have been proposed for a potential diagnostic criteria, including having episodes that are paroxysmal in nature [5, 26, 28] and having a certain frequency of episodes per day [8, 26] in addition to episodes that last for a certain number of days [8, 27, 28]. The combination of these findings has led to the development of a Consensus Working Group in 2014, which created an assessment measure yielding an 11-point probabilistic diagnostic scale that has been designed for both clinical and research settings (see Table 1) [4]. This clinical feature scale was then correlated with patients admitted for TBI and found that patients who met clinical criteria for PSH had higher scores than patients who did not have features of PSH [4].

Another approach that has been used in an effort to improve diagnostic accuracy has been to physiologically probe autonomic parameters of TBI patients who may be displaying signs of autonomic dysregulation. Heart rate variability (HRV) key measure has often been found to closely correlate with dysautonomia. Adding further credence to the notion of PSH as a paroxysmal phenomenon in the setting of painful stimuli, one study investigating HRV in the setting of nociceptive stimuli found that patterns of HRV and event-rated heart rate could be used to differentiate a group of patients with dysautonomia in the setting of the stimuli, but not at rest [6]. The authors suggest that this finding of over-responsiveness to nociceptive stimuli could be used as a clinical algorithm to help quickly screen or identify patients with dysautonomia. In addition to providing a quantifiable method of distinguishing patients with dysautonomia, this

Table 1 The paroxysmal sympathetic hyperactivity assessment measure (PSH-AM)—a diagnostic scale to determine the probability of PSH. Adapted from Consensus Working Group [4]

Clinical feature scale (CFS)					
Clinical feature	**0 point**	**1 point**	**2 points**	**3 points**	**Score**
Heart rate (beats per minute)	<100	100–119	120–139	≥140	
Respiratory rate (breaths per minute)	<18	18–23	24–29	≥30	
Systolic blood pressure (mm hg)	<140	140–159	160–179	≥180	
Temperature (°C)	<37	37–37.9	38–38.9	≥39.0	
Posturing during episodes	None	Mild	Moderate	Severe	
Sweating	None	Mild	Moderate	Severe	
CFS subtotal					
Diagnosis likelihood tool (DLT)					
Add 1 point for each feature present					**Score**
Simultaneously occurring clinical features (see above list)					
The nature of episodes is paroxysmal					
Normally non-painful stimuli evoke sympathetic over-reactivity					
Features continue for 3 or more consecutive days					
Features continue for 2 or more weeks after brain injury					
Features continue despite treatment of alternative differential diagnoses					
Medications are administered to decrease sympathetic features					
Two episodes or more daily					
Parasympathetic features are absent during episodes					
An absence of other presumed causes of features during episodes					
Antecedent-acquired brain injury					
DLT subtotal					
Combined total (CFS + DLT scores)					
Likelihood of PSH				Unlikely	<8
				Possible	8–16
				Probable	≥17

study also provided evidence that this syndrome is a result of an inability to control overactivity rather than a baseline hyperreactivity given that the measures were similar at rest. These findings are consistent with other research that has shown increases in heart rate and blood pressure following endotracheal intubation in TBI patients in the ICU [29]. Finally, a more comprehensive analysis of TBI patients in a persistent vegetative state with dysautonomia showed significantly divergent measures of autonomic parameters for these patients including a "non-dipper" blood pressure pattern (i.e., blood pressure does not decrease overnight), higher values of heart rate and blood pressure, and a decrease in the difference between day-night blood pressure and heart rate [30]. Altogether, these findings demonstrate that in addition to simply correlating clinical symptoms, autonomic parameters themselves may also be useful in order to elucidate which patients are at risk for PSH.

As an adjunct to these analyses that have taken place in the acute care setting, there have also been some attempts to investigate longer-term manifestations of PSH as well as other autonomic disturbances. Examining HRV variability at a 5-year follow-up in patients with PSH found that patients with dysautonomia following TBI had sympathetic overactivity in response to a painful stimulus (i.e., a botulinum injection for spasticity) when compared to TBI and non-TBI patients who did not suffer from dysautonomia [9]. As more time passed from their injuries, patients demonstrated decreased sympathetic overactivity, suggesting that the syndrome may diminish over time. Another long-term study described eight TBI patients without prior autonomic symptoms who later presented with symptoms resembling the autonomic disorder of postural orthostatic tachycardia syndrome (POTS). They were examined with tilt table testing, and all met the diagnostic criteria for the syndrome [31]. This appears to be a relatively late autonomic complication of TBI, and it likely differs from the long-term outcomes seen with patients initially diagnosed with PSH.

One final approach to diagnosis has been via radiological imaging, although the limited number of investigations in this area has led to a mixture of findings that precludes more conclusive results. While one study described an association between focal, intraparenchymal lesions and the development of dysautonomia [26], several other analyses have found a correlation between diffuse axonal injury (DAI) and PSH [5, 11]—findings that have also been corroborated by case reports [16, 32]. Thus, in the meantime, the balance of evidence favors an association of DAI with the development of autonomic dysfunction, although more analysis will be required to fully establish this link.

Prognosis

Patients with PSH often have an unclear prognosis, which is further complicated by the fact that recovery is often unpredictable for TBI patients, especially in the setting of autonomic dysfunction. Patients who meet the diagnostic criteria for PSH often have more complicated hospital stays because they require longer ICU and hospital stays, placing them at a further risk for other inpatient comorbidities. Patients with dysautonomia spend more days in a coma and require longer periods of mechanical ventilation, and so they typically take a longer amount of time to reach rehabilitation milestones compared with patients who are intact from an autonomic perspective [11]. The differences are especially notable in the short term. One study of 79 TBI patients found that those with autonomic dysfunction had a worse GCS and Disability Rating Scale score at both short and intermediate time points, in addition to a poorer performance on the Glasgow Outcome Scale (GOS) at the intermediate 6-month time point [10]. Nevertheless, it appears that the biggest differences may be seen earlier on, and there may be less severe long-term effects as time goes on. For example, one study found that patients with dysautonomia had a significantly lower level of consciousness when discharged from the ICU and significantly lower GCS score at time of discharge compared with control patients [26]. However, after 12 months of follow-up, the GCS appeared to be similar for both dysautonomic and control patients [26].

Corroborating these findings, an analysis of TBI patients both with and without PSH found that on admission to a rehabilitation hospital, these patients only differed significantly in terms of the Functional Independence Measure (FIM) and at discharge had similar scores on the DRS, FIM, and GOS-E. Interestingly, only patients with PSH (as opposed to non-PSH) showed a statistically significant improvement on the GOS-E, of all the measures examined [33]. This investigation showed a trend toward PSH patients spending a longer time in rehabilitation (consistent with other reports), suggesting that a longer time in rehab may allow these patients to achieve improvement in function comparable with control patients between the time of discharge from the rehabilitation setting and within a year following injury.

Even while outcomes may eventually become comparable with other TBI patients, there are still significant challenges for patients with PSH. One of the longest follow-ups in patients with dysautonomia (who were treated with intrathecal baclofen therapy [IBT]) found that only 12% of TBI patients with dysautonomia had attained a good long-term recovery (GOS 1), which is somewhat lower than measures of good outcomes found in other generalized studies of patients without dysautonomia [24]. These results may be confounded by the fact that PSH tends to occur in patients with the most severe injuries, and so to the extent that poorer outcomes have been found, they may be the result of the effects of a more severe initial injury rather than a particular complication of PSH (e.g., longer hospital stay, infection, or disruption of rehabilitation). Aside from functional outcomes, patients with PSH may also be at risk for further medical complications. HRV abnormalities, which have been found in dysautonomic patients both in the short term and as far out as 5 years following injury, are associated with other disease states such as ischemic heart disease, ventricular arrhythmias, and sudden death and have been postulated to be a possible factor associated with the decreased life expectancy seen for survivors of severe TBI [34].

One challenge in further predicting the prognosis of patients with PSH is that there is limited evidence following discharge from the hospital because most analyses of this topic are conducted in the acute inpatient portion of medical care in the ICU or neurosurgery units, with little follow-up in rehabilitation settings [33]. Therefore, in order to have a better sense of the outcomes for these patients, there will need to be follow-up studies that assess the outcomes of PSH patients following discharge from acute medical and rehabilitation care.

Treatment

The topic of treatment for patients with PSH is extremely challenging because there has been very little high-quality evidence for the treatment of dysautonomia following TBI. In fact, there currently are no class I studies regarding evidence for pharmaceutical intervention in treatment of dysautonomia following TBI, complicating the goal of evidence-based treatment [35]. This is in large part due to the fact that most reports of treatment efficacy are either case reports or small clinical series and there is little standardization of outcome measures or study designs [2].

With the wide-ranging effects of autonomic dysfunction seen following TBI, a large percentage of patients admitted with TBI experience autonomic symptoms, even if they do not go on to meet the criteria for PSH. Therefore, beta-blockers are one of the most widely used treatments for dysautonomia and are a well-suited treatment for symptomatic relief because of their ability to block the catecholamine surge that commonly follows TBI. This allows for the prevention of symptoms such as elevated high blood pressure and heart rate that frequently occur in the post-TBI patient. Although not studied strictly in the context of PSH, beta-blockers have been analyzed for their use in the care of the TBI patients with results strongly supporting a protective role for the medication class. One analysis of roughly 2600 patients who were admitted with TBI at one hospital during a 5-year period found that of the 20% of patients who received beta-blockers, despite being older and experiencing more severe injuries, they had no difference in mortality, suggesting that beta-blockers may have a protective effect in mitigating the initial effects of the catecholamine surge [36]. These findings have been corroborated by another study that analyzed 4117 trauma patients and found that the patient population who received beta-blockers was similarly older and more severely injured and also had no difference in mortality following treatment with beta-blockers. These results remained even after controlling for age, GCS, and blood pressure, among other factors [37].

These findings must be considered within the context of a possible survivor's bias, such that patients who end up receiving the beta-blockers may be different in some respect compared with patients who did not survive long enough to receive the medication. Furthermore, future studies would benefit from a prospective study design that would better address the question of a causal link between treatment with beta-blockers and survival. Additionally, there is limited evidence assessing which beta-blockers are most effective in treatment of TBI and autonomic symptoms. An analysis that examined TBI patients who had received atenolol, carvedilol, esmolol, labetalol, and other beta-blockers found that patients who received labetalol had the lowest mortality compared with patients who received other beta-blockers [38]. These findings were supported by another comparative study between metoprolol and labetalol, which found that only the latter medication was effective in regulating autonomic symptoms. This suggests that, in addition to beta-blockade, PSH patients may also benefit from blockade of the alpha-1 receptors, which have a crucial role in mediating blood pressure and thus are likely central to the development of hypertension seen in PSH [15].

Whether the benefits seen from beta-blockers are the result of actual suppression of PSH or merely symptomatic relief, possibly before the development of the syndrome itself, remains to be seen. Although not tested specifically in the context of dysautonomia, one study found that propranolol has a role in decreasing circulating catecholamines and lowering the amount of cardiac work—two mechanisms that would be beneficial in the setting

of PSH [39]. Intravenous (IV) propranolol has also been shown to decrease resting metabolic rate as a by-product of decreased heart rate translating to a decrease in hypermetabolism by about 25% for post-TBI patients [40]. Taken together, there is strong evidence for the use of beta-blockers in the post-TBI setting, with general benefits for survival and potential advantages for targeting the specific symptoms of autonomic dysregulation.

In addition to beta-blockers, there is a variety of other medication classes that has been tested in patients with autonomic dysfunction following TBI. However, virtually all studies of treatment efficacy specific to PSH are in the setting of either case reports or limited case series, and thus it is extremely difficult to extrapolate broader findings from this largely anecdotal evidence. Nevertheless, the evidence that does exist provides a foundation for future studies that can study different treatment regimens within the context of a more controlled experimental design. One of the first medications to be tested specifically for patients with PSH was the dopamine agonist bromocriptine. In a case series of three patients who were treated with bromocriptine, results demonstrated that in the short term the medication was capable of partially relieving hyperthermia and diaphoresis, while in the long term the symptoms either were reduced or abated completely [41]. However, this response has not been uniform, as other reports have failed to find an effect [22, 34]. While it was originally thought that the use of bromocriptine could imply a role of the dopaminergic system's involvement in the pathophysiology of dysautonomia [17], more recent research has made this theory less plausible [7].

Another medication that has been tested is gabapentin, a GABA analogue that is thought to modulate dysautonomia either at the spinal or cerebral level by interfacing at calcium channels found in the dorsal horn of the spinal cord [1]. One case series of six TBI patients with dysautonomia who were unresponsive to metoprolol and bromocriptine found that gabapentin was able to decrease the quantity and severity of dysautonomic paroxysms, which allowed other medications, such as IBT, to be decreased without the symptoms flaring up again [22]. The researchers in this study found that while IBT was able to alleviate symptoms of spasticity and the overall severity of autonomic symptoms, it did not have a substantial impact on how often the autonomic paroxysms occurred or on dystonic posturing, whereas gabapentin seemed to reduce or prevent the paroxysms altogether. As gabapentin is primarily a neuropathic pain medication, the authors speculate that it is possible that its mechanism of action is in promoting the inhibitory response of the spinal cord to pain, which allows for the direct modulation of nociceptive afferent activity as opposed to simply decreasing the subsequent sympathetic response.

In addition to pharmaceutical options, one more invasive treatment that has been tested is intrathecal baclofen therapy, which has been classically used for severe spasticity [42] and has been used in cases of dysautonomia when other treatment options have not been successful. While not firmly established, the mechanism of baclofen in the case of dysautonomia may be related to activation of GABA-B receptors on inhibitory interneurons in the spinal cord that are responsible for modulating autonomic afferents [43], and its properties are thought to have both antispasticity and antinociceptive properties [22]. An initial case series that looked at four patients found that the patients went from experiencing between four and ten paroxysmal episodes per day to no episodes by day 6 of the test period [32]. Another case series, also with four patients, demonstrated that IBT was able to immediately arrest symptoms of autonomic dysfunction in all but one of the patients tested, [44] and an additional case series corroborated these finding [45]. At a 10-year follow-up study for IBT, investigators found that around half of patients maintained a good recovery from TBI, many of whom had improvement in symptoms of dysautonomia and limb hypertonia [24]. These patients tended to be those who developed their symptoms later and required lower doses of the medication, suggesting that their symptoms were not as severe.

Given that it appears that nociceptive stimuli are a major trigger for paroxysmal dysautonomia episodes, it is unsurprising that pain control represents an effective method toward reducing autonomic symptoms. Case reports have indicated either partial or complete responses to morphine treatment, while another case series demonstrated that IV morphine could lead to decreases in temperature and heart rate (although these measures were seen to rise with the cessation of the medication) [16]. The effects of morphine are thought to be dose-dependent, with little effect seen at smaller doses [22].

While many medications have shown some degree of success in mitigating symptoms of PSH, clonidine, an alpha2-agonist, has shown relatively little capacity to modulate autonomic dysfunction. Even though it has been shown in TBI patients to decrease the level of circulating catecholamines as well as lowering heart rate without compromising cerebral blood flow [46], most case reports have found that patients with PSH are unresponsive to its effects [47].

Even with the relatively limited evidence described previously, there are still many other medications that have only been studied in a single case report. These include medications that have been found to be effective such as dexmedetomidine, prazosin, and oxycodone and medications that have not been effective such as trihexyphenidyl, diphenhydramine, and hydralazine [2]. Dexmedetomidine is a centrally acting alpha2-agonist that may have particular potential as it was found to control dysautonomic symptoms with a 72-h infusion protocol in a patient who was previously found to be unresponsive to a wide array of medications including morphine, fentanyl, and labetalol, among others [7]. However, larger case series will be needed to assess its clinical utility.

Common Treatments and a Discussion of Their Risks and Benefits

PSH is complicated from a management standpoint by the fact that there are currently no treatment guidelines and only limited evidence from case series and reports. Therefore, for each medication that has been used in treatment of PSH, there is extremely limited information regarding the risks and benefits.

Beta-blockers are one of the most common treatments used for autonomic dysregulation following TBI given their ability to moderate symptoms of autonomic dysfunction including tachycardia and hypertension and have been shown to decrease the severity of paroxysms [15, 16]. One downside to the use of beta-blockers is that they act to mitigate the sympathetic response in PSH but they do not necessarily have an impact on what may be the source of the sympathetic response in the first place—the allodynic over-reactivity of spinal afferents. As the excitatory/inhibitory model suggests, medications that target the pain response may be more useful than those that try to control autonomic symptoms. Nevertheless, given that it is not always possible to prevent triggers of autonomic symptoms (which can be as benign as turning or bathing), beta-blockers may be useful for the paroxysms that are unavoidable. Another potential benefit of beta-blockers is that there is some evidence showing that this medication is protective in the case of TBI, and so it may have wider advantages beyond simply treating symptoms of PSH [48]. Additionally, as cardiovascular risk represents a major non-neurologic source of organ dysfunction in TBI, beta-blockers may help mitigate some of the effects of the post-TBI hyperadrenergic state on cardiac work [48]. Aside from counteracting the high levels of catecholamines, there may be other benefits as well, including reducing the degree of immunosuppression and lowering levels of oxygen consumption [36] and producing decreases in thermal load by lowering heart rate, core temperature, and muscle tone [49]. One other benefit is that beta-blockers, compared with other more invasive options such as IBT, are highly cost-effective [36].

Morphine is another commonly used first-line agent, given that it is useful for both pain symptoms and pulmonary edema and it is also capable of decreasing autonomic symptoms such as tachycardia and tachypnea [7]. The major benefit of morphine is that, as an antinociceptive agent, it acts on the afferent response to nociceptive and non-nociceptive stimuli that are thought to provoke PSH, and so it is able to mitigate the potential source of sympathetic hyperactivity. One risk with morphine is that cessation of the medication has been found to lead to significant increases in heart and respiratory rates, a pattern that was seen similarly with midazolam, although these changes appear relatively isolated as changes in body temperature were not seen [49]. Additionally, morphine has many other well-documented risks including sedation, which can potentially interfere with the neurologic exam (although its effect is short-lived), as well as respiratory depression.

Even though intrathecal baclofen therapy has been shown to make a significant difference for symptoms of dysautonomia and limb hypertonia, it has an exceedingly high complication rate, as would be expected for an implanted medical device and continuous infusion of a potent central nervous system (CNS)-acting drug directly into the cerebrospinal fluid (CSF). In a 10-year follow-up study that looked at 43 patients treated with IBT, researchers found that 90% of patients experienced some form of complication, including operative site infections (20%), requirement of pump replacement (47%), and definitive device removal (14% due to device infection or meningitis) [24]. Another risk of intrathecal baclofen therapy is that upon withdrawal of the medication, it can potentially either worsen symptoms of dysautonomia [32] or it can produce a condition similar to dysautonomia in patients that were previously free of autonomic symptoms [50]. Finally, unintentional overdose can occur as well as pump failure resulting in withdrawal, both of which are potentially fatal.

For other medications used to treat symptoms of PSH, such as bromocriptine, gabapentin, and others, there is simply not enough evidence available to issue recommendations regarding risks and benefits. Because patients with PSH are often in very limited states of consciousness or comatose, it is difficult to truly appreciate the side effects or other risks of medications as patients often are unable to report adverse effects; and their medical condition is so complex that it is impossible to isolate which effects are a result of the medication itself versus simply a change due to the complicated nature of the post-TBI patient.

A Rational Approach to Treatment Given the Presence or Absence of Data

Given the absence of treatment guidelines or extensive data, there is no single approach that can be followed for patients with symptoms with PSH. Perhaps the most rational approach, proposed by Baguley et al., suggests starting with medications such as opioids, gabapentin, and benzodiazepines to limit the extent of nociceptive stimuli and beta-antagonists to mitigate the effects of the hyperadrenergic state [2]. Second-line medications could include other medications that have been less tested, for example, bromocriptine, which could be given in combination with morphine [2]. While IBT has been studied to the longest extent and has the most amount of evidence, given the high complication rate, it seems most reasonable to use this therapy as a second- or third-line treatment [2]. These recommendations have been echoed by others that say that in the absence of incontrovertible evidence, the best available evidence favors an approach of IV morphine, benzodiazepines, propranolol, or bromocriptine [49]. Based on limited evidence, clonidine does not appear to have substantial efficacy in the treatment of dysautonomia [1].

Other non-pharmacological treatment approaches include measures aimed at mitigating nociceptive stimuli. For example, splinting can be used to provide for better limb positioning, and other approaches can be used to limit the pain associated with movements during bathing, turning, and endotracheal tube suctioning [2]. Other conditions that are common in the post-TBI patient that should be monitored for include noxious stimuli; infection; kinking, obstruction or traction of bladder catheters; constipation; undiagnosed fractures; heterotopic ossification; and decubitus ulceration because these conditions can lead to an increase in sympathetic overactivity, especially in the context of PSH [49]. Another important multidisciplinary approach to treatment may be nutrition replacement therapy in order to replenish caloric energy lost as a result of hypermetabolism and insensible losses from diaphoresis [5].

The timing of medication administration has not been extensively researched. Although one report of 32 patients with dysautonomia found that medication was administered with wide onset interval, with medications such as chlorpromazine and benzodiazepines being administered around 2–6 days post-injury, while other medications that are more tailored toward autonomic symptoms typically were administered as much as 3–4 weeks later, often once the patient was already in the inpatient rehabilitation setting [49]. Many more resources will need to be devoted to this topic in order to assess what the optimal approaches are for treatment of TBI patients with PSH.

Conclusions

Future Directions and Questions That Need to Be Addressed Through Research

Given the large amount that remains unknown regarding dysautonomia following TBI, it is unsurprising that there is an extensive number of questions that still remain to be answered in order to develop improved diagnostic and treatment strategies. Although perhaps not the most significant issue, one subject that has moved in the direction of a solution is the nomenclature for the post-TBI dysautonomic clinical syndrome. As mentioned previously, the Consensus Working Group in 2014 recommended the term paroxysmal autonomic hyperactivity, and key attributes of this term include that it is specific, it does not endorse a specific pathophysiology, and it accurately portrays the syndrome [4]. Now that this term has been recommended for wider use, future studies will be able to rely upon this term to standardize diagnostic and treatment strategies, and it will be easier to conduct large multicenter studies when different research groups are able to rely on the same diagnostic nomenclature [6].

Earlier in this decade, several authors also began calling for a consensus group to meet and discuss the available evidence in order to develop a diagnostic framework that could be used to determine which patients meet clinical criteria for having autonomic symptoms [2]. As discussed earlier, a consensus group met in 2014 and developed the paroxysmal sympathetic hyperactivity assessment measure (PSH-AM), which is a critical first step in terms of standardizing the diagnostic methodology, which will, for one thing, allow treatment studies to have more rigorous criteria allowing for a better assessment of treatment efficacy [4]. Even with this recent development, however, there are still many developments that need to occur, including validating the measure in the clinical setting to better assess how well this measure can classify patients who may or may not have autonomic symptoms. In addition to the diagnostic guidelines, there is also a need for other consensus groups to develop guidelines on management and treatment efficacy [2].

With respect to the pathophysiology of dysautonomia following TBI, there is still significant progress to be made in order to understand the origins of the syndrome so that it can be treated more effectively. While at the moment it appears that the excitatory/inhibitory model may provide a better understanding compared with conventional disconnection theories or especially the epileptogenic theory of dysautonomia, many of the assumptions of the EIR model are untested and remain to be proven with further investigation [1]. Proponents of this theory have emphasized the need for more basic science research to investigate the putative targets in the brainstem and diencephalon that may be responsible for the syndrome. The authors emphasize that the lack of tools to quantify treatment response remains a great barrier for further investigation of the precise pathophysiology. Another potential method for studying this theory is through the development of treatments that have an inhibitory role at the level of the spinal cord (similar to IBT), which could allow for an improved assessment of the role of afferent activity that drives sympathetic activity in response [51].

In regard to imaging, there is still some controversy regarding which radiological findings are most predictive of the development of dysautonomia—whether diffuse axonal injury or discrete focal lesions. Some have suggested that functional magnetic resonance imaging (fMRI) could potentially add insights if imaging could occur during a paroxysm of autonomic symptoms and diffusion tensor imaging (DTI) could provide some clarification on the potential role of white matter disease following TBI [51]. For medication and treatment regimens, more research is needed using objective, quantitative measures in order to allow for a better assessment of treatment efficacy [2].

Finally, most of the research on PSH has been conducted in the adult population and very little has been conducted within the pediatric population. So, in addition to developing separate diagnostic measures, there will also be a need for more research into treating autonomic measures in the post-TBI pediatric population [4].

References

1. Baguley IJ, Heriseanu RE, Cameron ID, Nott MT, Slewa-Younan S. A critical review of the pathophysiology of dysautonomia following traumatic brain injury. Neurocrit Care. 2008;8(2):293–300.
2. Perkes I, Baguley IJ, Nott MT, Menon DK. A review of paroxysmal sympathetic hyperactivity after acquired brain injury. Ann Neurol. 2010;68(2):126–35.
3. Baguley IJ. Nomenclature of "paroxysmal sympathetic storms". Mayo Clin Proc. 1999;74(1):105
4. Baguley IJ, Perkes IE, Fernandez-Ortega J-F, Rabinstein AA, Dolce G, Hendricks HT, et al. Paroxysmal sympathetic hyperactivity after acquired brain injury: consensus on conceptual definition, nomenclature, and diagnostic criteria. J Neurotrauma. 2014;31(17):1515–20.
5. Baguley IJ, Nicholls JL, Felmingham KL, Crooks J, Gurka JA, Wade LD. Dysautonomia after traumatic brain injury: a forgotten syndrome? J Neurol Neurosurg Psychiatry. 1999;67(1):39–43.
6. Baguley IJ, Nott MT, Slewa-Younan S, Heriseanu RE, Perkes IE. Diagnosing dysautonomia after acute traumatic brain injury: evidence for overresponsiveness to afferent stimuli. Arch Phys Med Rehabil. 2009;90(4):580–6.
7. Goddeau RP, Silverman SB, Sims JR. Dexmedetomidine for the treatment of paroxysmal autonomic instability with dystonia. Neurocrit Care. 2007;7(3):217–20.
8. Blackman JA, Patrick PD, Buck ML, Rust RS. Paroxysmal autonomic instability with dystonia after brain injury. Arch Neurol. 2004;61(3):321–8.
9. Baguley IJ, Heriseanu RE, Nott MT, Chapman J, Sandanam J. Dysautonomia after severe traumatic

brain injury: evidence of persisting overresponsiveness to afferent stimuli. Am J Phys Med Rehabil. 2009;88(8):615–22.

10. Baguley IJ, Slewa-Younan S, Heriseanu RE, Nott MT, Mudaliar Y, Nayyar V. The incidence of dysautonomia and its relationship with autonomic arousal following traumatic brain injury. Brain Inj. 2007;21(11):1175–81.

11. Hendricks HT, Heeren AH, Vos PE. Dysautonomia after severe traumatic brain injury. Eur J Neurol. 2010;17(9):1172–7.

12. Rabinstein AA. Paroxysmal sympathetic hyperactivity in the neurological intensive care unit. Neurol Res. 2007;29(7):680–2.

13. Rutland-Brown W, Langlois JA, Thomas KE, Xi YL. Incidence of traumatic brain injury in the United States, 2003. J Head Trauma Rehabil. 2006;21(6):544–8.

14. Penfield W. Diencephalic autonomic epilepsy. Arch Neurol Psychiatr. 1929;22(2):358–74.

15. Do D, Sheen VL, Bromfield E. Treatment of paroxysmal sympathetic storm with labetalol. J Neurol Neurosurg Psychiatry. 2000;69(6):832–3.

16. Boeve BF, Wijdicks EF, Benarroch EE, Schmidt KD. Paroxysmal sympathetic storms ("diencephalic seizures") after severe diffuse axonal head injury. Mayo Clin Proc. 1998;73(2):148–52.

17. Bullard DE. Diencephalic seizures: responsiveness to bromocriptine and morphine. Ann Neurol. 1987;21(6):609–11.

18. Clifton GL, Ziegler MG, Grossman RG. Circulating catecholamines and sympathetic activity after head injury. Neurosurgery. 1981;8(1):10–4.

19. Grunsfeld A, Fletcher JJ, Nathan BR. Cardiopulmonary complications of brain injury. Curr Neurol Neurosci Rep. 2005;5(6):488–93.

20. Woiciechowsky C, Asadullah K, Nestler D, Eberhardt B, Platzer C, Schöning B, et al. Sympathetic activation triggers systemic interleukin-10 release in immunodepression induced by brain injury. Nat Med. 1998;4(7):808–13.

21. Mehta NM, Bechard LJ, Leavitt K, Duggan C. Severe weight loss and hypermetabolic paroxysmal dysautonomia following hypoxic ischemic brain injury: the role of indirect calorimetry in the intensive care unit. JPEN J Parenter Enteral Nutr. 2008;32(3):281–4.

22. Baguley IJ, Heriseanu RE, Gurka JA, Nordenbo A, Cameron ID. Gabapentin in the management of dysautonomia following severe traumatic brain injury: a case series. J Neurol Neurosurg Psychiatry. 2007;78(5):539–41.

23. Soukup J, Zauner A, Doppenberg EMR, Menzel M, Gilman C, Young HF, et al. The importance of brain temperature in patients after severe head injury: relationship to intracranial pressure, cerebral perfusion pressure, cerebral blood flow, and outcome. J Neurotrauma. 2002;19(5):559–71.

24. Hoarau X, Richer E, Dehail P, Cuny E. A 10-year follow-up study of patients with severe traumatic brain injury and dysautonomia treated with intrathecal baclofen therapy. Brain Inj. 2012;26(7–8):927–40.

25. Perkes IE, Menon DK, Nott MT, Baguley IJ. Paroxysmal sympathetic hyperactivity after acquired brain injury: a review of diagnostic criteria. Brain Inj. 2011;25(10):925–32.

26. Fernández-Ortega JF, Prieto-Palomino MA, Muñoz-López A, Lebron-Gallardo M, Cabrera-Ortiz H, Quesada-García G. Prognostic influence and computed tomography findings in dysautonomic crises after traumatic brain injury. J Trauma. 2006;61(5):1129–33.

27. Dolce G, Quintieri M, Leto E, Milano M, Pileggi A, Lagani V, et al. Dysautonomia and clinical outcome in vegetative state. J Neurotrauma. 2008:4.

28. Hendricks HT, Geurts ACH, van Ginneken BC, Heeren AJ, Vos PE. Brain injury severity and autonomic dysregulation accurately predict heterotopic ossification in patients with traumatic brain injury. Clin Rehabil. 2007;21(6):545–53.

29. Bilotta F, Branca G, Lam A, Cuzzone V, Doronzio A, Rosa G. Endotracheal lidocaine in preventing endotracheal suctioning-induced changes in cerebral hemodynamics in patients with severe head trauma. Neurocrit Care. 2008;8(2):241–6.

30. Pattoneri P, Tirabassi G, Pelá G, Astorri E, Mazzucchi A, Borghetti A. Circadian blood pressure and heart rate changes in patients in a persistent vegetative state after traumatic brain injury. J Clin Hypertens Greenwich Conn. 2005;7(12):734–9.

31. Kanjwal K, Karabin B, Kanjwal Y, Grubb BP. Autonomic dysfunction presenting as postural tachycardia syndrome following traumatic brain injury. Cardiol J. 2010;17(5):482–7.

32. Cuny E, Richer E, Castel JP. Dysautonomia syndrome in the acute recovery phase after traumatic brain injury: relief with intrathecal baclofen therapy. Brain Inj. 2001;15(10):917–25.

33. Laxe S, Terré R, León D, Bernabeu M. How does dysautonomia influence the outcome of traumatic brain injured patients admitted in a neurorehabilitation unit? Brain Inj. 2013;27(12):1383–7.

34. Baguley IJ, Heriseanu RE, Felmingham KL, Cameron ID. Dysautonomia and heart rate variability following severe traumatic brain injury. Brain Inj. 2006;20(4):437–44.

35. Gordon WA, Zafonte R, Cicerone K, Cantor J, Brown M, Lombard L, et al. Traumatic brain injury rehabilitation: state of the science. Am J Phys Med Rehabil. 2006;85(4):343–82.

36. Schroeppel TJ, Fischer PE, Zarzaur BL, Magnotti LJ, Clement LP, Fabian TC, et al. Beta-adrenergic blockade and traumatic brain injury: protective? J Trauma. 2010;69(4):776–82.

37. Arbabi S, Ahrns KS, Wahl WL, Hemmila MR, Wang SC, Brandt M-M, et al. Beta-blocker use is associated with improved outcomes in adult burn patients. J Trauma. 2004;56(2):265–269.271.

38. Schroeppel TJ, Sharpe JP, Magnotti LJ, Weinberg JA, Clement LP, Croce MA, et al. Traumatic brain injury and β-blockers: not all drugs are created equal. J Trauma Acute Care Surg. 2014;76(2):504–9. discussion 509

39. Robertson CS, Clifton GL, Taylor AA, Grossman RG. Treatment of hypertension associated with head injury. J Neurosurg. 1983;59(3):455–60.

40. Chioléro RL, Breitenstein E, Thorin D, Christin L, de Tribolet N, Freeman J, et al. Effects of propranolol on resting metabolic rate after severe head injury. Crit Care Med. 1989;17(4):328–34.

41. Rossitch E, Bullard DE. The autonomic dysfunction syndrome: aetiology and treatment. Br J Neurosurg. 1988;2(4):471–8.

42. Ivanhoe CB, Tilton AH, Francisco GE. Intrathecal baclofen therapy for spastic hypertonia. Phys Med Rehabil Clin N Am. 2001;12(4):923–38. viii–ix

43. Baguley IJ, Bailey KM, Slewa-Younan S. Prolonged anti-spasticity effects of bolus intrathecal baclofen. Brain Inj. 2005;19(7):545–8.

44. Becker R, Benes L, Sure U, Hellwig D, Bertalanffy H. Intrathecal baclofen alleviates autonomic dysfunction in severe brain injury. J Clin Neurosci. 2000;7(4):316–9.

45. François B, Vacher P, Roustan J, Salle JY, Vidal J, Moreau JJ, et al. Intrathecal baclofen after traumatic brain injury: early treatment using a new technique to prevent spasticity. J Trauma. 2001;50(1):158–61.

46. Payen D, Quintin L, Plaisance P, Chiron B, Lhoste F. Head injury: clonidine decreases plasma catecholamines. Crit Care Med. 1990;18(4):392–5.

47. Russo RN, O'Flaherty S. Bromocriptine for the management of autonomic dysfunction after severe traumatic brain injury. J Paediatr Child Health. 2000;36(3):283–5.

48. Heffernan DS, Inaba K, Arbabi S, Cotton BA. Sympathetic hyperactivity after traumatic brain injury and the role of beta-blocker therapy. J Trauma. 2010;69(6):1602–9.

49. Baguley IJ, Cameron ID, Green AM, Slewa-Younan S, Marosszeky JE, Gurka JA. Pharmacological management of dysautonomia following traumatic brain injury. Brain Inj. 2004;18(5):409–17.

50. Green LB, Nelson VS. Death after acute withdrawal of intrathecal baclofen: case report and literature review. Arch Phys Med Rehabil. 1999;80(12):1600–4.

51. Hinson HE, Sheth KN. Manifestations of the hyperadrenergic state after acute brain injury. Curr Opin Crit Care. 2012;18(2):139–45.

Use of Consciousness-Enhancing Medications in the Traumatic Brain Injury Patient

Justin R. Davanzo and Shelly D. Timmons

Introduction

After traumatic brain injury (TBI), patients often experience an altered level of consciousness for some period of time, and deeply altered levels of consciousness may be classified as comatose or vegetative states. Patients defined as comatose are those with no spontaneous eye opening and who cannot be awoken with vigorous stimulation [1]. Those patients defined as being in a vegetative state show no evidence of awareness of surroundings, but they have some spontaneous and stimulus-induced arousal and mainly maintained sleep-wake cycles [2]. Some patients do not fit either of these categories, due to some level of preservation of self-awareness, and are defined as being in a minimally conscious state; patients may progress to this state from coma or vegetative state after a TBI [3]. Understanding the criteria for each of these altered states is important for prognostication purposes [4]. While a large proportion of patients with prolonged coma after a TBI will "awaken" within 1 year, many researchers have focused on utilization of pharmaceutical agents to hasten recovery of consciousness due to the propensity for complications and other deleterious issues associated with prolonged coma [5]. However, as with all medications, the medications used have a side-effect profile that could certainly play a harmful role in recovery. In addition, limited data are available to suggest that these medications actually do aid TBI patients in their recovery. The goal of this chapter is to discuss the available evidence for conscious-enhancing medications for this use.

Basic Science

Methylphenidate

Animal models to determine the safety and potential efficacy of pharmacotherapy in post-TBI arousal have been conducted using bromocriptine, methylphenidate, and methamphetamine. Rodents injected with methylphenidate daily for 18 days post-injury ultimately showed improvement on Morris water maze swim latencies, but no improvement in overall motor function [6]. Animals subjected to daily bromocriptine therapy showed improvement in spatial and working memory but, once

J. R. Davanzo, MD
S. D. Timmons, MD, PhD, FACS, FAANS (✉)
Department of Neurosurgery, Penn State University
Milton S. Hershey Medical Center,
Hershey, PA, USA
e-mail: jdavanzo@pennstatehealth.psu.edu;
stimmons@mac.com

© Springer International Publishing AG, part of Springer Nature 2018
S. D. Timmons (ed.), *Controversies in Severe Traumatic Brain Injury Management*,
https://doi.org/10.1007/978-3-319-89477-5_15

again, no change in motor function [7]. A series of studies of methylphenidate in a rodent model, in which animals were subjected to controlled cortical injury or sham surgery and thereafter received methylphenidate daily, showed some improvement in motor function with methylphenidate administration, in addition to improved performance on the Morris water maze tests as shown with the other agents. Differences were noted between female and male rodents on water maze testing, with females demonstrating faster swim times and males demonstrating relatively more improvement in memory acquisition and retention [8]. Using voltammetry, this investigative group also demonstrated that these rodents had decreased striatal dopamine neurotransmission after controlled cortical injury but showed significant recovery of neurotransmission after daily methylphenidate administration [9]. Animals sustaining cortical injury showed a less robust increase in dopamine and dopamine metabolite levels after methylphenidate administration than controls, but if animals were pretreated with methylphenidate, the rodents showed comparable increases in dopamine neurotransmission when compared to control subjects [10].

Environmental enrichment has been studied in animal models of cognitive outcomes in TBI. Attempts to combine environmental enrichment with methylphenidate each led to improved cognitive outcomes, but the use of these interventions in combination was found to be of no greater benefit for cognitive function in a rodent model [11].

Rau et al. performed multiple animal studies in this topic as well. In all of these, methamphetamine was used as the pharmacotherapy. Using a fluid percussion model to induce severe TBI in rodents, they subsequently treated the subjects with either methamphetamine or placebo 3 h post-injury. Both clinical and histological testing were performed. Those subjects treated with methamphetamine showed improved clinical function. In addition, histological testing revealed lower rates of apoptosis and increased numbers of immature neurons in the methamphetamine-treated group [12]. This group went on to further characterize the therapeutic window of this medication, finding similar results even when the rodents were treated up to 12 h after the initial injury [13]. Using the data they obtained, the authors subsequently demonstrated that the plasma dose in rodents resulting in clinical differences was equivalent to the human dose acceptable to the current US Food and Drug Administration (FDA) guidelines [14].

Another class of medications of particular interest in TBI patients is the antipsychotic medication group, as TBI may lead to anxiety and agitation during coma emergence. The aforementioned rodent model designed was used to test the cognitive effects of some of these medications as well as the effects after their withdrawal. At 24 h after the injury or sham surgery, the rodents were given haloperidol, risperidone, bromocriptine, or placebo daily for 19 days. During the treatment phase, cognitive recovery was impaired for the haloperidol and risperidone groups, but bromocriptine was shown to improve cognitive outcomes. One month after the medication, both groups receiving antipsychotic medications had worse cognitive outcomes. This effect persisted at 3 months for haloperidol [15]. These data suggested that antipsychotic medications may have a significant effect on cognitive outcomes in TBI both during the treatment phase and after withdrawal and informed clinical studies.

Clinical Studies

Amantadine

Early case reports or case series were published on TBI patients in whom amantadine was used for a number of indications including agitation, cognitive failure, amotivational syndrome, minimally conscious state, mood lability, and aggression [16–21]. In order to test the effects of amantadine on executive dysfunction in post-TBI patients, Kraus et al. examined 22 post-TBI patients treated for 12 weeks with amantadine. All of the patients underwent pre- and posttreatment neuropsychological testing, and six patients underwent positron emission tomography (PET) scanning. While significant improvements in tests of executive function after treatment and increased glucose metabolism in the left frontal region were seen, there was no control group in this study [22].

Retrospective studies have also been published; in one such example, approximately 63% of pediatric patients who received amantadine were noted to have some degree of subjective improvement over those who did not in a retrospective case-control analysis. In addition, the amantadine group was noted to have a greater increase in their Ranchos Los Amigos Scale; however, the amantadine group started with lower scores. In addition, it was noted that 9% of patients had medication-related side effects (hallucinations, delusions, aggression) [23]. Another retrospective study of 123 patients showed no statistical difference between those who did receive amantadine and those who did not with regard to emergence from coma, but also noted that very few patients who received amantadine experienced side effects [24]. A third retrospective study in severe TBI patients noted greater improvements in the Glasgow Coma Scale (GCS) for the amantadine group in comparison to those who did not receive the medication (~5 point improvement vs. ~1 point improvement) [25].

The lack of side effects in retrospective studies should always be interpreted with caution, as clinicians documenting side effects may have overlooked them, attributed them to other issues, or introduced a variety of other biases. While such publications spawned interest in further investigation of amantadine in TBI patients, the level of evidence necessary to change the clinical practice was not present. In an effort to provide a higher level of evidence, randomized, controlled trials were performed.

A small, randomized, controlled trial was performed to study the effects on pediatric patients late after injury (as long as 36 months or more). Patients were randomized to either amantadine or placebo for 12 weeks. Some improvements in behavior were noted in the amantadine group, and, for those <2 years from injury, improvement in cognitive outcomes with amantadine treatment was also seen [26]. A second randomized, cross-over study in the pediatric population randomly assigned subjects to receive either pramipexole (a non-ergoline dopamine agonist) or amantadine. While all of the patients enrolled in this study remained in a low-response state, these medications led to significant improvements in Ranchos Los Amigos Scores ($p < 0.05$) [27]. Schneider et al. performed a small randomized, controlled, crossover trial of ten TBI patients. Their protocol included 2 weeks of amantadine or placebo, 2 weeks of washout, and 2 weeks of the opposite arm. No statistically significant impact on cognitive outcomes was noted with amantadine [28]. Another randomized trial focused specifically on patients who had suffered diffuse axonal injury. This was also a crossover study, consisting of 35 patients; however, the treatment period was longer at 12 weeks. Two groups were randomly assigned to receive either amantadine or placebo for 6 weeks and the alternative for the next 6 weeks. A consistent trend was seen toward a more rapid functional outcome in this patient population during the time they were on the drug arm, regardless of whether amantadine or placebo was received first. Particularly, improvements in scores on the Mini-Mental Status Examination (MMSE), Disability Rating Scale (DRS), Glasgow Outcome Scale scores (GOS), and Functional Independence Measure-Cognitive Domains were noted during amantadine treatment [29].

In 2012, Giacino et al. performed a large, randomized controlled trial in severe TBI patients who remained in a vegetative or minimally conscious state 4–16 weeks after their injury. In this study, 184 patients were randomized to receive either 4 weeks of amantadine or placebo and were followed for 2 weeks after completion of the protocol (a relatively short period vis-à-vis TBI recovery). Using the Disability Rating Scale (DRS), faster recovery trajectories in the amantadine group during the treatment period were observed. In the 2 weeks after treatment, the rate of recovery slowed significantly in the amantadine group and was actually significantly lower than that of the placebo group during this time. At the end of the 6 weeks, there was noted to be no difference in improvement in DRS scores between the two groups [30]. Thus, while amantadine seemed to speed the patient's recovery during treatment, the results were not durable and, in fact, a posttreatment decline was noted.

While the previous studies examined the effects of amantadine on overall neurologic outcomes, Hammond et al. performed a series of randomized trials specifically looking at its effects on irritability and aggressive symptoms in TBI patients more than 6 months from their injury. First, this investigative group performed a randomized study of 76 patients with 2 arms: amantadine vs. placebo for 28 days. All patients underwent pre-study testing for irritability and aggression via the Neuropsychiatric Inventory Irritability (NPI-I) and Aggression (NPI-A) scales. These same tests were performed at the completion of the study. They noted that patients who received amantadine had a mean improvement of their NPI-I of −4.3, while the placebo only showed an improvement of −2.3 ($p = 0.0016$). In addition, a decrease of −4.6 was noted on the NPI-A in the amantadine group, with the placebo group only showing a decrease of −2.5 (0.046). There were no differences noted in adverse effects between the groups [31]. The study group then performed a similar trial with longer treatment for 60 days. Patients were evaluated pre-study, at day 28 and at day 60. No statistical significance was noted between the groups with regard to NPI-I scores at day 60 [32]. These results again suggest a lack of durability of effect.

Multiple systematic reviews have been performed in an attempt to better elucidate the best use of amantadine in TBI—all noting trends in improvements on neuropsychiatric testing with the drug but noting the lack of large, randomized placebo-controlled trials and advising caution that more testing needs to be completed to confirm the efficacy of this treatment [33–35].

Considering all of the available information, the safety of amantadine has not been definitively demonstrated in post-TBI patients, and its efficacy remains questionable. While most of the studies available seem to show improvement in neuropsychometric testing, particularly with regard to speed of recovery, there is yet to be a large, multicenter, randomized controlled trial

addressing this medication and its use in TBI patients.

At this time, no consensus recommendation can be made with regard to the use of amantadine in post-TBI patients or which subsets of patients may benefit.

Methylphenidate

Methylphenidate is a central nervous system stimulant, the detailed mechanisms of action of which remain to be elucidated. It was originally suggested that methylphenidate caused an increase of dopamine efflux from the neuron and also prevented reuptake of dopamine at the synaptic cleft. It is now known that methylphenidate binds to the dopamine transporter, thus preventing reuptake of dopamine. This medication has received FDA approval for the treatment of attention deficit hyperactivity disorder (ADHD) and narcolepsy [36]. Due to its pharmacologic properties, there has been interest in its possible use for TBI.

While there are now a number of clinical trials available with regard to the use of methylphenidate in TBI, some of the earliest literature available was in the form of case reports and case series. Most of this work focused on cognitive and behavioral outcomes and arousal from coma [37–39]. One report specifically discussed the use of methylphenidate to treat narcolepsy in a post-TBI patient [40]. Yet another showed that methylphenidate actually had a paradoxical effect on a TBI patient, with the patient experiencing a decreased level of arousal [41].

Several retrospective studies have been published. One study of patients who had suffered cardiac arrest and cardiopulmonary resuscitation with neurologic injury showed nonsignificant trends in speed of return to following commands. However, the study consisted of only 16 patients, some of whom received methylphenidate, amantadine, both, or neither, making meaningful conclusions impossible [42]. A retrospective investigation into seizure rates in patients with an active seizure disorder receiving methylphenidate (which lowers seizure threshold) revealed that only 4 of the 30 patients studied had increased seizure activity and 3 of these patients were on tricyclic antidepressants as well. The authors concluded that methylphenidate could be used, even in patients at high risk for seizure activity, but again the small sample precludes broad adaptation [43]. The sleep-wake cycle of TBI patients was not affected by use of methylphenidate in 17 of 30 patients in the treatment arm [44].

Prospective trials, most of which were randomized and controlled, have been performed using methylphenidate in TBI patients, using a number of different outcomes measures. Many early studies focused on the effect of the medication on overall patient recovery and behavior, showing some promising results, albeit with small sample sizes [45–48]. Specifically, one study showed improvements in the Disability Rating Scale (DRS) for those who had received methylphenidate ($p < 0.02$), but the difference did not persist at 90 days. Furthermore, this particular study included a broad range of injury severities [48]. Mooney et al. demonstrated some reduction in anger symptoms with methylphenidate in TBI patients compared to placebo ($p = 0.002$) [47].

Specific symptoms have also been studied, such as fatigue, cognition, and symptoms of depression. Johansson et al. showed reduction in mental fatigue in mild TBI patients using multiple dosing regimens of methylphenidate, including low dose (15 mg/day) and normal dose (60 mg/day), as well as multiple durations of treatment (up to 6 months), with the greatest effect being seen in the normal-dose group. However, examination of long-term effects of methylphenidate by this investigative group was not a controlled study [49–51]. McAllister et al. conducted a trial of both TBI and posttraumatic stress disorder (PTSD) for effects of methylphenidate on cognition. While some improvement in cognition was observed in the treatment group, the sample size was small [52], and inclusion of both diagnostic groups is a confounder. Methylphenidate has been found to aid depressive symptoms in a similar manner to sertraline, a more conventional antidepressant [53].

Methylphenidate has a propensity to increase heart rate and blood pressure and has been dem-onstrated to decrease appetite in moderate to severe TBI patients [54]. In one trial, an increase in heart rate of 7 beats/min on average was seen with methylphenidate ($p < 0.001$); however, patients remained asymptomatic [54]. In another, significant increases in heart rate (12.3 beats/min, 95% CI 9.3–15.4), diastolic blood pressure (4.1 mmHg, 95% CI 2.1–6.1), and mean arterial pressure (3.75 mmHg, 95% CI 1.8–5.7) were all seen with the drug, but again, patients remained asymptomatic. Other adverse effects noted included irritability and sleep disturbance [55].

Very little work has been done on the effects of methylphenidate in the setting of acute TBI. Decreases in both intensive care unit (ICU) length of stay (23%: $p = 0.06$) and hospital length of stay (23%: $p = 0.029$) have been reported in severe TBI patients with methylphenidate administration [56], but administration in the acute phases after injury may have broader implications given autonomic effects. In moderate TBI patients, differences were only noted in ICU length of stay (26%: $p = 0.05$) [56].

Not surprisingly, methylphenidate effects on attention have garnered significant scientific interest. Preliminary studies conducted by Whyte et al. included a randomized controlled trial demonstrating improved mental processing speeds in TBI patients, but no differences in ability to orient to distractions or other symptoms of sustained attention [57]. A larger randomized controlled trial corroborated improved mental processing speeds and in the surrogate measure of caregiver ratings on attention symptoms [58]. Smaller studies of attentional effects in mixed TBI and non-TBI populations have had similar results [59]. The use of methylphenidate in the pediatric TBI population has been sparingly investigated. No differences have been observed on behavior, memory, and processing speed with methylphenidate compared to placebo [60], but the data on attention are mixed [61, 62].

Most of the data available on attentional effects relates to patients who are considerably remote in time from injury. Variations in treatment regimens have been investigated. Improvement in attention across multiple neuro-psychological tests has been shown when medication was initiated during the patient's posthospital rehabilitation [63], and even single-dose treatment has been utilized with some degree of success [64]. Extended-release methylphenidate showed no differences in attention symptoms when compared to a placebo group [65], but methylphenidate use concurrent with multiple cognitive rehabilitation techniques such as Memory and Attention Adaptation Training (MAAT) may improve not only attention but also memory and executive functions [66].

While one meta-analysis concluded that significant benefit for the use of methylphenidate to treat attention symptoms (standard mean difference = 0.45, 95% CI 0.1–0.8) exists, especially that of sustained attention (standard mean difference = 0.66, 95% CI 0.2–1.1), this analysis noted no differences in memory symptoms or processing speed [67]. Multiple systematic reviews have suggested that methylphenidate had shown some benefit in TBI patients, especially related to attention and cognitive symptoms [68–72]; however, the consensus is that further work is warranted prior to definitive recommendations being possible [73–76].

Questions remain about appropriate dosages and delivery formulas (e.g., extended release), the timing of treatment, the duration of treatment, and which subpopulations of TBI patients might benefit. While some of the smaller studies have suggested that this medication may be useful in treating other symptoms, such as fatigue and depression, larger studies need to be performed to confirm these findings.

The evidence is not yet compelling enough to make a recommendation regarding the use of methylphenidate in TBI.

Antipsychotics

While not specifically consciousness-enhancing, antipsychotic medications are often used to treat arousal state abnormalities such as agitation, so their use is reviewed here. Antipsychotic medications, both typical and atypical, have been used to treat agitation and aggressive behavior in post-TBI patients. Certainly, florid psychosis in the

face of prior TBI is sometimes effectively managed with these medications [72, 77, 78]. While post-TBI agitation, disinhibition, and aggressive behavior were not the initial indications for these medications, they have become commonly used clinically in TBI patients for these indications; however these medications are associated with a number of adverse effects. Thus, their role in the recovery of TBI patients needs to be carefully examined.

Several case reports on the use of antipsychotics in post-TBI patients for a variety of symptoms, including delirium, psychosis, self-injurious behavior, and aggression, [79–89] have been published, but very little prospective data is available.

Traditional antipsychotics such as haloperidol are generally contraindicated in TBI patients due not only to oversedation potential but also risk of extrapyramidal side effects such as acute dyskinesias and dystonic reactions, tardive dyskinesia, akinesia, akathisia, and Parkinsonism, all of which may be permanent, and even neuroleptic malignant syndrome (NMS), which can prove to be fatal. The constellation of symptoms in NMS includes muscle rigidity, autonomic instability, and fluctuating levels of consciousness [90]. Multiple case reports are available in which NMS was noted in TBI patients who received antipsychotics [91–93]. Without early recognition and treatment, NMS can lead to rapid death. Furthermore, as in the animal studies previously described, antipsychotics have been shown to have a negative impact on arousal states and slowing of ultimate recovery in humans after TBI. Early studies showed negative effects with longer periods of posttraumatic amnesia [94], no benefit with regard to rehabilitation success [94], and negative impact on cognition [95]. Therefore, the use of haloperidol has largely been appropriately abandoned in acute and subacute phases after TBI.

Quetiapine, a so-called novel antipsychotic, has been used in varying doses to treat symptoms of irritability and aggression in post-TBI patients. Medication use led to significant improvement in Overt Aggression Scale (OAS-M) scores (84.5%, $p = 0.002$) and Clinical Global Impression (CGI) scores (4.14 vs. 2.29, $p = 0.002$) in a small, open-label (and therefore subject to biased outcome reporting), uncontrolled (albeit prospectively conducted) study [96]. Behavioral reporting is especially prone to bias when subjects are aware of treatment, and placebo-controlled studies are critically important in this type of investigation.

A number of review studies have been done on the use of antipsychotics in post-TBI patients. While insufficient data are available for meta-analyses on this subject due to the heterogeneity of trial design, thorough systemic reviews have recommended the use of antipsychotics in acute settings for protection of the patient and staff members in the lowest effective dose and frequency. However, the level of evidence for such recommendations remains at the level of consensus, and further research is needed [97–100].

While antipsychotics may be helpful in the treatment of acute agitation and aggressive behavior, they do not appear to be satisfactory long-term solutions for these symptoms due in large part to possible serious adverse effects. Furthermore, not only do they not appear to have a significant long-term benefit in TBI patients, but they may actually have detrimental effects on cognition in this patient population. If used, they should only be used briefly and with caution, with preference toward the more novel antipsychotics for their theoretically lower side-effect profiles.

Other Medications

While amantadine and methylphenidate are the most well-studied consciousness-enhancing medications in TBI patients, there have been numerous other medications studied in this population.

Modafinil is a neurostimulant (the exact mechanism of action of which is again unknown) that has been used to treat narcolepsy and symptoms of excessive daytime sleepiness, so it has been proposed as a potential treatment for post-TBI fatigue. Two randomized trials have been published with conflicting results. A randomized, crossover trial showed no significant differences in fatigue and daytime sleepiness between modafinil and placebo [101]. On the contrary, a noncrossover study of lower-dose modafinil did show an improvement in daytime sleepiness with modafinil but no difference in symptoms of fatigue [102]. Interestingly, meta-analysis of the data available from both studies derived a significant mean difference in fatigue scores of -0.82 (95% CI -0.11, -1.54). However, when the data for daytime sleepiness was pooled, no significant difference was found (MD -1.77, 95% CI 0.72, -4.26) [103].

Armodafinil is an enantiomeric formulation of modafinil. Only one study has been performed on armodafinil in post-TBI patients. While this study began as a randomized, controlled, double-blind trial, it was eventually converted to an open-label trial. During the controlled portion of the study, armodafinil was noted to have a significant (undesirable) effect on sleep latency ($+7.2$ min vs. $+2.4$ min, $p = 0.0010$) but not on daytime sleepiness [104].

Bromocriptine is a dopamine agonist that is often used to treat pituitary tumors and Parkinson's disease. Due to its mechanism of action and some preclinical studies in animal models as discussed previously, it has been proposed as a possible agent for use in post-TBI patients to enhance arousal [105]. One small clinical study of bromocriptine's effects on multiple post-TBI symptoms showed accelerated rates of return to arousal in 47% of the small cohort given bromocriptine and improvements in hemiparesis and aphasia [106]. However, bromocriptine was not found to be helpful with symptoms of inattention, which were actually worse than placebo and caused lower blood pressure (asymptomatic) in a separate randomized crossover study [107].

Carbidopa/levodopa, a dopamine agonist commonly used in the treatment of Parkinson's disease, has been discussed in a handful of case reports, with mixed results [108, 109]. One cohort study demonstrated functional and behavioral improvements in a small group of patients, but no control group was provided for comparison [110].

Donepezil, a cholinesterase inhibitor used for improvement of memory symptoms in Alzheimer's disease, has undergone limited study in a case report [111] and cohort study [112]. In the latter, 22 patients had both baseline IQ testing as well as at some point during follow-up. A 2.5 point improvement in overall IQ scores was seen in these subjects, the significance of which could certainly be called into question.

Larger, well-controlled studies are needed to draw definitive conclusions regarding all of these agents.

Conclusions

Stimulant medications may play some role in certain long-term sequelae of traumatic brain injury, particularly inattention and information processing speed [113–118]. However, definitive conclusions about the use of these medications in post-TBI patients are difficult to draw from the available data [119, 120]. Compelling evidence for the use of these medications to improve cognitive outcomes is lacking, as is the delineation of any effect on levels of arousal in the acute phase of TBI recovery [114–120]. The adverse effects from these medications are not trivial, and the screening processes for capturing the incidence of adverse effects in most of the published literature have been sparse [120].

There is not enough evidence to support the routine use of stimulant medications in post-TBI patients to improve functional or cognitive outcomes or return to higher levels of consciousness or arousal. However, neurostimulants may be useful in the post-TBI patient to treat symptoms of inattention. Certainly, further large-scale, randomized trials are warranted.

References

1. Posner JB, Plum F. Plum and posner's diagnosis of stupor and coma. 4th ed. Oxford: Oxford University Press; 2007.
2. Jennett B, Plum F. Persistent vegetative state after brain damage. A syndrome in search of a name. Lancet. 1972;1(7753):734–7.
3. Giacino JT, Ashwal S, Childs N, Cranford R, Jennett B, Katz DI, et al. The minimally conscious state: definition and diagnostic criteria. Neurology. 2002;58(3):349–53.
4. Giacino JT, Kalmar K. Diagnostic and prognostic guidelines for the vegetative and minimally conscious states. Neuropsychol Rehabil. 2005;15(3–4):166–74.
5. Lombardi F, Taricco M, De Tanti A, Telaro E, Liberati A. Sensory stimulation for brain injured individuals in coma or vegetative state. Cochrane Database Syst Rev 2002(2):CD001427.
6. Kline AE, Yan HQ, Bao J, Marion DW, Dixon CE. Chronic methylphenidate treatment enhances water maze performance following traumatic brain injury in rats. Neurosci Lett. 2000;280(3):163–6.
7. Kline AE, Massucci JL, Marion DW, Dixon CE. Attenuation of working memory and spatial acquisition deficits after a delayed and chronic bromocriptine treatment regimen in rats subjected to traumatic brain injury by controlled cortical impact. J Neurotrauma. 2002;19(4):415–25.
8. Wagner AK, Kline AE, Ren D, Willard LA, Wenger MK, Zafonte RD, et al. Gender associations with chronic methylphenidate treatment and behavioral performance following experimental traumatic brain injury. Behav Brain Res. 2007;181(2):200–9.
9. Wagner AK, Drewencki LL, Chen X, Santos FR, Khan AS, Harun R, et al. Chronic methylphenidate treatment enhances striatal dopamine neurotransmission after experimental traumatic brain injury. J Neurochem. 2009;108(4):986–97.
10. Wagner AK, Sokoloski JE, Chen X, Harun R, Clossin DP, Khan AS, et al. Controlled cortical impact injury influences methylphenidate-induced changes in striatal dopamine neurotransmission. J Neurochem. 2009;110(3):801–10.
11. Leary JB, Bondi CO, LaPorte MJ, Carlson LJ, Radabaugh HL, Cheng JP, et al. The therapeutic efficacy of environmental enrichment and methylphenidate alone and in combination after controlled cortical impact injury. J Neurotrauma. 2017;34(2):444–50.
12. Rau TF, Kothiwal AS, Rova AR, Brooks DM, Poulsen DJ. Treatment with low-dose methamphetamine improves behavioral and cognitive function after severe traumatic brain injury. J Trauma Acute Care Surg. 2012;73(2 Suppl 1):S165–72.
13. Rau TF, Kothiwal AS, Rova AR, Brooks DM, Rhoderick JF, Poulsen AJ, et al. Administration of low dose methamphetamine 12 h after a severe traumatic brain injury prevents neurological dysfunction and cognitive impairment in rats. Exp Neurol. 2014;253:31–40.
14. Rau T, Ziemniak J, Poulsen D. The neuroprotective potential of low-dose methamphetamine in preclinical models of stroke and traumatic brain injury. Prog Neuro-Psychopharmacol Biol Psychiatry. 2016;64:231–6.
15. Phelps TI, Bondi CO, Ahmed RH, Olugbade YT, Kline AE. Divergent long-term consequences of chronic treatment with haloperidol, risperidone, and bromocriptine on traumatic brain injury-induced cognitive deficits. J Neurotrauma. 2015;32(8):590–7.

16. Chandler MC, Barnhill JL, Gualtieri CT. Amantadine for the agitated head-injury patient. Brain Inj. 1988;2(4):309–11.

17. Andersson S, Berstad J, Finset A, Grimsmo J. Amantadine in cognitive failure in patients with traumatic head injuries. Tidsskr Nor Laegeforen. 1992;112(16):2070–2.

18. Van Reekum R, Bayley M, Garner S, Burke IM, Fawcett S, Hart A, et al. N of 1 study: amantadine for the amotivational syndrome in a patient with traumatic brain injury. Brain Inj. 1995;9(1):49–53.

19. Zafonte RD, Watanabe T, Mann NR. Amantadine: a potential treatment for the minimally conscious state. Brain Inj. 1998;12(7):617–21.

20. Gwynette MF, Beck B, VandenBerg A, Stocking N. Under arrest: the use of amantadine for treatment-refractory mood lability and aggression in a patient with traumatic brain injury. J Clin Psychopharmacol. 2015;35(1):102–4.

21. Wu TS, Garmel GM. Improved neurological function after amantadine treatment in two patients with brain injury. J Emerg Med. 2005;28(3):289–92.

22. Kraus MF, Smith GS, Butters M, Donnell AJ, Dixon E, Yilong C, et al. Effects of the dopaminergic agent and nmda receptor antagonist amantadine on cognitive function, cerebral glucose metabolism and d2 receptor availability in chronic traumatic brain injury: a study using positron emission tomography (pet). Brain Inj. 2005;19(7):471–9.

23. Green LB, Hornyak JE, Hurvitz EA. Amantadine in pediatric patients with traumatic brain injury: a retrospective, case-controlled study. Am J Phys Med Rehabil. 2004;83(12):893–7.

24. Hughes S, Colantonio A, Santaguida PL, Paton T. Amantadine to enhance readiness for rehabilitation following severe traumatic brain injury. Brain Inj. 2005;19(14):1197–206.

25. Saniova B, Drobny M, Kneslova L, Minarik M. The outcome of patients with severe head injuries treated with amantadine sulphate. J Neural Transm (Vienna). 2004;111(4):511–4.

26. Beers SR, Skold A, Dixon CE, Adelson PD. Neurobehavioral effects of amantadine after pediatric traumatic brain injury: a preliminary report. J Head Trauma Rehabil. 2005;20(5): 450–63.

27. Patrick PD, Blackman JA, Mabry JL, Buck ML, Gurka MJ, Conaway MR. Dopamine agonist therapy in low-response children following traumatic brain injury. J Child Neurol. 2006;21(10):879–85.

28. Schneider WN, Drew-Cates J, Wong TM, Dombovy ML. Cognitive and behavioural efficacy of amantadine in acute traumatic brain injury: an initial double-blind placebo-controlled study. Brain Inj. 1999;13(11):863–72.

29. Meythaler JM, Brunner RC, Johnson A, Novack TA. Amantadine to improve neurorecovery in traumatic brain injury-associated diffuse axonal injury: a pilot double-blind randomized trial. J Head Trauma Rehabil. 2002;17(4):300–13.

30. Giacino JT, Whyte J, Bagiella E, Kalmar K, Childs N, Khademi A, et al. Placebo-controlled trial of amantadine for severe traumatic brain injury. N Engl J Med. 2012;366(9):819–26.

31. Hammond FM, Bickett AK, Norton JH, Pershad R. Effectiveness of amantadine hydrochloride in the reduction of chronic traumatic brain injury irritability and aggression. J Head Trauma Rehabil. 2014;29(5):391–9.

32. Hammond FM, Sherer M, Malec JF, Zafonte RD, Whitney M, Bell K, et al. Amantadine effect on perceptions of irritability after traumatic brain injury: results of the amantadine irritability multisite study. J Neurotrauma. 2015;32(16):1230–8.

33. Leone H, Polsonetti BW. Amantadine for traumatic brain injury: does it improve cognition and reduce agitation? J Clin Pharm Ther. 2005;30(2):101–4.

34. Sawyer E, Mauro LS, Ohlinger MJ. Amantadine enhancement of arousal and cognition after traumatic brain injury. Ann Pharmacother. 2008;42(2):247–52.

35. Williams SE. Amantadine treatment following traumatic brain injury in children. Brain Inj. 2007;21(9):885–9.

36. Challman TD, Lipsky JJ. Methylphenidate: its pharmacology and uses. Mayo Clin Proc. 2000;75(7):711–21.

37. Weinberg RM, Auerbach SH, Moore S. Pharmacologic treatment of cognitive deficits: a case study. Brain Inj. 1987;1(1):57–9.

38. Hornyak JE, Nelson VS, Hurvitz EA. The use of methylphenidate in paediatric traumatic brain injury. Pediatr Rehabil. 1997;1(1):15–7.

39. Worzniak M, Fetters MD, Comfort M. Methylphenidate in the treatment of coma. J Fam Pract. 1997;44(5):495–8.

40. Francisco GE, Ivanhoe CB. Successful treatment of post-traumatic narcolepsy with methylphenidate: a case report. Am J Phys Med Rehabil. 1996;75(1):63–5.

41. Grønborg P, Liljegren J, Jansen J. Paradoxical effect of methylphenidate in the treatment of a patient with severe traumatic brain injury. Ugeskr Laeger. 2009;171(26):2201–2.

42. Reynolds JC, Rittenberger JC, Callaway CW. Methylphenidate and amantadine to stimulate reawakening in comatose patients resuscitated from cardiac arrest. Resuscitation. 2013;84(6):818–24.

43. Wroblewski BA, Leary JM, Phelan AM, Whyte J, Manning K. Methylphenidate and seizure frequency in brain injured patients with seizure disorders. J Clin Psychiatry. 1992;53(3):86–9.

44. Al-Adawi S, Burke DT, Dorvlo AS. The effect of methylphenidate on the sleep-wake cycle of brain-injured patients undergoing rehabilitation. Sleep Med. 2006;7(3):287–91.

45. Gualtieri CT, Evans RW. Stimulant treatment for the neurobehavioural sequelae of traumatic brain injury. Brain Inj. 1988;2(4):273–90.

46. Speech TJ, Rao SM, Osmon DC, Sperry LT. A double-blind controlled study of methylpheni-

date treatment in closed head injury. Brain Inj. 1993;7(4):333–8.

47. Mooney GF, Haas LJ. Effect of methylphenidate on brain injury-related anger. Arch Phys Med Rehabil. 1993;74(2):153–60.

48. Plenger PM, Dixon CE, Castillo RM, Frankowski RF, Yablon SA, Levin HS. Subacute methylphenidate treatment for moderate to moderately severe traumatic brain injury: a preliminary double-blind placebo-controlled study. Arch Phys Med Rehabil. 1996;77(6):536–40.

49. Johansson B, Wentzel AP, Andréll P, Odenstedt J, Mannheimer C, Rönnbäck L. Evaluation of dosage, safety and effects of methylphenidate on post-traumatic brain injury symptoms with a focus on mental fatigue and pain. Brain Inj. 2014;28(3):304–10.

50. Johansson B, Wentzel AP, Andréll P, Mannheimer C, Rönnbäck L. Methylphenidate reduces mental fatigue and improves processing speed in persons suffered a traumatic brain injury. Brain Inj. 2015;29(6):758–65.

51. Johansson B, Wentzel AP, Andréll P, Rönnbäck L, Mannheimer C. Long-term treatment with methylphenidate for fatigue after traumatic brain injury. Acta Neurol Scand. 2017;135(1):100–7.

52. McAllister TW, Zafonte R, Jain S, Flashman LA, George MS, Grant GA, et al. Randomized placebo-controlled trial of methylphenidate or galantamine for persistent emotional and cognitive symptoms associated with ptsd and/or traumatic brain injury. Neuropsychopharmacology. 2016;41(5):1191–8.

53. Lee H, Kim SW, Kim JM, Shin IS, Yang SJ, Yoon JS. Comparing effects of methylphenidate, sertraline and placebo on neuropsychiatric sequelae in patients with traumatic brain injury. Hum Psychopharmacol. 2005;20(2):97–104.

54. Alban JP, Hopson MM, Ly V, Whyte J. Effect of methylphenidate on vital signs and adverse effects in adults with traumatic brain injury. Am J Phys Med Rehabil. 2004;83(2):131–7. quiz 138-141, 167

55. Willmott C, Ponsford J, Olver J, Ponsford M. Safety of methylphenidate following traumatic brain injury: impact on vital signs and side-effects during inpatient rehabilitation. J Rehabil Med. 2009;41(7):585–7.

56. Moein H, Khalili HA, Keramatian K. Effect of methylphenidate on icu and hospital length of stay in patients with severe and moderate traumatic brain injury. Clin Neurol Neurosurg. 2006;108(6):539–42.

57. Whyte J, Hart T, Schuster K, Fleming M, Polansky M, Coslett HB. Effects of methylphenidate on attentional function after traumatic brain injury. A randomized, placebo-controlled trial. Am J Phys Med Rehabil. 1997;76(6):440–50.

58. Whyte J, Hart T, Vaccaro M, Grieb-Neff P, Risser A, Polansky M, et al. Effects of methylphenidate on attention deficits after traumatic brain injury: a multidimensional, randomized, controlled trial. Am J Phys Med Rehabil. 2004;83(6):401–20.

59. Kaelin DL, Cifu DX, Matthies B. Methylphenidate effect on attention deficit in the acutely brain-injured adult. Arch Phys Med Rehabil. 1996;77(1):6–9.

60. Williams SE, Ris MD, Ayyangar R, Schefft BK, Berch D. Recovery in pediatric brain injury: is psychostimulant medication beneficial? J Head Trauma Rehabil. 1998;13(3):73–81.

61. Mahalick DM, Carmel PW, Greenberg JP, Molofsky W, Brown JA, Heary RF, et al. Psychopharmacologic treatment of acquired attention disorders in children with brain injury. Pediatr Neurosurg. 1998;29(3):121–6.

62. Ekinci O, Direk M, Gunes S, Teke H, Ekinci N, Yıldırım F, et al. Short-term efficacy and tolerability of methylphenidate in children with traumatic brain injury and attention problems. Brain and Development. 2017;39(4):327–36.

63. Willmott C, Ponsford J. Efficacy of methylphenidate in the rehabilitation of attention following traumatic brain injury: a randomised, crossover, double blind, placebo controlled inpatient trial. J Neurol Neurosurg Psychiatry. 2009;80(5):552–7.

64. Kim YH, Ko MH, Na SY, Park SH, Kim KW. Effects of single-dose methylphenidate on cognitive performance in patients with traumatic brain injury: a double-blind placebo-controlled study. Clin Rehabil. 2006;20(1):24–30.

65. Dymowski AR, Ponsford JL, Owens JA, Olver JH, Ponsford M, Willmott C. The efficacy and safety of extended-release methylphenidate following traumatic brain injury: a randomised controlled pilot study. Clin Rehabil. 2017;31(6):733–41.

66. McDonald BC, Flashman LA, Arciniegas DB, Ferguson RJ, Xing L, Harezlak J, et al. Methylphenidate and memory and attention adaptation training for persistent cognitive symptoms after traumatic brain injury: a randomized, placebo-controlled trial. Neuropsychopharmacology. 2017;42(9):1766–75.

67. Huang CH, Huang CC, Sun CK, Lin GH, Hou WH. Methylphenidate on cognitive improvement in patients with traumatic brain injury: a meta-analysis. Curr Neuropharmacol. 2016;14(3):272–81.

68. Kraus MF. Neuropsychiatric sequelae of stroke and traumatic brain injury: the role of psychostimulants. Int J Psychiatry Med. 1995;25(1):39–51.

69. Kajs-Wyllie M. Ritalin revisited: does it really help in neurological injury? J Neurosci Nurs. 2002;34(6):303–13.

70. Siddall OM. Use of methylphenidate in traumatic brain injury. Ann Pharmacother. 2005;39(7–8):1309–13.

71. Whyte J, Vaccaro M, Grieb-Neff P, Hart T. Psychostimulant use in the rehabilitation of individuals with traumatic brain injury. J Head Trauma Rehabil. 2002;17(4):284–99.

72. Lee HB, Lyketsos CG, Rao V. Pharmacological management of the psychiatric aspects of traumatic brain injury. Int Rev Psychiatry. 2003;15(4):359–70.

73. Jin C, Schachar R. Methylphenidate treatment of attention-deficit/hyperactivity disorder secondary to traumatic brain injury: a critical appraisal of treatment studies. CNS Spectr. 2004;9(3):217–26.

74. Forsyth R, Jayamoni B, Paine T, Mascarenhas S. Monoaminergic agonists for acute traumatic brain injury. Cochrane Database Syst Rev. 2006;(1):CD003984.

75. Tenovuo O. Pharmacological enhancement of cognitive and behavioral deficits after traumatic brain injury. Curr Opin Neurol. 2006;19(6):528–33.

76. Maksimowski MB, Tampi RR. Efficacy of stimulants for psychiatric symptoms in individuals with traumatic brain injury. Ann Clin Psychiatry. 2016;28(3):156–66.

77. Elovic EP, Lansang R, Li Y, Ricker JH. The use of atypical antipsychotics in traumatic brain injury. J Head Trauma Rehabil. 2003;18(2):177–95.

78. Arciniegas DB, McAllister TW. Neurobehavioral management of traumatic brain injury in the critical care setting. Crit Care Clin. 2008;24(4):737–65. viii

79. Krieger D, Hansen K, McDermott C, Matthews R, Mitchell R, Bollegala N, et al. Loxapine versus olanzapine in the treatment of delirium following traumatic brain injury. NeuroRehabilitation. 2003;18(3):205–8.

80. Temple MJ. Use of atypical anti-psychotics in the management of post-traumatic confusional states in traumatic brain injury. J R Army Med Corps. 2003;149(1):54–5.

81. Freeman T, High WM. Treatment of a patient with traumatic brain injury-related severe self-injurious behavior. J Head Trauma Rehabil. 2009;24(4):292–6.

82. Trémeau F, Mauro CJ, Shope C, Riber LM, Dhami S, Citrome L. High dose quetiapine in the treatment of psychosis due to traumatic brain injury: a case report. Prog Neuro-Psychopharmacol Biol Psychiatry. 2011;35(1):280–1.

83. Viana BM, Prais HA, Nicolato R, Caramelli P. Posttraumatic brain injury psychosis successfully treated with olanzapine. Prog Neuro-Psychopharmacol Biol Psychiatry. 2010;34(1):233–5.

84. Richardson JK. Psychotic behavior after right hemispheric cerebrovascular accident: a case report. Arch Phys Med Rehabil. 1992;73(4):381–4.

85. Silva JA, Leong GB, Wine DB. Misidentification delusions, facial misrecognition, and right brain injury. Can J Psychiatr. 1993;38(4):239–41.

86. Sipahimalani A, Masand PS. Use of risperidone in delirium: case reports. Ann Clin Psychiatry. 1997;9(2):105–7.

87. Umansky R, Geller V. Olanzapine treatment in an organic hallucinosis patient. Int J Neuropsychopharmacol. 2000;3(1):81–2.

88. Noe E, Ferri J, Trenor C, Chirivella J. Efficacy of ziprasidone in controlling agitation during post-traumatic amnesia. Behav Neurol. 2007;18(1):7–11.

89. Michals ML, Crismon ML, Roberts S, Childs A. Clozapine response and adverse effects in nine brain-injured patients. J Clin Psychopharmacol. 1993;13(3):198-203.

90. American Psychiatric Association. DSM-5 task force. Diagnostic and statistical manual of mental disorders: DSM-5. 5th ed. Arlington, VA: American Psychiatric Association; 2013.

91. Wilkinson R, Meythaler JM, Guin-Renfroe S. Neuroleptic malignant syndrome induced by haloperidol following traumatic brain injury. Brain Inj. 1999;13(12):1025–31.

92. Kadyan V, Colachis SC, Depalma MJ, Sanderson JD, Mysiw WJ. Early recognition of neuroleptic malignant syndrome during traumatic brain injury rehabilitation. Brain Inj. 2003;17(7):631–7.

93. Bellamy CJ, Kane-Gill SL, Falcione BA, Seybert AL. Neuroleptic malignant syndrome in traumatic brain injury patients treated with haloperidol. J Trauma. 2009;66(3):954–8.

94. Rao N, Jellinek HM, Woolston DC. Agitation in closed head injury: haloperidol effects on rehabilitation outcome. Arch Phys Med Rehabil. 1985;66(1):30–4.

95. Stanislav SW. Cognitive effects of antipsychotic agents in persons with traumatic brain injury. Brain Inj. 1997;11(5):335–41.

96. Kim E, Bijlani M. A pilot study of quetiapine treatment of aggression due to traumatic brain injury. J Neuropsychiatry Clin Neurosci. 2006;18(4):547–9.

97. Levy M, Berson A, Cook T, Bollegala N, Seto E, Tursanski S, et al. Treatment of agitation following traumatic brain injury: a review of the literature. NeuroRehabilitation. 2005;20(4):279–306.

98. Lombard LA, Zafonte RD. Agitation after traumatic brain injury: considerations and treatment options. Am J Phys Med Rehabil. 2005;84(10):797–812.

99. Luauté J, Plantier D, Wiart L, Tell L, SOFMER Group. Care management of the agitation or aggressiveness crisis in patients with tbi. Systematic review of the literature and practice recommendations. Ann Phys Rehabil Med. 2016;59(1):58–67.

100. Plantier D, Luaute J, SOFMER Group. Drugs for behavior disorders after traumatic brain injury: systematic review and expert consensus leading to French recommendations for good practice. Ann Phys Rehabil Med. 2016;59(1):42–57.

101. Jha A, Weintraub A, Allshouse A, Morey C, Cusick C, Kittelson J, et al. A randomized trial of modafinil for the treatment of fatigue and excessive daytime sleepiness in individuals with chronic traumatic brain injury. J Head Trauma Rehabil. 2008;23(1):52–63.

102. Kaiser PR, Valko PO, Werth E, Thomann J, Meier J, Stocker R, et al. Modafinil ameliorates excessive daytime sleepiness after traumatic brain injury. Neurology. 2010;75(20):1780–5.

103. Sheng P, Hou L, Wang X, Huang C, Yu M, Han X, et al. Efficacy of modafinil on fatigue and excessive daytime sleepiness associated with neurological disorders: a systematic review and meta-analysis. PLoS One. 2013;8(12):e81802.

104. Menn SJ, Yang R, Lankford A. Armodafinil for the treatment of excessive sleepiness associated with mild or moderate closed traumatic brain injury: a 12-week, randomized, double-blind study followed by a 12-month open-label extension. J Clin Sleep Med. 2014;10(11):1181–91.

105. Passler MA, Riggs RV. Positive outcomes in traumatic brain injury-vegetative state: patients treated with bromocriptine. Arch Phys Med Rehabil. 2001;82(3):311–5.

106. Munakomi S, Bhattarai B, Mohan Kumar B. Role of bromocriptine in multi-spectral manifestations of traumatic brain injury. Chin J Traumatol. 2017;20(2):84–6.

107. Whyte J, Vaccaro M, Grieb-Neff P, Hart T, Polansky M, Coslett HB. The effects of bromocriptine on attention deficits after traumatic brain injury: a placebo-controlled pilot study. Am J Phys Med Rehabil. 2008;87(2):85–99.

108. Haig AJ, Ruess JM. Recovery from vegetative state of six months' duration associated with sinemet (levodopa/carbidopa). Arch Phys Med Rehabil. 1990;71(13):1081–3.

109. Wolf AP, Gleckman AD. Sinemet and brain injury: functional versus statistical change and suggestions for future research designs. Brain Inj. 1995;9(5):487–93.

110. Lal S, Merbtiz CP, Grip JC. Modification of function in head-injured patients with sinemet. Brain Inj. 1988;2(3):225–33.

111. Taverni JP, Seliger G, Lichtman SW. Donepezil medicated memory improvement in traumatic brain injury during post acute rehabilitation. Brain Inj. 1998;12(1):77–80.

112. Whelan FJ, Walker MS, Schultz SK. Donepezil in the treatment of cognitive dysfunction associated with traumatic brain injury. Ann Clin Psychiatry. 2000;12(3):131–5.

113. Richer E, Tell L. Indications, efficacy and tolerance of drug therapy in view of improving recovery of consciousness following a traumatic brain injury. Ann Readapt Med Phys. 2003;46(4):177–83.

114. Arciniegas DB, Silver JM. Pharmacotherapy of posttraumatic cognitive impairments. Behav Neurol. 2006;17(1):25–42.

115. Chew E, Zafonte RD. Pharmacological management of neurobehavioral disorders following traumatic brain injury--a state-of-the-art review. J Rehabil Res Dev. 2009;46(6):851–79.

116. Writer BW, Schillerstrom JE. Psychopharmacological treatment for cognitive impairment in survivors of traumatic brain injury: a critical review. J Neuropsychiatry Clin Neurosci. 2009;21(4):362–70.

117. Sivan M, Neumann V, Kent R, Stroud A, Bhakta BB. Pharmacotherapy for treatment of attention deficits after non-progressive acquired brain injury. A systematic review. Clin Rehabil. 2010;24(2):110–21.

118. Cossu G. Therapeutic options to enhance coma arousal after traumatic brain injury: state of the art of current treatments to improve coma recovery. Br J Neurosurg. 2014;28(2):187–98.

119. Napolitano E, Elovic EP, Qureshi AI. Pharmacological stimulant treatment of neurocognitive and functional deficits after traumatic and non-traumatic brain injury. Med Sci Monit. 2005;11(6):RA212–20.

120. Frenette AJ, Kanji S, Rees L, Williamson DR, Perreault MM, Turgeon AF, et al. Efficacy and safety of dopamine agonists in traumatic brain injury: a systematic review of randomized controlled trials. J Neurotrauma. 2012;29(1):1–18.

Management of Traumatic Brain Injury in the Face of Antithrombotic Medication Therapy

Jonathan H. DeAntonio, Kimberly N. Means, Sudha Jayaraman, and Gretchen M. Brophy

Introduction

Traumatic brain injury (TBI) has long been associated with coagulopathy. Both hypercoagulable (microthrombi and ischemia) and hypocoagulable (progressive or acute hemorrhage) states are observed following TBI; however, the causes of each are not well understood. Multiple factors have been described as potential sources of this coagulopathy including tissue factor release, hyperfibrinolysis, activated protein C, and decreased number of platelets along with decreased platelet function [1]. Patients who are

J. H. DeAntonio, MD
Department of Surgery, Virginia Commonwealth University Health System, VCU School of Medicine, Richmond, VA, USA
e-mail: jonathan.deantonio@vcuhealth.org

K. N. Means, PharmD, BSN, RN
Department of Pharmacy Services, Medical College of Virginia, Richmond, VA, USA
e-mail: newtonk@vcu.edu

S. Jayaraman, MD, MSc, FACS
Division of Acute Care Surgical Services, Virginia Commonwealth University Health System, Richmond, VA, USA
e-mail: Sudha.jayaraman@vcuhealth.org

G. M. Brophy, PharmD, BCPS, FCCP, FCCM, FNCS (✉)
Department of Pharmacotherapy and Outcomes Science and Neurosurgery, Virginia Commonwealth University, Richmond, VA, USA
e-mail: gbrophy@vcu.edu

on therapeutic anticoagulation have further increased risk for poor clinical outcome in the setting of trauma-induced coagulopathy. A significant portion of the US population, especially older adults, is on anticoagulation or antiplatelet agents for atrial fibrillation, venous thromboembolism, stroke, or other thrombotic diseases [2]. These numbers have increased with the development of direct-acting oral anticoagulants (DOACs), such as rivaroxaban, apixaban, edoxaban, and dabigatran, which are being used with increasing frequency because of their reliable pharmacokinetic profiles [2]. In order to manage these patients properly, in the setting of brain trauma, there must be an understanding of the pathophysiology of coagulopathy following TBI and how this is further altered in patients who are on therapeutic antithrombotic agents.

Predictors of Outcome and Timing of Trauma-Induced Coagulopathy

Coagulopathy can have significant short-term and long-term impact on the management of TBI patients. The International Mission for Prognosis and Analysis of Clinic Trials in TBI (IMPACT Trial—2007) identified prolongation of prothrombin time (PT) as an independent risk factor for poor outcome following TBI [3]. Coagulopathy (international normalized ratio [INR] > 1.3/platelets <100 k) on admission was

© Springer International Publishing AG, part of Springer Nature 2018
S. D. Timmons (ed.), *Controversies in Severe Traumatic Brain Injury Management*,
https://doi.org/10.1007/978-3-319-89477-5_16

also shown to be associated with an increase in the rate of intubation, single- and multi-system organ failure, intensive care unit (ICU) length of stay, overall length of stay, and overall hospital mortality from 17.3 to 50.4% (adjusted odds ratio of 2.97) [4, 5]. Increased rates of sepsis and diabetes insipidus have also been reported in coagulopathic TBI patients [4]. Elevated mortality rates in coagulopathic trauma patients take on a greater significance when the overall incidence of acute coagulopathy of trauma (independent of TBI) has been shown to be as high as 86% [5, 6]. Early coagulopathy, when it began at least 24 h following admission, has been associated with a 55% mortality compared to 23%, even when controlled for severity of TBI [4].

Regardless of mechanism, the loss of equilibrium in the coagulation cascade following trauma can lead to hypocoagulable or hypercoagulable states. These coagulopathic states may frequently be demonstrated by increases in prothrombin time (PT), international normalized ratio (INR) and partial thromboplastin time (PTT), decreased platelet count or fibrinogen, or thromboelastography (TEG) abnormalities. Independent risk factors for acute (<24 h) coagulopathy after TBI include severity of injury (as measured by the abbreviated injury scale, AIS_{head}, 0–6 with 6 being worst), low pre-resuscitation Glasgow Coma Scale (GCS < 8) score, hypotension (systolic blood pressure < 90), amount of prehospital intravenous fluids (IVF > 2000 mL), and age > 75 years [7]. Others have confirmed the same independent risk factors for poor prognosis following TBI and additionally elevated PTT (> 30.2 s) and D-dimer [8]. AIS_{head} of 3–6 have been associated with coagulopathy rates ranging from 14 to 77%, across several studies [4, 7]. A meta-analysis has shown the prevalence of TBI-associated coagulopathy to be 32.7–35.2% [5].

Several studies have discussed the timing of the coagulopathy following TBI and the association between this timing and subsequent morbidity and prognosis [4, 8]. An increased risk of coagulopathy and hyperfibrinolysis has been seen within the first 3 h of injury based on elevated PTT and D-dimer levels [8]. Hyperfibrinolysis has even been shown to start within the first hour

following injury [8]. This same study also identified elevated D-dimer level within 12 h or an upward trend of PTT within 3 h of injury as significant negative prognostic indicators [8].

Pathophysiology of Trauma-Induced Coagulopathy

Historically, trauma-induced coagulopathy (TIC) has been attributed to the classic triad of hypothermia, acidosis, and the dilution of coagulation factors. While the cause is still not entirely known, several hypotheses have been proposed in the literature to describe the underlying mechanism by which this coagulopathy occurs in the setting of trauma or TBI.

The first suggests that tissue factor (TF) released into the systemic circulation following TBI activates the extrinsic coagulation cascade [1]. TF expression is particularly high in the central nervous system, with a high concentration within astrocytes. In addition, it has been hypothesized that, by overactivating the extrinsic pathway, TF causes hyperfibrinolysis, leading to a hypocoagulable state [1, 9, 10]. Fibrinolysis is a negative feedback loop response when the coagulation cascade is activated; however, in this instance it is overactivated, causing hyperfibrinolysis. This was also shown in another study where the most severely injured and shocked patients had decreased fibrinogen concentration and increased fibrinolytic activation [10].

Another possible cause of coagulopathy following TBI is platelet dysfunction [11]. Adenosine diphosphate (ADP) and arachidonic acid receptor inhibition occurs following trauma prior to resuscitation. ADP receptor inhibition correlates strongly with the severity of injury based on GCS scoring [12, 13]. Whole blood analysis with thrombelastography (TEG) showed platelet dysfunction despite no observable abnormalities in TEG parameters, suggesting that the first hematologic abnormality following TBI may be platelet dysfunction at the ADP receptor site [13]. Less ADP receptor inhibition has also been noted in trauma survivors when compared to non-survivors who both suffered life-threatening injuries [14, 15].

Protein C and tissue plasminogen activator (tPA) have also been shown to cause coagulopathy following trauma. Activation of protein C initially causes a hypocoagulable state but can also lead to a hypercoagulable state. Brohi et al. showed that hypoperfusion states induce the release of soluble thrombomodulin, which binds to thrombin, and then this bound thrombin activates protein C (aPC), which creates an "anticoagulant thrombin" [16]. Thrombin complexed with thrombomodulin also activates thrombin activatable fibrinolysis inhibitor (TAFI). aPC in excess decreases plasminogen activator inhibitor-1 (PAI-1) leading to continued conversion of plasminogen to plasmin. Lastly, patients in shock have an increased release of tissue plasminogen activator (tPA) from endothelial walls [6, 16]. Post-traumatic inflammation can lead to a depletion of protein C, which may shift this delicate balance to an acute hypercoagulable state [1].

Special Clinical Scenarios and Considerations in Coagulopathic Patients

Pregnancy

Significant physiological changes occur throughout pregnancy that affect coagulopathy. These include, but are not limited to, a 40% increase in plasma volume with only a 25% increase in red blood cell volume. This leads to a dilutional decrease in hemoglobin concentration known as the physiological anemia of pregnancy. Platelet counts decrease from this dilutional state and from consumption by the uteroplacental unit [17]. These physiological changes (Table 1) prepare women for childbirth and the associated blood loss; however, it vastly impacts the physiological response to trauma [17]. There is very limited published data on the management of pregnant trauma patients, with or without TBI, and in the setting of therapeutic anticoagulation. Trauma surgery, obstetric, and pharmacy consultations are highly recommended in the acute setting to help interpret these physiological changes, manage the TIC, and adjust medication regimens.

Table 1 Hemostatic changes that occur during pregnancy (Adapted from Katz [17])

Coagulopathy of pregnancy	
Fibrinogen	Increases by more than 100%
Factor VII	Increases up to 1000%
Factor VII, IX, X, XII, and Von Willebrand factor	Increases greater than 100%
D-dimer	Increases by up to 400%
Factor XIII	Decreases by up to 50%
Protein S	Decreases by up to 50%
Platelets	Decreases by up to 20%
Factor II, V; Factor XI; Protein C	No change; Variable; No change

Older Adult Patients

Age greater than 75 has been shown to be an independent risk factor for predicting coagulopathy following TBI [7, 18]. Older adult trauma patients are also more likely to be on oral anticoagulants, which can complicate their care and prognoses [2]. Clinicians should be cognizant of the combination of risk factors for bleeding in this patient population post-TBI and be ready to promptly reverse oral anticoagulant agents, when appropriate. Older adults may also have renal or hepatic dysfunction, comorbidities, and multiple medications (including anticoagulant, antiplatelet, anti-inflammatory, and herbal medications) that complicate the use of anticoagulant reversal agents. Obtaining pharmacy and geriatric consultations may be invaluable in effectively managing older adult TBI patients who are on therapeutic anticoagulation prior to admission.

Hypothermia

Hypothermia is frequently found in polytrauma patients with an incidence rate of up to 40% [19]. Hypothermia affects the enzymatic activity of clotting factors (a decrease of 1 °C leads to a 10% reduction in coagulation factor activity), changes platelet function, and also modifies fibrinogen synthesis oftentimes causing hyperfibrinolysis [19]. Hypothermia can be very detrimental in TBI patients on oral anticoagulant agents, as this may enhance the effects of the medication in addition to exacerbating the acute TIC. Hepatic metabolism is also reduced in the hypothermic state, which may lead to prolonged effects of select antithrombotic agents that rely on this mechanism of clearance. Therapeutic hypothermia is sometimes initiated for the treatment of elevated intracranial pressure in TBI patients and would pose similar threats for coagulopathy and reduced drug metabolism.

Prevention remains the best course of action in accidental hypothermia from trauma, and temperatures should be closely monitored throughout the resuscitation efforts. Passive methods of external warming include removing cold or wet clothing and warming the trauma bay. Active methods included forced-air warming blankets and can include adjuncts, such as extracorporeal circulation in severe cases.

Anticoagulation Agents and Their Associated Risks of Major Bleeding

The use of vitamin K antagonists (VKA) (Table 2) continues to increase as the older adult population continues to enlarge [20]. VKA are associated with approximately 12–14% of all intraparenchymal hemorrhages [21]. The functional outcomes and mortality are worse for patients with VKA-related intraparenchymal hemorrhages compared to those unrelated to VKA use. In patients taking VKA therapy, 0.3–1.1% will have an intraparenchymal hemorrhage at some point during their treatment, resulting in 90% of all VKA-related deaths [21]. In particular, warfarin is associated with an annual 15–20% risk of major bleeding and 1–3% risk of life-threatening hemorrhages [22]. These worse outcomes may be due to several factors including larger hemorrhage volumes, increased risk of hematoma expansion, and increased comorbidities of these patients. Most patients who suffer from an intraparenchymal hemorrhage while on VKA are within the recommended INR range.

Direct-acting oral anticoagulants (DOACs) are alternatives to warfarin for various indications. These newer agents have the advantage of having predictable pharmacokinetics in those without renal insufficiency and do not require routine monitoring. Their anticoagulant effect weakens within 24–48 h after the last ingested dose in patients with normal renal function [23]. Older adult patients or those with renal dysfunction may experience a prolonged anticoagulant effect, which could be detrimental in patients with acute traumatic injuries or requiring emergency surgery. These drugs as well as their mechanism of actions, route of elimination, and half-life are listed in Table 2 [20].

There are some data available comparing the outcomes of patients suffering from intracranial injuries taking either warfarin or a DOAC. The Trauma Quality Improvement Project (TQIP) was a retrospective review of patients from a registry who presented with blunt traumatic intracranial hemorrhage while using either warfarin or a DOAC. The included patients suffered a fall and experienced either a subdural hematoma (SDH), subarachnoid hemorrhage (SAH), intraparenchymal hemorrhage (IPH), or intraventricular hemorrhage (IVH). The patients were divided into two groups: 61 patients taking a DOAC and 101 patients taking warfarin. There were no significant differences between groups in terms of proportions of patients with SDH, SAH, IPH, or IVH. The study found that the DOAC group had significantly lower rate of mortality 3/61, 4.9% (95% CI 1.1–14.0%) when compared to patients taking warfarin 23/101, 20.8% (95% CI 15.6–31.9%); $p < 0.008$ [24]. Additionally, the authors concluded that there was also a significantly lower rate of operative intervention in the DOAC group (5/61, 8.2% [95% CI 3.2–18.2%]) when compared with the warfarin group 27/101, 26.7% (95% CI 19–36.1%; $p = 0.02$) [24]. Please refer to Table 3 for the relative risk of bleeding with DOACs compared to warfarin [13].

In Tables 4 and 5, antiplatelet medications and pain medications with platelet-inhibiting properties are listed as well as their mechanism of action, route of elimination, and half-life [20].

Table 2 Anticoagulation agent characteristics [20]

Medication	Mechanism of action	Elimination	Half-life
Oral vitamin K antagonist (VKA)			
Warfarin (Coumadin®, Jantoven®)	Competitively inhibits a subunit of VKOR complex, depleting vitamin K reserves and reducing synthesis of clotting factors	Renal: 92%	20–60 h
Direct-acting oral factor Xa inhibitors			
Rivaroxaban[a] (Xarelto®)	Selective, reversible FXa inhibition	Renal: 66% Fecal: 28%	5–9 h Older adults: 11–13 h
Apixaban[a] (Eliquis®)	Selective, reversible FXa inhibition (free and clot-bound FXa)	Renal: 27% Fecal: majority	12 h
Edoxaban[a] (Savaysa®)	Selective FXa inhibition	Renal: 50%	10–14 h
Factor Xa inhibitor (injectable agent)			
Fondaparinux[a] (Arixtra®)	Selective FXa inhibition	Renal: Up to 77%	17–21 h Prolonged in renal impairment and older adults
Direct-acting oral thrombin inhibitors (DTI)			
Dabigatran Etexilate[a] (Pradaxa®)	Reversible direct thrombin inhibitor (inhibits free and fibrin-bound thrombin)	Renal: 80%	12–17 h Renal impairment: Mild-moderate: 15–18 h Severe: 28 h Older adults: 14–17 h
Thrombin inhibitors (injectable agents)			
Argatroban[b]	Reversibly binds to free and clot-bound thrombin	Renal: 22% Fecal: 65%	39–51 min Hepatic impairment: 181 min
Bivalirudin[a] (Angiomax®)	Reversibly binds to free and clot-bound thrombin	Renal: 20%	25 min Renal impairment: Severe: 57 min
UFH (injectable agent)			
Heparin	Inactivates thrombin and prevents conversion of fibrinogen to fibrin	Renal	90 min
LMWHs (injectable agents)			
Enoxaparin[a] (Lovenox®)	Enhances inhibition of clotting proteases by antithrombin III and inhibition of FXa	Renal: 40%	4.5–7 h
Dalteparin (Fragmin®)	Inhibits FXa and factor IIa (thrombin)	Renal	IV: 40 unit/kg/dose: 2.1 ± 0.3 h 60 unit/kg/dose: 2.3 ± 0.4 h Prolonged in chronic renal impairment
Nadroparin[a] (Fraxiparine®, Fraxiparine Forte®)	Inhibits FXa and factor IIa (thrombin)	Renal	3.5 h Prolonged in renal impairment
Tinzaparin (Innohep®)	Inhibits FXa and factor IIa (thrombin)	Renal	82 min Prolonged in renal impairment
Heparinoid (injectable agent)			
Danaparoid[a] (Orgaran®)	Inhibits FXa and factor IIa (thrombin)	Renal	25 h Renal impairment: 29–35 h

[a]Requires renal dosing adjustment
[b]Requires hepatic dosing adjustment

Table 3 DOAC relative risk of mortality and major bleeding compared to warfarin [confidence interval] (Adapted from Maegele et al. [13])

	Apixaban	Rivaroxaban	Edoxaban	Dabigatran
Atrial fibrillation				
Mortality	0.50 [0.34; 0.74]	0.69 [0.45; 1.04]	No data	0.56 [0.36; 0.86]
Fatal bleeding (includes intracranial hemorrhage)	0.88 [0.44; 1.76]	0.48 [0.30; 0.76]	0.45 [0.31; 0.65]	0.69 [0.37; 1.27]
Venous thromboembolism				
Mortality	0.79 [0.53; 1.19]	0.95 [0.64; 1.42]	1.05 [0.83; 1.33]	1.00 [0.67; 1.42]
Intracranial bleeding	0.50 [0.13; 2.01]	0.40 [0.11; 1.47]	0.08 [0.00; 1.37]	0.28 [0.07; 1.13]
Fatal bleeding	0.50 [0.05; 5.54]	0.20 [0.02; 1.70]	0.20 [0.02; 1.70]	0.20 [0.02; 1.70]

Modified table of a meta-analysis on A-fib with >43,000 patients and 2 meta-analyses on venous thromboembolism with >27,000 patients

Table 4 Antiplatelet agent characteristics [20]

Medication	Mechanism of action	Elimination	Half-life
Oral antiplatelet agents			
Aspirin (Bufferin®, Ecotrin®)	Irreversibly inhibits cyclooxygenase-1 and 2 (COX-1 and 2) and inhibits thromboxane A2	Renal	20 min
Dipyridamole (Persantine®)	Inhibits adenosine deaminase and phosphodiesterase	Fecal	10–12 h
Cilostazol (Pletal®)	Reversibly inhibits phosphodiesterase (PDE) III inhibitor and increases cAMP	Renal: 74% Fecal: 20%	11–13 h
Anagrelide[a] (Agrylin®)	Inhibits cyclic nucleotide phosphodiesterase and release of arachidonic acid, possibly inhibiting phospholipase A_2	Renal	1.5 h
Vorapaxar (Zontivity®)	Protease-activated receptor-1 (PAR-1) receptor antagonist	Renal: 25% Fecal: 58%	3–4 h Terminal half-life elimination: 8 days Long half-life makes this agent effectively irreversible
P2Y$_{12}$ platelet inhibitors (injectable agent)			
Cangrelor (Kengreal®)	Reversibly and selectively binds directly to P2Y$_{12}$ platelet receptor and blocks adenosine diphosphate (ADP)-induced platelet activation and aggregation	Renal: 58% Fecal: 35%	3–6 min
P2Y$_{12}$ platelet inhibitors (oral agents)			
Clopidogrel (Plavix®)	Irreversible inhibition of P2Y$_{12}$ ADP receptor	Renal: 50% Fecal: 46%	6–8 h
Ticlopidine	Irreversible inhibition of P2Y$_{12}$ ADP receptor	Renal: 60% Fecal: 23%	13 h
Prasugrel (Effient®)	Irreversible inhibition of P2Y$_{12}$ ADP receptor	Renal: 68% Fecal: 27%	2–15 h
Ticagrelor (Brilinta®)	Reversible and noncompetitive inhibition of P2Y$_{12}$ ADP receptor	Renal: 26% Fecal: 58%	7–9 h

[a]Requires hepatic dosing adjustment

Table 5 Pain medications with platelet inhibition properties [20]

Medication	Mechanism of action	Elimination	Half-life
Oral agents			
Ibuprofen (Advil®, Motrin®)	Reversible COX-1 and 2 enzyme inhibitor	Renal: 45–80%	2 h
Naproxen (Aleve®, Naprosyn®)	Reversible COX-1 and 2 enzyme inhibitor	Renal: 95% Fecal: 3%	12–17 h Moderate-severe renal impairment: 15–21 h
Ketorolac* (Toradol®)	Reversible COX-1 and 2 enzyme inhibitor	Renal: 92% Fecal: 6%	5 h Prolonged in renal impairment and elderly

*Requires renal dosing adjustment

Anticoagulation Reversal Agents

There are few reversal agents currently available specifically for the reversal of DOACs; however, studies are ongoing to develop such agents (Table 6 [20] and Table 7 [23]). Vitamin K antagonists, such as warfarin, are reversed by phytonadione (vitamin K). Phytonadione has some disadvantages in that it can take up to 6–12 h to produce meaningful reversal. Idarucizumab (Praxbind®) has recently been approved for the reversal of dabigatran. Andexanet alfa is currently in early trials to gain approval for the reversal of factor Xa (FXa) inhibitors. Four-factor and three-factor prothrombin concentrates are currently used for reversal of life-threatening anticoagulant-related bleeding in patients taking warfarin and FXa inhibitors. Blood products, such as platelets and fresh frozen plasma, are sometimes used in life-threatening bleeds to attempt to reverse the effects of antiplatelet and anticoagulant agents, respectively, but have been associated with worse outcomes [7, 25]. Tranexamic acid, an antifibrinolytic agent, may also be considered as it was shown to reduce hematoma expansion without serious adverse effects in patients with TBI [26].

A recent small study compared the effects of 4-factor prothrombin complex concentrate (4F-PCC) and fresh frozen plasma (FFP) [27]. Adult patients with VKA-related intracranial hemorrhage were randomized to receive 20 mL/kg of IV FFP or 30 IU/kg of IV 4F-PCC. These patients had an INR $\geq$ 2.0 and had presented within 12 h of symptom onset. Nine percent of patients in the FFP group compared to sixty-seven percent of patients in the 4F-PCC group reached the primary endpoint of an INR $\leq$ 1.2 within 3 h of initiation of treatment (adjusted odds ratio 30.6, 95% CI 4.7–197.9, $p = 0.0003$). Eight patients (35%) of twenty-three in the FFP group died due to hematoma expansion and five (19%) of twenty-seven patients in the 4F-PCC group (none from hematoma expansion). Additionally, 83% of patients in the FFP group received 4F-PCC as the INR had not normalized at 3 h. Three thromboembolic events occurred within the first 3 days, and six occurred after day 12. Four-factor PCC was found to be superior to FFP in normalizing the INR in patients with a VKA-related intracranial hemorrhage [27].

Additional evidence has been reported comparing platelet transfusions plus standard care to standard care alone in patients with an intracerebral hemorrhage (ICH) taking antiplatelet agents. The PATCH study compared death rates and dependence of patients who had an acute spontaneous primary intracerebral hemorrhage [25]. The patients were randomized to receive either standard care alone or to receive standard care and platelet transfusion [25]. These were adult patients who had received antiplatelet therapy with a COX

Table 6 Anticoagulant reversal agents [20]

Medication/MOA	Indications	PK	Others
Phytonadione (Vitamin K1)	Warfarin-induced prothrombin deficiency	IV: onset of action in 1–2 h; normalized INR may be obtained in 12–14 h PO: onset of action in 6–10 h; normalized INR in 24–48 h	– If given IV, should not exceed 1 mg/min – SQ absorption is variable and not recommended – Risk of anaphylactic reaction after IM or IV administration
4-factor prothrombin complex concentrate (Kcentra®) Factors II, IV, IX, X	Reversal of warfarin in patients with acute major bleeding or need for an urgent procedure/surgery *(Off-label uses: Xa Inhibitor reversal)*	Onset: INR decline within 10 min – Duration ~6–8 h – Half-life elimination: depends on factor Factor II: 48–60 h Factor VII: 1.5–6 h Factor IX: 20–24 h Factor X: 24–48 h Protein C: 1.5–6 h Protein S: 24–48 h	– Consider giving with vitamin K – Repeat dosing not recommended – Dosing based on INR and body weight – Use weight of 100 kg if patient weights >100 kg – Product contains 8–40 units of heparin per 500-unit vial – Risk of thromboembolic complications – Contraindicated: in patients with HIT, DIC
Factor IX complex (Profilnine®) Factors II, IX, X	Prevention and control of bleeding in patients with hemophilia B (factor IX deficiency) *(Off-label uses: warfarin/Xa Inhibitor reversal)*	– Combination of factors II, IX, X, and low levels of factor VII Half-life: IX ~19–25 h	– Thrombotic risk – Vasomotor reactions can result from administration faster than 10 mL/min
Idarucizumab (Praxbind®) Humanized monoclonal antibody fragment	Reversal of dabigatran	– Onset: immediate – Duration: reduction of dabigatran concentrations were observed up to 24 h	– Thrombotic risk – Additional 5 g dose may be given if an additional emergent procedure/surgery or reappearance of clinically relevant bleeding occurs
Protamine sulfate	Treatment of heparin and LMWH overdose	– Neutralization of heparin occurs within 5 min – Each 1 mg of protamine sulfate neutralizes 100 units of heparin given in the previous 2–3 h or 1 mg of enoxaparin given in the previous 8 h – Administer as slow IV injection over 10 min – Do not exceed 50 mg	– Anaphylactoid reactions and hypotension may occur if given too quickly – May cause bleeding in overdose of protamine – Dose of protamine sulfate may decrease as heparin activity decreases over time
Coagulation factor VIIa (recombinant) (Novoseven RT®)	Treatment of bleeding and perioperative management of hemophilia A or B with inhibitors, congenital factor VII deficiency, Glanzmann's thrombasthenia refractory to platelet transfusions, treatment of bleeding episodes, and perioperative management in adults with acquired hemophilia *(Off-label uses: warfarin/Xa inhibitor reversal)*	– Hemophilia A or B: terminal half-life in adults 2.9–3.1 h – Factor VII deficiency: terminal half-life 2.8–3.1 h	– Thrombotic risk – Dosing depends on indication

Table 7 Reversal agents for direct oral anticoagulants (DOACs) currently in development [23]

Medication	Reversal agent	MOA of reversal agent
Direct and indirect FXa inhibitors	Andexanet alfa	– Modified recombinant protein – Binds with direct FXa inhibitors, LMWH, and activated antithrombin III – Partial LMWH reversal
DOACs (edoxaban, rivaroxaban, apixaban, dabigatran), UFH, LMWH, fondaparinux	Ciraparantag	– Binds to DOACs, UFH, and LMWH

inhibitor (aspirin, 78%), ADP inhibitor, or adenosine reuptake inhibitor for at least 7 days prior to the intracerebral hemorrhage. The odds of death or dependence at 3 months were 2.05 times higher in the platelet transfusion group when compared to the standard care alone group (adjusted common odds ratio 2.05, 95% CI 1.18–3.56; $p = 0.0114$). Therefore, platelet transfusion was not recommended for this indication, as it appeared to be inferior to standard care alone for these patients.

The recently published RE-VERSE AD trial studied idarucizumab as a reversal agent for dabigatran. Dabigatran is an oral thrombin inhibitor used for stroke prevention in patients with non-valvular atrial fibrillation and prevention and treatment of venous thromboembolism [5, 28]. Idarucizumab is a monoclonal antibody fragment that binds free and thrombin-bound dabigatran and neutralizes its activity. In the RE-VERSE AD trial, 5 g of IV idarucizumab was given to patients with uncontrollable or life-threatening bleeding or patients who required surgery or an invasive procedure that required normal hemostasis. Of 90 patients, 18 had intracranial bleeding and 9 had trauma-related bleeding. The median maximum percentage reversal of dabigatran was 100% in both groups of patients as measured by dilute

thrombin time and ecarin clotting time [28]. Idarucizumab was found to rapidly and completely reverse anticoagulant activity in 88–98% of patients [28]. Thrombotic events including deep vein thrombosis (DVT), pulmonary embolism (PE), left atrial thrombus, non-ST-segment elevation myocardial infarction (MI), and ischemic stroke were found to have occurred in five patients [28].

A new agent, andexanet alfa, is currently being studied for the reversal of FXa inhibitors [29]. The ANNEXA-4 study evaluated andexanet alfa for use in patients with potentially life-threatening acute major bleeding from FXa inhibitors. Andexanet alfa is a recombinant modified human FXa decoy protein that binds to direct and indirect FXa inhibitors. This study included adult patients who had received either apixaban, rivaroxaban, or enoxaparin within 18 h prior to enrollment. Andexanet alfa decreased the FXa activity by 89% from baseline in patients taking rivaroxaban. In patients taking apixaban, the FXa activity decreased by 93% from baseline [29]. After 12 h, 79% of patients had achieved excellent or good hemostasis [29]. During the 30-day follow-up period, 18% of patients had suffered a thrombotic event [29].

TBI patients are at an increased risk for DVT and PE after injury and require preventative measures. However, initiating venous thromboembolism (VTE) prophylaxis in patients who have not achieved hemostasis could potentially lead to bleeding complications that further complicate patient care and recovery following a TBI. The Neurocritical Care Society recommends initiating low-molecular-weight heparin (LMWH) or unfractionated heparin (UFH) for VTE prophylaxis within 24–48 h of presentation in patients with TBI or ICH [30]. Intermittent pneumatic compression devices are recommended to be initiated within 24 h of presentation or within 24 h after craniotomy [30]. The Brain Trauma Foundation recommends using LMWH or low-dose UFH in addition to mechanical prophylaxis for the prevention of VTE as a level III recommendation [31]. However, they do note that there may be an increased risk for expansion of intracranial hemorrhage.

A multicenter retrospective cohort evaluated the safety of LMWH on patients with traumatic intracranial hemorrhage. In this study, hemorrhage progression occurred in 93 of 220 patients that received LMWH while only occurring in 239 of 995 patients who did not receive LMWH (42% vs. 24%, $p < 0.001$) [32].

Testing and Monitoring

Several tests have been used to monitor coagulopathy in post-trauma and TBI patients. Traditionally, tests such as prothrombin time (PT) or international normalized ratio (INR), partial thromboplastin time (PTT), platelet count, fibrinogen level, or D-dimer are used; these are often referred to as conventional coagulation assays (CCA). Increasingly, TEG or rotational thromboelastography (ROTEM), which has been used extensively by anesthesiologists and perfusionists in cardiac surgery, is being employed in trauma resuscitation. ROTEM measures standard TEG parameters and intrinsic and extrinsic pathway activation, fibrin component of clot and aprotinin (a fibrinolysis inhibitor with extrinsic activation). ROTEM and TEG parameters are shown in Table 8 [33] and Table 9 [17, 34], respectively.

TEG and ROTEM can be used as point-of-care tests to help achieve hemostatic resuscitation in TBI patients (Table 9) and those whose resuscitation is further complicated by anticoagulants. A complete TEG takes approximately 30 min, but the results can be observed in real time, which allows rapid support for treatment decisions—especially for post-traumatic resuscitations. As a point-of-care test, which can be followed continuously, TEG can be used to monitor resuscitation efforts as the patient's care transitions from the emergency department to the operating room or the intensive

care unit [33]. A recent randomized control trial showed that TEG-guided resuscitation compared to CCA resulted in significantly higher survival despite a decrease in plasma and platelets used during the first 2 h of resuscitation in the TEG group [35]. Walsh et al., have provided recommendations for TEG-based resuscitation (Table 9) [34]. Figure 1 shows normal and abnormal TEG tracings in a coagulopathic TBI patient (see also Table 10).

TEG and ROTEM have several limitations. They do not measure the interactions that occur between fluid phase and endothelial cell surface during coagulation, only the final product of clot formation [33]. Also, platelet function or its inhibition is not measured with either TEG or ROTEM. Platelet mapping with ADP and arachidonic acid inhibition must be used in addition to

Table 8 ROTEM parameters (Created with information from Gonzalez et al. [33])

Parameter	Dysfunction
Clotting time (CT) $_{IN}$	Heparin or intrinsic factor
CT $_{EX}$	Extrinsic factor
Amplitude10 (A10) $_{IN, EX}$	Poor firmness of clot: platelets, fibrinogen, and/or FXIII
Max clot firmness (MCF) $_{IN, EX}$	Poor firmness of clot: platelets, fibrinogen, and/or FXIII
MCF $_{FIB}$	Fibrin
Maximum lysis $_{IN, EX, FIB}$	Hyperfibrinolysis

Reference ranges for each parameter of ROTEM vary based on which activator is used: INTEM (IN), EXTEM (EX), HEPTEM, APTEM, FIBTEM (FIB). Commonly used abbreviations are included in the table. Amplitude10 (A10) is amplitude at 10 min following clotting time. Please visit manufacturers Website for reference ranges.

Table 9 TEG-guided resuscitation with product recommendations based on TEG parameter abnormalities (Created from Katz [17] and Walsh [34])

Abnormal parameter	Normal values (range)	Dysfunction	Product-guided resuscitation
Prolonged R	5–10 min	Clotting factors	Fresh frozen plasma
Prolonged K/reduced α(alpha) angle	*K time*: 1–3 min *α(alpha) angle*: 53–72°	Fibrinogen	Cryoprecipitate, fibrinogen concentrate
Low maximum amplitude (MA)	50–70 mm	Platelets, fibrinogen	Platelets ± DDAVP
Increased lysis of clot at 30 min	0–8%	Hyperfibrinolysis	Antifibrinolytic: tranexamic acid and/or aminocaproic acid

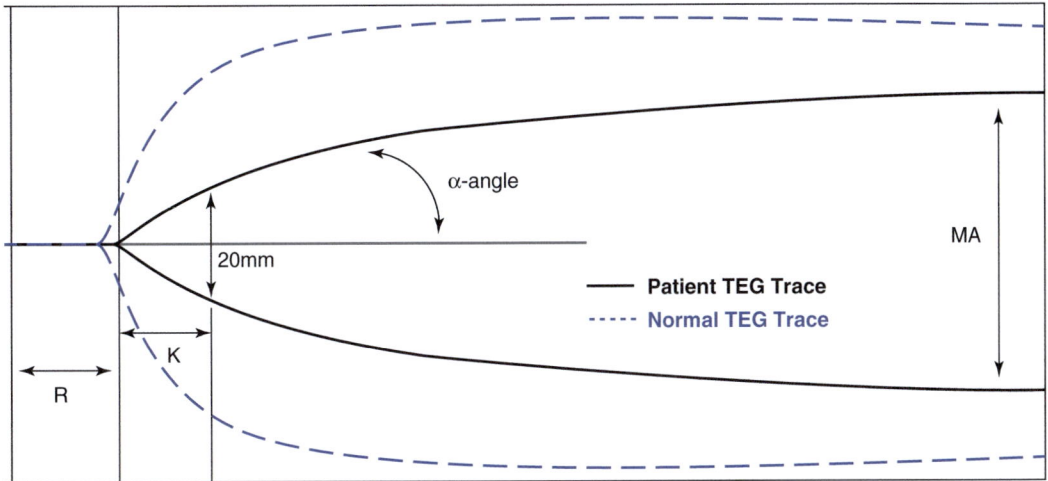

Fig. 1 Normal and coagulopathic TEG tracing. Table 10 shows the clinical data and laboratory values that corresponded to this coagulopathic TEG tracing from a TBI patient

Table 10 Clinical data and laboratory values that corresponded to the coagulopathic TEG tracing from a TBI patient in Fig. 1

Clinical data and TEG parameters for one patient with coagulopathy		Reference range
Injury Severity Score (ISS)	26	0–75
Glasgow Coma Scale (GCS)	3	3–15
Revised Trauma Score (RTS)	2.2	0–7.8
Lactate (mmol/L)	0.4	0.5–2.2
Base excess (mEq/L)[a]	−14	(−2)–(+2)
International normalized ratio (INR)	5.2	0.9 1.1
Partial thromboplastin time (PTT) (seconds)	110.5	20–35
Hematocrit (%)	27	35–50
Platelet (PLT) count (×10^9/L)	137	150–450
Fibrinogen (mg/dL)	100	200–450
R (min)	7	2–8
K (min)	6.4	1–3
Angle (degrees)	40	55–78
MA (mm)	38.8	51–69

R time to clot formation, *K* initial speed of clot formation, *Angle* rate of clot formation (speed of fibrin buildup and cross-linking), *MA* maximum clot strength
[a]$HCO_3 < 10$ mmol/L

TEG or ROTEM to measure platelet function [13]. Lastly, TEG is very operator-dependent, with up to an 80% coefficient of variation from institution to institution and suffers from sampling and/or processing errors [33].

Recommended Monitoring Test(s) per Anticoagulant Class

Due to the risk of serious, life-threating complications with supra- and sub-therapeutic anticoagulation, numerous tests have been developed to monitor these medications and their effects. Table 11 shows the recommended laboratory test for various anticoagulant classes. Also, please refer to Tables 3 and 4 for the mechanism of action, mode of excretion, and half-life for each drug.

Vitamin K antagonists (coumarins) are monitored by prothrombin/international normalized ratio (PT/INR) due to their ability to measure the extrinsic cascade that includes factors affected by coumarins (II, VII, IX, X, proteins C and S). Unfractionated heparin affects factor II (thrombin) and is monitored by prothrombin time (PT) because it measures the internal clotting cascade. Low-molecular-weight heparins (enoxaparin) affect factor Xa and can be measured by testing for anti-factor Xa activity levels (institutional availability varies). Intravenous direct thrombin inhibitors (bivalirudin, argatroban) are monitored by measuring the thrombin time (TT) and often titrated by PTT in the inpatient setting.

Oral direct thrombin inhibitors (dabigatran) and direct factor Xa inhibitors (apixaban, rivaroxaban, edoxaban) are monitored by different

Table 11 Recommended test for each anticoagulant class

Anticoagulant class	Laboratory test
Vitamin K antagonists (warfarin, coumarins)	PT/INR
Direct factor Xa inhibitor (apixaban, rivaroxaban, edoxaban)	Anti-factor Xa activity[a]
Oral direct thrombin inhibitor (dabigatran)	Thrombin time (TT), dilute TT, ecarin clotting time
IV direct thrombin inhibitor (bivalirudin, argatroban)	PT
Unfractionated heparin	PTT
Low-molecular-weight heparin (enoxaparin)	Anti-factor Xa activity[a]

[a]Depends on institutional availability of chromogenic assay for each specific agent

measures depending on drug level and timing of administration. For oral direct thrombin inhibitors, if the timing and amount of most recent dose is unknown, a normal thrombin time, ecarin clotting time, and diluted thrombin time would show absence of dabigatran at clinically relevant concentration; however, ecarin clotting time and diluted thrombin time testing have limited clinical availability [36]. For direct factor Xa inhibitors, a normal anti-Xa activity likely excludes clinically relevant anticoagulation levels. Anti-Xa activity can also provide a linear correlation with drug concentration but has limited clinical availability [36].

Restarting Antithrombotic Agents After Traumatic Brain Injury

The decision to restart antithrombotic agents, including DOACs, after a TBI, should be based on the risk versus the benefit for each individual patient. Patients at high risk of clotting (e.g., mechanical valve) and low risk of bleeding should be considered for anticoagulation 7–10 days after injury, if the patient is stabilized. However, in patients in whom the risk of bleeding far outweighs the risk of clotting, it is reasonable to wait 6–10 weeks before restarting anticoagulants. A VKA may take up to 1 week to

reach full anticoagulant effects, while DOACs would take effect within a few hours of administration.

A single-center, retrospective study of 72 mild to moderate TBI patients who received therapeutic anticoagulation within 60 days after injury showed that 6 of 25 patients that had a repeat head computed tomography (CT) scan developed progression of hemorrhagic TBI [8, 37]. Atrial fibrillation was the most common pre-injury indication for therapeutic anticoagulation, while new-onset VTE was the most common indication post-TBI. Therapeutic anticoagulation agents post-TBI included unfractionated heparin, low-molecular-weight heparin, fondaparinux, and warfarin. Interestingly, hemorrhagic complications were not found to be related to therapeutic anticoagulation in these patients [37]. Additionally, after a multiple logistic regression analysis, age ≥ 65 years was associated with progression of hemorrhagic TBI on repeat head CT [37]. The median number of days after injury of initiation of therapeutic anticoagulation was 5.5 days in the group that had progression of hemorrhagic TBI and 10 days in the groups without progression [37]. This suggests that shorter periods off anticoagulants than those commonly used may be safe.

A study of 26 patients with traumatic intracranial hemorrhage and therapeutic anticoagulation with enoxaparin or unfractionated heparin concluded that 96% of patients had no extension of their hemorrhage after anticoagulation was started [38]. For the single patient that had minimal hemorrhagic extension, it was not felt to alter the clinical course for this patient [38]. The therapeutic anticoagulation was initiated an average of 13 days after injury [38]. The recently published CHIRONE study examined the risk of recurrence of ICH after resuming VKA therapy in patients that had previously survived an ICH [39]. In this study, 20 of 267 (7.5%) patients suffered from a recurrent ICH after receiving anticoagulation with a VKA [39]. The median time to recurrence was 16.5 months and was fatal in 5 patients [39]. The Delayed Versus Early Enoxaparin Prophylaxis I (DEEP I) study conducted in 62 patients with low-risk TBI, found that enoxaparin 30 mg twice daily initiated 24 h after injury resulted in a subclinical, radiographic progression on CT scan of 5.9% (95% CI, 0.7–19.7%) versus 3.6% (95% CI, 0.1–18.3%) for the placebo group [40]. Antiplatelet agents (Table 4) have less data to suggest appropriate timing for reinitiating therapy. It may be reasonable in patients with a high risk of clotting (e.g., recent MI) but without elevated ICP or planned surgeries, to start these agents a few days after hemostasis is achieved.

In order to determine the risk versus benefit of reinitiating antithrombotic therapy, the use of published risk assessment scoring tools is suggested. The risk of spontaneous (nontraumatic) bleeding in patients receiving oral anticoagulation for atrial fibrillation can be assessed with the HAS-BLED score, while the risk of stroke in patients with atrial fibrillation can be estimated with $CHADS_2$ or CHA_2DS_2-VASC scores. The HAS-BLED score takes into consideration several factors including systolic blood pressure > 160 mm Hg, abnormal renal or liver function, stroke, bleeding history, predisposition for bleeding, INR, age > 65 years, antiplatelet or nonsteroidal anti-inflammatory drug (NSAID) use, and alcohol use >8 servings/week [41]. A HAS-BLED sore of 0 is associated with a low risk of bleeding, a score of 1–2 is associated with a moderate risk of bleeding, and a score of ≥3 is associated with a high risk of bleeding [41]. The $HEMORR_2HAGES$ score considers hepatic or renal disease, ethanol use, malignancy, age > 75 years, reduced platelet count or function, rebleeding, uncontrolled hypertension, anemia, genetic factors, elevated fall risk, neuropsychiatric disease, and stroke factors [41]. The risk of bleeding is low with a score of 0–1, moderate with a score of 2–3, and high with a score of ≥4 [41]. The $CHADS_2$ score considers whether the patient has congestive heart failure, hypertension, age ≥ 75 years, diabetes, and a history of stroke or transient ischemic attack [41]. The CHA_2DS_2-VASC considers the same factors as the $CHADS_2$ score but also includes left ventricular dysfunction, history of thromboembolism, vascular disease, age 65–74 years, and female sex [41]. A score of 0 on either scale is associated with low risk, a score of 1 is associated with intermediate risk, and a score of ≥2 is associated with high risk of stroke [41].

Conclusions

Traumatic brain injury and its associated coagulopathies provide ever-challenging clinical scenarios. These coagulopathies are further complicated by antithrombotic medications being taken by TBI patients prior to their injury. Monitoring laboratory, clinical, and radiographic changes are essential in these patients, taking into account the timing of trauma-induced coagulopathy, along with special clinical scenarios that may complicate the management of these patients. There are many antithrombotic agents currently available, and clinicians must be aware of the various mechanisms of action, pharmacokinetic characteristics, and reversal strategies for TBI patients needing emergent surgery due to life-threatening bleeding. It is also important to consider the risks of thrombosis and bleeding when, or if, restarting these medications after TBI.

References

1. Laroche M, Kutcher ME, Huang MC, Cohen MJ, Manley GT. Coagulopathy after traumatic brain injury. Neurosurgery. 2012;70(6):1334–45.
2. Barnes GD, Lucas E, Alexander GC, Goldberger ZD. National trends in ambulatory oral anticoagulant use. Am J Med. 2015;128(12):1300–5.e2.
3. Murray GD, Butcher I, McHugh GS, Lu J, Mushkudiani NA, Maas AI, et al. Multivariable prognostic analysis in traumatic brain injury: results from the IMPACT study. J Neurotrauma. 2007;24(2):329–37.
4. Lustenberger T, Talving P, Kobayashi L, Inaba K, Lam L, Plurad D, et al. Time course of coagulopathy in isolated severe traumatic brain injury. Injury. 2010;41(9):924–8.
5. Epstein DS, Mitra B, O'Reilly G, Rosenfeld JV, Cameron PA. Acute traumatic coagulopathy in the setting of isolated traumatic brain injury: a systematic review and meta-analysis. Injury. 2014;45(5):819–24.
6. Brohi K, Cohen MJ, Ganter MT, Schultz MJ, Levi M, Mackersie RC, et al. Acute coagulopathy of trauma: hypoperfusion induces systemic anticoagulation and hyperfibrinolysis. J Trauma. 2008;64(5):1211–7; discussion 1217.

7. Wafaisade A, Lefering R, Tjardes T, Wutzler S, Simanski C, Paffrath T, et al. Acute coagulopathy in isolated blunt traumatic brain injury. Neurocrit Care. 2010;12(2):211–9.

8. Nakae R, Takayama Y, Kuwamoto K, Naoe Y, Sato H, Yokota H. Time course of coagulation and fibrinolytic parameters in patients with traumatic brain injury. J Neurotrauma. 2016;33(7):688–95.

9. Kushimoto S, Shibata Y, Yamamoto Y. Implications of fibrinogenolysis in patients with closed head injury. J Neurotrauma. 2003;20(4):357–63.

10. White NJ, Contaifer D Jr, Martin EJ, Newton JC, Mohammed BM, Bostic JL, et al. Early hemostatic responses to trauma identified with hierarchical clustering analysis. J Thromb Haemost. 2015;13(6):978–88.

11. Brophy GM, Mohammed BM, Contaifer D, Newton JC, Martin EJ, Pusateri AE, et al. Defining platelet function in polytrauma patients with traumatic brain injury upon admission to the Emergency Department. A podium flash presentation and poster presentations at the International Neurotrauma Society Symposia 2014, Budapest, Hungary. J Neurotrauma; 2014.

12. Wohlauer MV, Moore EE, Thomas S, Sauaia A, Evans E, Harr J, et al. Early platelet dysfunction: an unrecognized role in the acute coagulopathy of trauma. J Am Coll Surg. 2012;214(5):739–46.

13. Davis PK, Musunuru H, Walsh M, Cassady R, Yount R, Losiniecki A, et al. Platelet dysfunction is an early marker for traumatic brain injury-induced coagulopathy. Neurocrit Care. 2013;18(2):201–8.

14. Solomon C, Traintinger S, Ziegler B, Hanke A, Rahe-Meyer N, Voelckel W, et al. Platelet function following trauma. A multiple electrode aggregometry study. Thromb Haemost. 2011;106(2):322–30.

15. Brophy GM, Contaifer D, Mohammed BM, White NJ, Newton JC, Martin EJ, et al. Multimodality monitoring of platelet function in traumatic brain injury patients with trauma induced coagulopathy. A poster presentation at the 32nd Annual National Neurotrauma Symposium, San Francisco, California, June 30, 2014. J Neurotrauma; 2014.

16. Brohi K, Cohen MJ, Ganter MT, Matthay MA, Mackersie RC, Pittet JF. Acute traumatic coagulopathy: initiated by hypoperfusion: modulated through the protein C pathway? Ann Surg. 2007;245(5):812–8.

17. Katz D, Beilin Y. Disorders of coagulation in pregnancy. Br J Anaesth. 2015;115(Suppl 2):ii75–88.

18. Oertel M, Kelly DF, McArthur D, Boscardin WJ, Glenn TC, Lee JH, et al. Progressive hemorrhage after head trauma: predictors and consequences of the evolving injury. J Neurosurg. 2002;96(1):109–16.

19. Vardon F, Mrozek S, Geeraerts T, Fourcade O. Accidental hypothermia in severe trauma. Anaesth Crit Care Pain Med. 2016;35(5):355–61.

20. Frontera JA, Lewin JJ, Rabinstein AA, Aisiku IP, Alexandrov AW, Cook AM, et al. Guideline for reversal of antithrombotics in intracranial hemorrhage: a statement for healthcare professionals from the Neurocritical Care Society and Society of Critical Care Medicine. Neurocrit Care. 2016;24(1):6–46.

21. Al-Majzoub O, Rybak E, Reardon DP, Krause P, Connors JM. Evaluation of warfarin reversal with 4-factor prothrombin complex concentrate compared to 3-factor prothrombin complex concentrate at a Tertiary Academic Medical Center. J Emerg Med. 2016;50(1):7–13.

22. Gulseth MP. Overview of direct oral anticoagulant therapy reversal. Am J Health Syst Pharm. 2016;73(10 Suppl 2):S5–S13.

23. Feeney JM, Santone E, DiFiori M, Kis L, Jayaraman V, Montgomery SC. Compared to warfarin, direct oral anticoagulants are associated with lower mortality in patients with blunt traumatic intracranial hemorrhage: a TQIP study. J Trauma Acute Care Surg. 2016;81(5):843–8.

24. Maegele M, Grottke O, Schochl H, Sakowitz OA, Spannagl M, Koscielny J. Direct oral anticoagulants in emergency trauma admissions. Dtsch Arztebl Int. 2016;113(35–36):575–82.

25. Baharoglu MI, Cordonnier C, Al-Shahi Salman R, de Gans K, Koopman MM, Brand A, et al. Platelet transfusion versus standard care after acute stroke due to spontaneous cerebral haemorrhage associated with antiplatelet therapy (PATCH): a randomised, open-label, phase 3 trial. Lancet. 2016;387(10038):2605–13.

26. Yutthakasemsunt S, Kittiwatanagul W, Piyavechvirat P, Thinkamrop B, Phuenpathom N, Lumbiganon P. Tranexamic acid for patients with traumatic brain injury: a randomized, double-blinded, placebo-controlled trial. BMC Emerg Med. 2013;13:20.

27. Steiner T, Poli S, Griebe M, Hüsing J, Hajda J, Freiberger A, et al. Fresh frozen plasma versus prothrombin complex concentrate in patients with intracranial haemorrhage related to vitamin K antagonists (INCH): a randomised trial. The Lancet Neurology. 2016;15(6):566–73.

28. Pollack CV, Reilly PA, Eikelboom J, Glund S, Verhamme P, Bernstein RA, et al. Idarucizumab for dabigatran reversal. New Engl J Med. 2015;373(6):511–20.

29. Connolly SJ, Milling TJ, Eikelboom JW, Gibson CM, Curnutte JT, Gold A, et al. Andexanet Alfa for acute major bleeding associated with factor Xa inhibitors. N Engl J Med. 2016;375:1131–41.

30. Nyquist P, Bautista C, Jichici D, Burns J, Chhangani S, DeFilippis M, et al. Prophylaxis of venous thrombosis in neurocritical care patients: an evidence-based guideline: a statement for healthcare professionals

from the Neurocritical Care Society. Neurocrit Care. 2016;24(1):47–60.

31. Carney N, Totten AM, O'Reilly C, Ullman JS, Hawryluk GW, Bell MJ, et al. Guidelines for the management of severe traumatic brain injury, fourth edition. Neurosurgery. 2017;80(1):6–15.

32. Kwiatt ME, Patel MS, Ross SE, Lachant MT, MacNew HG, Ochsner MG, et al. Is low-molecular-weight heparin safe for venous thromboembolism prophylaxis in patients with traumatic brain injury? A Western Trauma Association multicenter study. J Trauma Acute Care Surg. 2012;73(3):625–8.

33. Gonzalez E, Moore EE, Moore HB. Management of trauma-induced coagulopathy with thrombelastography. Crit Care Clin. 2017;33(1):119–34.

34. Walsh M, Thomas SG, Howard JC, Evans E, Guyer K, Medvecz A, et al. Blood component therapy in trauma guided with the utilization of the perfusionist and thromboelastography. J Extra Corpor Technol. 2011;43(3):162–7.

35. Gonzalez E, Moore EE, Moore HB, Chapman MP, Chin TL, Ghasabyan A, et al. Goal-directed hemostatic resuscitation of trauma-induced coagulopathy: a pragmatic randomized clinical trial comparing a viscoelastic assay to conventional coagulation assays. Ann Surg. 2016;263(6):1051–9.

36. Cuker A, Siegal DM, Crowther MA, Garcia DA. Laboratory measurement of the anticoagulant activity of the non-vitamin K oral anticoagulants. J Am Coll Cardiol. 2014;64(11):1128–39.

37. Matsushima K, Inaba K, Cho J, Mohammed H, Herr K, Leichtle S, et al. Therapeutic anticoagulation in patients with traumatic brain injury. J Surg Res. 2016;205(1):186–91.

38. Byrnes MC, Irwin E, Roach R, James M, Horst PK, Reicks P. Therapeutic anticoagulation can be safely accomplished in selected patients with traumatic intracranial hemorrhage. World J Emerg Surg. 2012;7(1):25.

39. Poli D, Antonucci E, Dentali F, Erba N, Testa S, Tiraferri E, et al. Recurrence of ICH after resumption of anticoagulation with VK antagonists: CHIRONE study. Neurology. 2014;82(12):1020–6.

40. Phelan HA, Wolf SE, Norwood SH, Aldy K, Brakenridge SC, Eastman AL, et al. A randomized, double-blinded, placebo-controlled pilot trial of anticoagulation in low-risk traumatic brain injury: the Delayed Versus Early Enoxaparin Prophylaxis I (DEEP I) study. J Trauma Acute Care Surg. 2012;73(6):1434–41.

41. Nutescu EA. Oral anticoagulant therapies: balancing the risks. Am J Health Syst Pharm. 2013;70(10 Suppl 1):S3–11.

Use of Guidelines in the Management of Traumatic Brain Injury

Ilyas Eli, Evan Joyce, and Gregory W. J. Hawryluk

Introduction

Clinical practice guidelines (CPGs) are systematically developed manuals intended to assist healthcare professionals with recommendations on best care practices. CPGs have been defined as "any statement that promotes or advocates a particular course of action in clinical care" [1]. In the guidelines, experts evaluate the current literature and translate the wide range of evidence into practice recommendations. The goal is to reduce harm and allow for maximal evidence-proven benefit. The principal benefit of CPGs is to improve the quality of care and outcomes of patients. Additionally, CPGs promote the application of interventions of proven benefit, especially those that reduce morbidity and mortality. Implementation of guidelines can improve consistency of care of patients. Furthermore, CPGs are intended to be utilized to provide a systematic approach that guides complex medical decision-making.

The process for developing guidelines has progressed incrementally over the last several decades. In 1977, the National Institute of Health Consensus Development Program introduced its methods for developing practice guidelines, which consisted of an expert panel reaching consensus on recommendations based on a several-day conference consisting of sessions and open discussion followed by a press conference on a third day [2]. In its Clinical Efficacy Assessment Project in the 1980s, the American College of Physicians developed guidelines based on the evaluation of existing evidence by expert consultants [3]. A more explicit guideline development process pioneered by Eddy proposed the use of explicit methods that included specification of the benefits, harms, and costs of intervention [4, 5]. In the 1990s, the Institute of Medicine (IOM) issued several reports on CPGs. The first report Clinical Practice Guidelines: Directions for a New Program [6]—emphasized the use of a systematic, evidence-based process for guideline development. It further detailed the need for careful documentation of assumptions, evidence, and rationale for recommendations. Subsequent interest and surge in the production of CPGs led to the publication of *Guidelines for Clinical Practice* by the IOM, which advised on the responsibilities for guideline development [7]. Emphasis in this report was on the role of systematically developed, evidence-based guidelines as part of the infrastructure of healthcare in the United States in improving quality of care, reducing healthcare costs, and discouraging dangerous care. The following years resulted in a proliferation in the production of CPGs. The Agency for Healthcare

I. Eli, MD · E. Joyce, MD, MS
G. W. J. Hawryluk, MD, PhD (✉)
Department of Neurosurgery, University of Utah,
Clinical Neurosciences Center,
Salt Lake City, UT, USA
e-mail: Ilyas.Eli@hsc.utah.edu; Evan.Joyce@hsc.
utah.edu; Gregory.Hawryluk@hsc.utah.edu

© Springer International Publishing AG, part of Springer Nature 2018
S. D. Timmons (ed.), *Controversies in Severe Traumatic Brain Injury Management*,
https://doi.org/10.1007/978-3-319-89477-5_17

Research and Quality's National Guideline Clearinghouse contains close to 2700 CPGs. The development of CPGs expanded to other countries resulting in the preparation of more than 3700 CPGs listed in the Guidelines International Network's database. The IOM, at the request of the US Congress, developed a set of standards for developing rigorous, reliable CPGs in 2011 [8]. The standards discuss aspects that are paramount for developing CPGs, such as establishing evidence foundations supporting strength of recommendations, clarity of recommendations, external reviews, updating, development of group composition, intersection between CPGs and system reviews, transparency, and conflict of interest.

Traumatic brain injury (TBI) is the leading cause of death and disability in children and adults ages 1–44 years, with 2.5 million individuals in the United States every year incurring injuries, of which approximately 50,000 result in death and more than 80,000 experience permanent disability. This translates to a cost of $76.5 billion annually to society [9]. Additionally, TBI is one of the leading causes of death around the world [10, 11]. The burden of TBI, especially as a result of closed head injury, continues to increase worldwide as a consequence of growth and urbanization.

CPGs have been a crucial component in the management of traumatic brain injury. Guideline implementation has been shown to decrease mortality, improve outcomes, and reduce the length of hospital stay. Several guidelines published in the United States—the Brain Trauma Foundation (BTF) Guidelines, the Penetrating Brain Injury Guidelines, the Surgical Management of Traumatic Brain Injury guidelines, the Neurocritical Care Society (NCS) Guidelines, and the American College of Surgeons (ACS) Trauma Quality Improvement Program (TQIP)—encompass a broad spectrum of management before and after injury.

Understanding the Context

American Association of Neurological Surgeons

The American Association of Neurological Surgeons (AANS), founded in 1931 as the Harvey Cushing Society, whose mission is to promote the highest quality of patient care and advance the specialty of neurological surgery, was the first neurosurgical organization to coproduce (with the BTF) evidence-based guidelines. The AANS, together with the Congress of Neurological Surgeons (CNS), supports the ongoing guidelines development primarily through the activities of the Joint Guidelines Committee of the Washington Committee.

American College of Surgeons

Established in 1913, the American College of Surgeons (ACS) is the largest scientific and educational group of surgeons in the world. With the mission statement to "improve the care of the surgical patient and to safeguard standards of care in an optimal and ethical practice environment," the ACs has several efforts aimed at surgical education, including clinical practice guidelines and quality improvement programs. One such effort by the ACS Committee on Trauma is the TQIP.

Brain Trauma Foundation

The BTF, founded in 1986, is a multinational consortium of experts in neurological trauma dedicated to improving outcomes from TBI by establishing evidence-based guidelines through meticulous review, synthesis, and application of relevant, current literature. The BTF simultaneously fosters clinical research partnerships and provides educational outreach opportunities.

Congress of Neurological Surgeons

The CNS was founded in 1951, and its mission is to enhance health and improve lives through the advancement of neurosurgical education and scientific exchange. The CNS has an independent CNS Guidelines Committee that reviews and approves nominations to develop new internally generated evidence-based guidelines and also oversees the development task forces and methodological processes used to develop these internally produced guidelines.

Joint Guidelines Committee/ Washington Committee of AANS/CNS

In recent years, the Joint Guidelines Committee (JGC) has been the responsible entity for the evaluation of both internally generated and externally produced clinical practice guidelines that are relevant to neurosurgical practice. Organizationally, the JGC is a subcommittee of the advocacy and health policy Washington Committee (WC) of the AANS/CNS. The committee has volunteer members appointed by the WC with representation from the AANS and CNS and each of the neurosurgical subspecialty AANS/CNS joint sections, including the Section on Neurotrauma and Critical Care. Membership requires training and expertise in evidence-based medicine techniques and evaluation of clinical practice guidelines. The committee reviews submissions and provides recommendations for endorsement or review for substantive feedback to the submitting agency.

Neurocritical Care Society

Since its founding in 2002, the Neurocritical Care Society (NCS) has been dedicated to the values of quality patient care, professional collaboration, research, training and education, and advocacy. A substantial undertaking of the NCS is publishing guideline documents through its Guidelines Committee, the focus of which is to "determine topics suitable for guideline development, identify key experts in the chosen topic, facilitate the development of 'best practice' clinical management guidelines, and review the final document."

History of Guidelines Development for Traumatic Brain Injury

Since the initial publication of the first Guidelines for the Management of Traumatic Brain Injury in 1995 by the BTF and the AANS, subsequent editions of the Guidelines have evolved as new data pertaining to TBI treatment and management were elucidated and validated [12]. In 2000, a revised 2nd edition was published in the *Journal of Neurotrauma* [13]. This was followed by a 3rd edition, updated in 2007, as a joint project between the BTF, the AANS, and the CNS, again published and disseminated in the *Journal of Neurotrauma* [14]. Transition from the 2nd to the 3rd edition saw the addition of six new evidence-based topics, a more stringent and well-defined methodology for evaluation and critique of available evidence, and publication of adjuvant sets of guideline documents focused on unique subsets of patient populations, treatment venues, and phases of patient care. Published in 2016, the 4th edition Guidelines for the Management of Severe TBI is the most current and inclusive publication by the BTF on management of patients with TBI [15].

Several additional evidence-based guidelines from the BTF on coma prognostication and management have been developed where peculiarities in etiology, presentation, and treatment diverge to an appreciable degree. These include the 2nd edition Guidelines for the Prehospital Management of TBI; 2nd edition Guidelines for Severe TBI in Infants, Children, and Adolescents; Early Indicators of Prognosis in Severe TBI; and Guidelines for Field Management of Combat-Related Head Trauma [16–19]. These guidelines reflect an ever-shifting medical environment presented with challenges related to the evolving evidence-based care of select patient populations in new hospital and prehospital environments, which may have been previously nonexistent, underappreciated, or unrecognized.

Traumatic Brain Injury Guidelines

4th Edition Guidelines for the Management of Severe TBI

The 4th edition of the Guidelines for the Management of Severe TBI, published in September 2016, incorporates 102 new studies since publication of the 3rd edition in 2007 and has been endorsed by both the AANS and the CNS via the JGC review process [15]. Funding for research, development, and publication of these guidelines was derived from the US Army Contracting Command, Aberdeen Proving Ground, and Natick Contracting Division, as well as grants awarded to Stanford University, contracts to the BTF, and subcontracts through the Oregon Health & Science University. Evidence from a total of 189 publications—5 with Class 1 evidence, 46 with Class 2 evidence, 136 with Class 3 evidence, and 2 meta-analyses—is organized into logical, sequential sections on TBI-specific treatments, monitoring, and thresholds. (The BTF has also established the Brain Trauma Evidence-Based Consortium [B-TEC], with support from the US Army Contracting Command, to help establish further infrastructure for clinical trials and future guidelines development.)

Three overarching TBI-specific sections—treatments, monitoring, and thresholds, each with appropriate subsections—shape the 4th edition guidelines. The first section, Treatments, is subdivided into Decompressive Craniectomy; Prophylactic Hypothermia; Hyperosmolar Therapy; Cerebrospinal Fluid Drainage; Ventilation Therapies; Anesthetics, Analgesics, and Sedatives; Steroids; Nutrition; Infection Prophylaxis; Deep Vein Thrombosis Prophylaxis; and Seizure Prophylaxis. Next, subdivisions of Monitoring are Intracranial Pressure (ICP), Cerebral Perfusion Pressure (CPP), and Advanced Cerebral Monitoring. Lastly, Thresholds is organized in a similar fashion to monitoring with subdivisions on Blood Pressure, Intracranial Pressure, Cerebral Perfusion Pressure, and Advanced Cerebral Monitoring.

Each subsection is a logically organized chapter, guiding the reader through rationale, recommendations, and review of the studies providing data for evidence. Chapters open with a brief summary of the historical perspective, physiology, pathophysiology, and current practices related to that section. Recommendations are presented in concise, bulleted form as Level I, II, or III. When relevant, a brief summary of changes from the 3rd edition guidelines follows the recommendations. Next, each study used as evidence for the recommendations is deconstructed into components of overall quality and rated by

the authors (i.e., number of studies, meta-analysis, number of subjects, class of studies, consistency, directness, precision, quality of evidence). This is followed by appraisal of the quality and applicability of the aggregated studies in that chapter. A table-based summary of the evidence, consisting of study design, outcomes, data class (described later), results, and conclusions is then utilized to highlight the key elements of each study used to draw conclusions in the form of recommendations. Finally, a list of appropriate references is provided for each chapter. Table 1 summarizes the compiled recommendations from each subsection.

As compared with the 3rd edition, revisions were made to numerous subsections including Cerebrospinal Fluid Drainage (new topic), Decompressive Craniectomy (new topic), Deep Vein Thrombosis (indirect evidence included), Intracranial Pressure Technology (technology assessment no longer included), Hyperventilation (renamed "Ventilation Therapies"), Brain Oxygen Monitoring (renamed "Advanced Cerebral Monitoring" and divided into risks/benefits of monitoring and targeted thresholds sections), Infection Prophylaxis (focus narrowed to ventilator-associated pneumonia and external ventricular drain infections), and Intracranial Pressure Monitoring and Cerebral Perfusion Pressure (divided into risks/benefits of monitoring and targeted thresholds sections).

The BTF does not intend to produce a 5th edition of the guidelines. Instead, the foundation's intent is for the 4th edition to be a transitional, living set of recommendations, referred to as a "living guidelines model," which will be permanently available online. This novel paradigm will allow the BTF to continually monitor the literature and make appropriate adjustments based on the availability and synthesis of new data as it emerges. With the near-constant flux of new information in the current digital age of data acquisition, this is a necessary model to optimize patient care. The notion of a living guideline is referenced throughout the 4th edition. For example, the authors acknowledge the results of the recently published RESCUEicp (Randomized Evaluation of Surgery with Craniectomy for

Table 1 A summary table with compiled recommendations from each subsection of the BTF's Guidelines for the Management of Severe Traumatic Brain Injury, 4th edition. Reproduced with permission from Carney N, Totten AM, O'Reilly C, Ullman JS, Hawryluk GW, Bell MJ, et al. Guidelines for the Management of Severe Traumatic Brain Injury, Fourth Edition. Neurosurgery. 2017;80(1):6–15

Topic	Recommendations
Decompressive craniectomy	Level IIA
	• **Bifrontal DC is not recommended to improve outcomes as measured by the GOS-E score at 6-mo post-injury in severe TBI patients with diffuse injury (without mass lesions) and with ICP elevation to values >20 mm Hg for more than 15 min within a 1-h period that are refractory to first-tier therapies. However, this procedure has been demonstrated to reduce ICP and to minimize days in the ICU**
	• **A large frontotemporoparietal DC (not less than 12 × 15 cm or 15 cm diameter) is recommended over a small frontotemporoparietal DC for reduced mortality and improved neurologic outcomes in patients with severe TBI**
	• The committee is aware that the results of the RESCUEicp trial were released soon after the completion of these guidelines. The results of this trial may affect these recommendations and may need to be considered by treating physicians and other users of these guidelines. We intend to update these recommendations if needed. Updates will be available at https://braintrauma.org/coma/guidelines
Prophylactic hypothermia	Level IIB
	• **Early (within 2.5 h), short-term (48 h post-injury), prophylactic hypothermia is not recommended to improve outcomes in patients with diffuse injury**
Hyperosmolar therapy	Recommendations from the prior (Third) Edition not supported by evidence meeting current standards
	Mannitol is effective for control of raised ICP at doses of 0.25–1 g/kg body weight. Arterial hypotension (systolic blood pressure <90 mm Hg) should be avoided
	Restrict mannitol use prior to ICP monitoring to patients with signs of transtentorial herniation or progressive neurologic deterioration not attributable to extracranial causes
Cerebrospinal fluid drainage	Level III
	• **An EVD system zeroed at the midbrain with continuous drainage of CSF may be considered to lower ICP burden more effectively than intermittent use**
	• **Use of CSF drainage to lower ICP in patients with an initial GCS <6 during the first 12 h after injury may be considered**
Ventilation therapies	Level IIB
	• Prolonged prophylactic hyperventilation with $PaCO_2$ of ≤25 mm Hg is not recommended
	Recommendations from the prior (Third) Edition not supported by evidence meeting current standards
	Hyperventilation is recommended as a temporizing measure for the reduction of elevated ICP
	Hyperventilation should be avoided during the first 24 h after injury when CBF often is reduced critically
	If hyperventilation is used, SjO_2 or $BtpO_2$ measurements are recommended to monitor oxygen delivery
Anesthetics, analgesics, and sedatives	Level IIB
	• Administration of barbiturates to induce burst suppression measured by EEG as prophylaxis against the development of intracranial hypertension is not recommended

(continued)

Table 1 (continued)

Topic	Recommendations
	• High-dose barbiturate administration is recommended to control elevated ICP refractory to maximum standard medical and surgical treatment. Hemodynamic stability is essential before and during barbiturate therapy
	• Although propofol is recommended for the control of ICP, it is not recommended for improvement in mortality or 6-month outcomes. Caution is required as high-dose propofol can produce significant morbidity
Steroids	Level I
	• The use of steroids is not recommended for improving outcome or reducing ICP. In patients with severe TBI, high-dose methylprednisolone was associated with increased mortality and is contraindicated
Nutrition	Level IIA
	• **Feeding patients to attain basal caloric replacement at least by the fifth day and at most by the seventh day post-injury is recommended to decrease mortality**
	Level IIB
	• **Transgastric jejunal feeding is recommended to reduce the incidence of ventilator-associated pneumonia**
Infection prophylaxis	Level IIA
	• Early tracheostomy is recommended to reduce mechanical ventilation days when the overall benefit is thought to outweigh the complications associated with such a procedure. However, there is no evidence that early tracheostomy reduces mortality or the rate of nosocomial pneumonia
	• **The use of PI oral care is not recommended to reduce ventilator-associated pneumonia and may cause an increased risk of acute respiratory distress syndrome**
	Level III
	• **Antimicrobial-impregnated catheters may be considered to prevent catheter-related infections during external ventricular drainage**
Deep vein thrombosis prophylaxis	Level III
	• LMWH or low-dose unfractionated heparin may be used in combination with mechanical prophylaxis. However, there is an increased risk for expansion of intracranial hemorrhage
	• In addition to compression stockings, pharmacologic prophylaxis may be considered if the brain injury is stable and the benefit is considered to outweigh the risk of increased intracranial hemorrhage
	• There is insufficient evidence to support recommendations regarding the preferred agent, dose, or timing of pharmacologic prophylaxis for deep vein thrombosis
Seizure prophylaxis	Level IIA
	• Prophylactic use of phenytoin or valproate is not recommended for preventing late PTS
	• Phenytoin is recommended to decrease the incidence of early PTS (within 7 days of injury), when the overall benefit is thought to outweigh the complications associated with such treatment. However, early PTS have not been associated with worse outcomes
	• **At the present time, there is insufficient evidence to recommend levetiracetam compared with phenytoin regarding efficacy in preventing early post-traumatic seizures and toxicity**

Bold: new or revised recommendations

BtpO₂ brain tissue O_2 partial pressure, *CBF* cerebral blood flow, *CSF* cerebrospinal fluid drainage, *DC* decompressive craniectomy, *EEG* electroencephalogram, *EVD* external ventricular drainage, *GCS* Glasgow Coma Scale, *GOS-E* Glasgow Outcome Scale—extended, *ICP* intracranial pressure, *ICU* intensive care unit, *LMWH* low-molecular-weight heparin, *PaCO₂* partial pressure of arterial carbon dioxide, *PI* povidone-iodine, *PTS* post-traumatic seizures, *RESCUEicp trial* randomized evaluation of surgery with craniectomy for uncontrollable elevation of ICP trial, *SjO₂* jugular venous oxygen saturation, *TBI* traumatic brain injury

Uncontrollable Elevation of ICP) study may necessitate adjustment of the document's recommendations for the Decompressive Craniectomy and Intracranial Pressure Thresholds chapters within the Treatments and Thresholds sections, respectively [20].

Additional Brain Trauma Foundation Guidelines

As discussed earlier, the BTF has four other coma-related guidelines. While in-depth discussion of these documents is beyond the scope of this chapter, it is nevertheless important for their content to be briefly summarized herein.

2nd Edition Guidelines for the Prehospital Management of Traumatic Brain Injury

The 2nd edition Guidelines for the Prehospital Management of TBI, current as of July 2006, is intended to be used by emergency medical service (EMS) personnel coming from a spectrum of experience, knowledge, and scope of practice [16]. It includes streamlined recommendations, applicable to all levels of EMS, to help mitigate secondary injury in TBI by improving early coma assessment, treatment, and transport for adult and pediatric patients before definitive care is rendered. The publication is broadly categorized into three sections: Assessment, Treatment, and Decision-Making. It also includes an introductory preamble on prevention, since EMS providers are uniquely positioned at the junction of "public health, public safety, and individual patient care." The Assessment section includes chapters on oxygenation and blood pressure, Glasgow Coma Scale (GCS) score, and pupil examination. The Treatment section is subdivided into airway/ventilation/oxygenation, fluid resuscitation, and cerebral herniation. Finally, Decision-making has one chapter titled "Dispatch, Scene, Transportation, and Destination." Each chapter is organized as follows: recommendations, evidence tables, overview, process, scientific foundations, key issues for future

investigation, and references. Recommendations are no longer assigned levels of evidence, but new discussions on the strength of the recommendations and quality of evidence have been added (compared with the 1st edition, published in 2000) [21].

2nd Edition Guidelines for Severe TBI in Infants, Children, and Adolescents

Published in 2012, the second edition Guidelines for Severe TBI in Infants, Children, and Adolescents [18] provides an evidence-based series of recommendations for the pediatric patient population—a patient group where the leading cause of death is consistently, and by a wide margin, unintentional injury (http://www.cdc.gov/injury/wisqars/leadingcauses.html). A rigorous new set of inclusion and exclusion criteria saw the addition of 27 new studies and removal of 25 studies previously included in the 1st edition from 2003 [22]. Despite drawing endorsement from a litany of pediatric, neurological, and critical care professional societies, the 2nd edition guidelines readily acknowledges a relative paucity of high-quality studies, mostly stemming from a lack of standardization within pediatric TBI data collection, which has hampered the ability to draw strong conclusions and make Level I recommendations. However, these trends appear to be changing, as new data on neuromonitoring and neuroimaging as well as multicentered randomized controlled trials (RCTs) in pediatric TBI have been published. The guidelines outline their methodology for selection, assessment, and rating evidence used to form and grade recommendations. This is followed by chapters on Indication for Intracranial Pressure Monitoring; Threshold for Treatment of Intracranial Hypertension; Cerebral Perfusion Pressure Thresholds; Advanced Neuromonitoring; Neuroimaging; Hyperosmolar Therapy; Temperature Control; Cerebrospinal Fluid Drainage; Barbiturates; Decompressive Craniectomy for the Treatment of Intracranial Hypertension; Hyperventilation; Corticosteroids; Analgesics, Sedatives, and Neuromuscular Blockade; Glucose and Nutrition; and Antiseizure Prophylaxis. Each chapter has a list of recommendations stratified by level of evidence (i.e., I, II, or

III), an evidence table to compare each study, an overview of the chapter topic, discussion of the process used to survey the literature, the scientific foundation highlighting key questions within the chapter scope, discussion of information from other sources touching on adult guidelines and information that was excluded, and finally a summary and future investigation section.

Early Indicators of Prognosis in Severe Traumatic Brain Injury

Early and accurate appraisal of TBI prognosis enables clinicians to set realistic goals of care and facilitates earnest, open dialogue and counseling with patients and families. The BTF published Early Indicators of Prognosis in Severe TBI to clarify prognostic uncertainty and avoid ambiguity after head injury [17]. The goal of this publication is to highlight objective patient and injury characteristics that portend consistent probabilistic outcome estimations, of which relatively few have been recognized. Examples include patient age, clinical rating of severity of brain injury, trends in intracranial pressure, and features observed on computed tomographic (CT) imaging. Chapters are divided into GCS Score, Age, Pupillary Diameter and Light Reflex, Hypotension, and CT Scan Features. Studies were classified qualitatively based on the presence of prospective inclusion criteria and whether Bayesian analysis on individual study data was used to calculate sensitivity, specificity, positive and negative predictive value, and likelihood ratios. Each chapter first emphasizes final conclusions and recommendations, followed by a topic overview, discussion of the literature search process, explanation of scientific foundation and rationale, and a concise summary of the prognosticator as related to clinical outcomes. Key issues needing future investigation are also addressed. Finally, Bayesian evidentiary tables are presented for each study included in the chapter.

Guidelines for Field Management of Combat-Related Head Trauma

In 2005, the BTF developed the Guidelines for Field Management of Combat-Related Head Trauma through multidisciplinary collaboration among health professionals from both the civilian and the military sectors [19]. Funding was supplied by a grant from the Defense and Veterans Brain Injury Center through the Henry M. Jackson Foundation for the Advancement of Military Medicine, Inc. The publication acknowledges the inherent systemic challenges unique to military medical practice, such as extrapolation of medical data derived from controlled civilian studies, consideration of tactical scenarios and logistical limitations that may hinder rendering certain aspects of medical aid in active combat zones, differences in scope of practice between civilian and military medics, alterations in human physiology during combat, and an understanding of the importance of communication between the medic and the chain of command. The guidelines were developed in a patient-centered manner with full consideration of these impositions and are divided into sections on assessment, treatment, and triage and transport decisions. Chapters in the assessment section provide "conclusions" related to diagnosis or prognostication rather than "recommendations" provided for specific treatments in the treatment section. Assessment is divided into two chapters: (1) Oxygenation and Blood Pressure, and (2) Glasgow Coma Scale and Pupils. The Treatment section includes four chapters: (1) Airway, Ventilation, and Oxygenation, (2) Fluid Resuscitation, (3) Pain Management and the Use of Analgesics for Sedation, and (4) Brain-Targeted Therapies. Finally, Triage and Transport Decisions is a single chapter. In closing, the publication consolidates the conclusions and recommendations into a Field Management of Combat-related Head Trauma algorithm to guide medics in the combat theater.

Guidelines for the Management of Penetrating Brain Injury

In 1998, the International Brain Injury Association, the Brain Injury Association, USA, and the AANS/CNS acknowledged the lack of clinical guidance for management of penetrating brain injuries (PBI)—an injury that shares management considerations similar to those of blunt TBI. Therefore, a two-part PBI-specific, evidence-based guideline document based on the literature from January 1966 to January 2000 was published in 2001 as the Guidelines for Management of Penetrating Brain Injury [23]. These guidelines were endorsed by the Section on Neurotrauma and Critical Care of the AANS and CNS, the AANS, the CNS, the American Society on Neuroradiology, the Society of Critical Care Medicine, and the American Academy of Neurology.

These guidelines encompass treatment, diagnosis, clinical assessment, prognosis, and prognostic factors of PBI, providing specific therapy recommendations and more general prognosis conclusions in Parts 1 and 2, respectively. Part 1 of the guidelines focuses on management of PBI and provides recommendations for the following sections: Neuroimaging, Intracranial Pressure Monitoring, Surgical Management, Vascular Complications, Management of Cerebrospinal Fluid Leaks, Antibiotic Prophylaxis, and Antiseizure Prophylaxis. In contrast, Part 2 provides conclusions regarding the data on prognosis in PBI [24]. Chapters in Part 2 include Prognostic Indicators; Demographic Factors, Age; Epidemiology: Cause of Injury; Epidemiology: Mode of Injury; Epidemiology: Caliber of Weapon; Systemic Measures: Hypotension; Systemic Measures: Coagulopathy; Systemic Measures: Respiratory Distress; Neurologic Measures: Level of Consciousness and GCS; Neurologic Measures: Pupillary Size and Light Reflex; Neurologic Measures ICP; Features on CT Scanning; and Key Issues for

Future Research in Prognosis in PBI. Because of the lack of available PBI-specific data, the authors highlight that until more relevant data become available for review and evaluation, practicing clinicians are best served by defaulting to recommendations from the BTF TBI guidelines, as previously discussed in detail.

Guidelines for Surgical Management of Traumatic Brain Injury

Development of intracranial lesions related to trauma complicates 25–45% of severe traumatic brain injuries [25]. Surgical intervention plays an important role in the management of this subset of TBI patients and can transform an otherwise morbid condition into a benign clinical course. Because of the lack of guidelines in this area, in 2006, the Guidelines for the Surgical Management of Traumatic Brain Injury were published in *Neurosurgery*. These guidelines are a meticulous review of the literature for surgical management of post-traumatic intracranial mass lesions. The focus is on acute lesions (≤10 days of injury) related to closed TBI. The guidelines discuss literature-based classification of post-traumatic mass lesions, including epidural hematoma, acute subdural hematoma, intraparenchymal lesions (contusion and intracerebral hematoma), acute posterior fossa mass lesions, and depressed cranial fractures (Table 2). The guidelines do not address the management of chronic subdural hematomas, hygromas, and post-traumatic hydrocephalus. The published guidelines are limited in both quality and scope. Out of 700 papers reviewed by the authors, no controlled clinical trials were discovered to support surgical management versus medical management. As a result of lacking Class 1 evidence, recommendations at the standard level could not be made. All the recommendations are supported by Class 3 evidence and considered at the option level. Because of the limited available evidence, this guideline highlights areas where new research

Table 2 A summary table with compiled recommendations from the *Surgical Management of Traumatic Brain Injury*

	Indications for surgery	Timing	Methods
Acute epidural hematomas	• An epidural hematoma (EDH) greater than 30 cm³ should be surgically evacuated regardless of the patient's Glasgow Coma Scale (GCS) score • An EDH less than 30 cm³ and with less than a 15-mm thickness and with less than a 5-mm midline shift (MLS) in patients with a GCS score greater than 8 without focal deficit can be managed nonoperatively with serial computed tomographic (CT) scanning and close neurological observation in a neurosurgical center	• It is strongly recommended that patients with an acute EDH in coma (GCS score 9) with anisocoria undergo surgical evacuation as soon as possible	• There are insufficient data to support one surgical treatment method. However, craniotomy provides a more complete evacuation of the hematoma
Acute subdural hematomas	• An acute subdural hematoma (SDH) with a thickness greater than 10 mm or a midline shift greater than 5 mm on computed tomography (CT) scan should be surgically evacuated, regardless of the patient's Glasgow Coma Scale (GCS) score • All patients with acute SDH in coma (GCS score less than 9) should undergo intracranial pressure (ICP) monitoring • A comatose patient (GCS score less than 9) with an SDH less than 10 mm thick and a midline shift less than 5 mm should undergo surgical evacuation of the lesion if the GCS score decreased between the time of injury and hospital admission by 2 or more points on the GCS and/or the patient presents with asymmetric or fixed and dilated pupils and/or the ICP exceeds 20 mm Hg	• In patients with acute SDH and indications for surgery, surgical evacuation should be performed as soon as possible	• If surgical evacuation of an acute SDH in a comatose patient (GCS 9) is indicated, it should be performed using a craniotomy with or without bone flap removal and duraplasty

Table 2 (continued)

	Indications for surgery	Timing	Methods
Depressed cranial fractures	• Patients with open (compound) cranial fractures depressed greater than the thickness of the cranium should undergo operative intervention to prevent infection • Patients with open (compound) depressed cranial fractures may be treated nonoperatively if there is no clinical or radiographic evidence of dural penetration, significant intracranial hematoma, depression greater than 1 cm, frontal sinus involvement, gross cosmetic deformity, wound infection, pneumocephalus, or gross wound contamination • Nonoperative management of closed (simple) depressed cranial fractures is a treatment option	• Early operation is recommended to reduce the incidence of infection	• Elevation and debridement is recommended as the surgical method of choice • Primary bone fragment replacement is a surgical option in the absence of wound infection at the time of surgery • All management strategies for open (compound) depressed fractures should include antibiotics
Posterior fossa mass	• Patients with mass effect on computed tomographic (CT) scan or with neurological dysfunction or deterioration referable to the lesion should undergo operative intervention. Mass effect on CT scan is defined as distortion, dislocation, or obliteration of the fourth ventricle, compression or loss of visualization of the basal cisterns, or the presence of obstructive hydrocephalus • Patients with lesions and no significant mass effect on CT scan and without signs of neurological dysfunction may be managed by close observation and serial imaging	• In patients with indications for surgical intervention, evacuation should be performed as soon as possible because these patients can deteriorate rapidly, thus, worsening their prognosis	• Suboccipital craniectomy is the predominant method reported for evacuation of posterior fossa mass lesions, and is therefore recommended

(continued)

Table 2 (continued)

	Indications for surgery	Timing	Methods
Traumatic parenchymal lesions	• Patients with parenchymal mass lesions and signs of progressive neurological deterioration referable to the lesion, medically refractory intracranial hypertension, or signs of mass effect on computed tomographic (CT) scan should be treated operatively • Patients with Glasgow Coma Scale (GCS) scores of 6–8 with frontal or temporal contusions greater than 20 cm^3 in volume with midline shift of at least 5 mm and/or cisternal compression on CT scan and patients with any lesion greater than 50 cm^3 in volume should be treated operatively • Patients with parenchymal mass lesions who do not show evidence for neurological compromise have controlled intracranial pressure (ICP), and no significant signs of mass effect on CT scan may be managed nonoperatively with intensive monitoring and serial imaging	• Bifrontal decompressive craniectomy within 48 h of injury is a treatment option for patients with diffuse, medically refractory post-traumatic cerebral edema and resultant intracranial hypertension	• Craniotomy with evacuation of mass lesion is recommended for those patients with focal lesions and the surgical indications listed above, under indications • Decompressive procedures, including subtemporal decompression, temporal lobectomy, and hemispheric decompressive craniectomy, are treatment options for patients with refractory intracranial hypertension and diffuse parenchymal injury

questions can be formulated that may be resolved by future clinical trials. As new evidence becomes available, future editions of these guidelines will address those changes [26].

Neurocritical Care Guidelines

At present, there are eight NCS guideline documents covering a range of unique patient management considerations as they pertain to care of the neurocritical care patient. With the exception of Recommendations for the Critical Care Management of Devastating Brain Injury: Prognostication, Psychosocial, and Ethical Management, the NCS publications do not explicitly nor entirely focus on management of patients with TBI. Rather, they present recommendations for any patient in need of neurointensive care, with TBI patients only being one subset of such patients [27]. However, many of the best practice recommendations include aspects of care that are inevitably and intrinsically necessary in the immediate and delayed management of patients with TBI. These include The Insertion and Management of External Ventricular Drains: An Evidence-Based Consensus Statement; Guideline for Reversal of Antithrombotics in Intracranial Hemorrhage; Prophylaxis of Venous Thrombosis in Neurocritical Care Patients; and a Consensus Summary Statement of the International Multidisciplinary Consensus Conference on Multimodality Monitoring in Neurocritical Care

[28–31]. Furthermore, a statement on targeted temperature management is in process but at the time of publication is not available for review.

The care of patients with TBI does not exist in a vacuum, and patients frequently have confounding medical comorbidities, both neurological and non-neurological. Therefore, TBI-related patient management considerations are neither singular nor mutually exclusive, and they must be interpreted in the appropriate clinical context for proper application of recommendations. Although the focus of this chapter is TBI, related guidelines may be useful in certain subsets of TBI patients. For example, the NCS has published Evidence-Based Guidelines for the Management of Large Hemispheric Infarction, Guidelines for the Evaluation and Management of Status Epilepticus, and Critical Care Management of Patients Following Aneurysmal Subarachnoid Hemorrhage [32–34].

Traumatic Brain Injury-Related Neurocritical Care Society Guidelines

As discussed earlier, five of the NCS guidelines have significant utility in management of patients with TBI and will be summarized as follows. These documents provide recommendations related to psychosocial and ethical decision considerations, therapeutic procedures to manage ICP, pharmacological treatments related to the coagulation cascade, and neuromonitoring.

Recommendations for the Critical Care Management of Devastating Brain Injury: Prognostication, Psychosocial, and Ethical Management

The NCS published its Recommendations for the Critical Care Management of Devastating Brain Injury: Prognostication, Psychosocial, and Ethical Management in 2015 to address these aspects of patient care during the first 72 h post-injury [27]. The authors first provide a definition for "devastating brain injury," explaining their rationale for using such terminology, which identifies an exceedingly vulnerable patient population with imminent threat to life due to their brain injury. The guidelines are then divided into three sections: (1) prognostication, (2) psychosocial management, and (3) ethics. Each section is presented as a series of clinical questions, followed by a brief discussion and a series of recommendations. Within the Prognostication section, questions addressed include: "How accurate is prognostication in devastating brain injury?" "What is the impact of prognostication before 72 hours?" and "What factors identify patients at high risk for death due to their injury?" The Psychosocial Management section builds upon itself, first focusing on identifying the needs of family members and then highlighting ways for clinicians to effectively meet those needs. Next, the role of surrogate decision-makers is discussed, both in terms of how they arrive at treatment decisions and also how clinicians can best assist with this extremely personal and monumental task. Lastly, Ethics questions are addressed, including who should be resuscitated, how donor status affects patient care, and how the ethical principles of justice and autonomy should be applied to patient care.

Insertion and Management of External Ventricular Drains: An Evidence-Based Consensus Statement

Preventing elevations in ICP is widely believed to mitigate secondary brain injury related to cerebral hypoperfusion, thereby improving neurological outcomes after TBI. This is typically achieved through ICP monitoring and tightly regulated drainage of cerebrospinal fluid using an extraventricular drain (EVD). The Insertion and Management of External Ventricular Drains: An Evidence-Based Consensus Statement is an evidence-based set of recommendations, published in 2016, based on numerous clinical questions surrounding EVD placement and management [29]. The section on EVD placement addresses clinician preparation for performance of the procedure, the impact of placement setting on deleterious mechanical or infectious events, risk of hemorrhage and catheter malposition, and timing of venous thromboembolism (VTE) prophylaxis. Next, risks, prevention, and management of ventriculostomy-related infections are explored. Specifically, evidence is outlined for how duration of placement and the use of antibiosis with systemic antimicrobials, antimicrobial-impregnated catheters, or intraventricular antimicrobials contribute to the incidence of ventriculostomy-related infections. Finally, general EVD management considerations are discussed. Topics such as the impact of routinely sampling cerebrospinal fluid and prophylactically changing catheter/tubing/collection devices on incidence of ventriculostomy-related infections, how weaning parameters influence the incidence of developing hydrocephalus requiring ventriculoperitoneal shunting, and role of EVD management bundles in reducing EVD-related infections are discussed.

Guideline for Reversal of Antithrombotics in Intracranial Hemorrhage

Treating coagulopathy is a double-edged sword of increasing complexity in modern medicine. Rapid reversal of hypocoagulable states secondary to antithrombotic therapy (i.e., anticoagulants, antiplatelet agents, and thrombolytics) is essential in minimizing intracranial hemorrhage expansion, when present, in early TBI management. Conversely, preventing morbidity and mortality from VTE due to hypercoagulability, limited mobility or paralysis, and inflammation-promoted endothelial injury is paramount in the later stages of neurocritical TBI care.

An aging patient demographic combined with increasing availability and frequency of antithrombotic use necessitates a set of guidelines to inform clinical practice. The NCS Guideline for Reversal of Antithrombotics in Intracranial Hemorrhage provides recommendations for reversal of anticoagulants (i.e., vitamin K antagonists, oral direct factor Xa inhibitors, direct thrombin inhibitors, unfractionated heparin, low-molecular-weight heparin, pentasaccharides), thrombolytics (i.e., plasminogen activators), and antiplatelet agents (i.e., COX inhibitors, ADP receptor inhibitors, phosphodiesterase inhibitors, glycoprotein IIB/IIIA antagonists, thromboxane receptor antagonists, PAR-1 antagonists) [30]. Additionally, data are presented in tabular form on pharmacokinetic parameters for common anticoagulants and antiplatelet agents, compositions of prothrombin complex concentrates, and antidotes in development for novel oral anticoagulants. In closing, a summary table is presented with compiled recommendations for reversal of antithrombotic agents in patients with intracranial hemorrhage.

Prophylaxis of Venous Thrombosis in Neurocritical Care Patients

Initiation of the proper pharmacological prophylaxis agent against VTE (i.e., deep vein thrombosis and pulmonary embolism) in patients with TBI is of critical importance. TBI is an independent risk factor for deep vein thrombosis, likely related to the immobility, prolonged mechanical ventilation, and increased activation of pro-inflammatory mediators in these patients [35]. The 2016 publication of Prophylaxis of Venous Thrombosis in Neurocritical Care Patients includes recommendations for VTE prophylaxis in myriad neurological ailments, with a section specific to VTE prophylaxis in TBI [31]. The guidelines draft recommendations based on data derived primarily from the 2001 Eastern Association for the Surgery of Trauma Guidelines, the 8th edition of the American College of Chest Physicians Guidelines, and the 2007 BTF Guidelines as well as data from neurologic, but non-TBI, research [14, 36, 37].

Consensus Summary Statement of the International Multidisciplinary Consensus Conference on Multimodality Monitoring in Neurocritical Care

Heavy reliance is placed on objective, quantifiable data derived from bedside neuromonitoring for making diagnostic and management decisions in the neurocritical care setting. The use of multiple monitors, termed "multimodality monitoring," as an augmentation to clinical examination alone, is addressed in the Consensus Summary Statement of the International Multidisciplinary Consensus Conference on Multimodality Monitoring in

Neurocritical Care [28]. Emphasis is placed on multimodality monitoring data interpretation and integration into the decision-making scheme, rather than suggesting recommended therapies. The publication is divided into sections based on a key physiologic parameter being measured, followed by a list of questions addressed, a written summary of the data, and numerical recommendations drawn from the data. Physiological parameters include the Clinical Evaluation, Systemic Hemodynamics, ICP and Cerebral Perfusion Pressure, Cerebral Autoregulation, Systemic and Brain Oxygenation, Cerebral Blood Flow, Electrophysiology, Cerebral Metabolism, Glucose and Nutrition, Hemostasis and Hemoglobin, Temperature and Inflammation, and Cellular Damage and Degeneration. Systems level decision questions are addressed in a section on ICU processes of care and quality assurance. Metrics of the data collection and abstraction are discussed in multimodality monitoring: informatics, data integration, display, and analysis. Finally, resource limitations and utilization are the focus of the chapter monitoring in emerging economies. The summary statement is closed with an overview of future directions and emerging technologies.

American College of Surgeons Trauma Quality Improvement Program

The Trauma Quality Improvement Program (TQIP) is a comprehensive program with an overarching goal to "elevate the care for trauma patients at trauma centers." Currently, more than 500 trauma centers in the United States are enrolled in the fee-based program, which provides center-by-center data collection and feedback. Areas of patient care necessitating improvement are identified, and institutional plans to bring about positive changes are recommended. Data from these centers are also used to provide national comparisons on a risk-adjusted basis to participating centers. Finally, TQIP contributes education and training to trauma staff, hosts annual scientific meetings, and has published four best practice guidelines to date, including Geriatric Trauma Management [38], massive transfusion in trauma [39], management

of orthopedic trauma [40], and management of traumatic brain injury. The focus of this chapter will be on the ACS TQIP Best Practices in Management of Traumatic Brain Injury.

ACS TQIP Best Practices in Management of Traumatic Brain Injury

Published in January 2015, ACS TQIP Best Practices in Management of Traumatic Brain Injury [41] is a set of evidence-based recommendations produced by a multidisciplinary expert panel to improve the care of trauma patients with TBI. Panel participants include members from the ACS, the AANS/CNS Joint Section of Neurotrauma and Critical Care, the NCS, and the American College of Emergency Medicine. Recommendations are provided based on available evidence and expert consensus opinion.

The best practices document is divided into 15 chapters, highlighting many of the common treatment and management challenges encountered during the treatment of patients with TBI. These chapters include Using the GCS, Triage and Transport, Goals of Treatment, Intracranial Pressure Monitoring, Management of Intracranial Hypertension, Advanced Neuromonitoring, Surgical Management, Nutritional Support, Tracheostomy, Timing of Secondary Procedures, Timing of Pharmacologic VTE Prophylaxis, Management Considerations for Pediatric Patients with TBI, Management Considerations for Elderly Patients with TBI, Prognostic Decision-Making and Withdrawal of Medical Support, and Outcome Assessment and Quality Improvement in TBI.

Each chapter begins with a section on key messages, summarizing the take-home points of the section, followed by a brief description of the relevant physiology, pathophysiology, evidence, and rationale for the recommendations. The Goals of Treatment, Management of Intracranial Hypertension, and Timing of Pharmacologic VTE Prophylaxis chapters include a table of specific numerical treatment ranges, a management algorithm with a three-tiered management of ICP (adapted from the National Institute of

Table 3 Three-tiered management of intracranial pressure (ICP)

Tier 1
• Head of bed elevated at 30° (reverse Trendelenburg) to improve cerebral venous outflow
• Sedation and analgesia using recommended short-acting agents (e.g., propofol, fentanyl, midazolam) in intubated patients
• Ventricular drainage performed intermittently. Continuous drainage is not recommended unless an additional ICP monitor is placed, as when the drain is open, it does not accurately reflect true ICP
• Repeat computed tomography (CT) imaging and neurological examination should be considered to rule out the development of a surgical mass lesion and guide treatment
If ICP remains ≥ 20–25 mm Hg, proceed to Tier 2

Tier 2
• In patients with a parenchymal ICP monitor, an extraventricular drain (EVD) should be considered to allow for intermittent cerebrospinal fluid (CSF) drainage
• Hyperosmolar therapy should be given intermittently as needed for ICP elevation and not on a routine schedule
– Mannitol should be administered in intermittent boluses (0.25–1 gm/kg body weight). Caution should be taken in the hypovolemic patient when osmotic diuresis is instituted with mannitol. The serum sodium and osmolality must be assessed frequently (every 6 h) and additional doses should be held if serum osmolality exceeds 320 mOsm/L. Mannitol may also be held if there is evidence of hypovolemia
– Hypertonic saline may be administered in intermittent boluses of 3% sodium chloride solution (250 mL over 1/2 h) or other concentrations (e.g., 30 ml of 23.4%). Serum sodium and osmolality must be assessed frequently (every 6 h), and additional doses should be held if serum sodium exceeds 160 mEq/L
• Cerebral autoregulation should be assessed. If the patient is not autoregulating, the cerebral perfusion pressure (CPP) goal should be lowered to reduce ICP (to no less than 50 mm Hg). Additional neuromonitoring (e.g., pB_tO_2, $SjvO_2$, CBF) may help determine optimal CPP
• $PaCO_2$ goal of 30–35 mm Hg should be maintained, as long as brain hypoxia is not encountered. Additional neuromonitoring (e.g., pB_tO_2, $SjvO_2$, CBF) may help determine optimal $PaCO_2$
• Repeat CT imaging and neurological examination should be considered to rule out the development of a surgical mass lesion and guide treatment
• Neuromuscular paralysis achieved with a bolus "test dose" of a neuromuscular-blocking agent should be considered if the above measures fail to adequately lower ICP and restore CPP. If there is a positive response, continuous infusion of neuromuscular-blocking agent should be employed (Tier 3)
If ICP remains ≥ 20–25 mm Hg, proceed to Tier 3

Table 3 (continued)

Tier 3 (includes salvage therapies)
• Decompressive hemicraniectomy or bilateral craniectomy should only be performed if treatments in Tiers 1 and 2 are not sufficient or are limited by the development of side effects of medical treatment
• Neuromuscular paralysis via continuous infusion of neuromuscular blocking agent can be employed if there is a positive response to a bolus dose. The infusion should be titrated to maintain at least two twitches (out of a train of four) using a peripheral nerve stimulator. Adequate sedation must be utilized
• Barbiturate or propofol (anesthesia dosage) coma may be induced for those patients who have failed to respond to aggressive measures to control malignant intracranial hypertension; however, it should only be instituted if a test dose of barbiturate or propofol results in a decrease in ICP, thereby identifying the patient as a "responder." Hypotension is a frequent side effect of high-dose therapy with these agents. Meticulous volume resuscitation should be ensured and infusion of vasopressor/inotropes may be required. Prolonged use or high dose of propofol can lead to propofol infusion syndrome. Continuous electroencephalography may be used to ensure targeting of the infusion to burst suppression
• Hypothermia (≤36 °C) is not currently recommended as an initial TBI treatment. Hypothermia should be reserved for "rescue" or salvage therapy after reasonable attempts at ICP control via the previous Tier 3 treatments have failed

pB_tO_2 brain tissue oxygen tension, $PaCO_2$ partial pressure of arterial carbon dioxide, $SjvO_2$ jugular venous oxygen saturation, *CBF* cerebral blood flow

Neurological Disorders and Stroke of the NIH ProTECT III clinical trial protocol) based on ACS expert consensus-refined BTF guidelines (discussed earlier) and the Modified Berne-Norwood Criteria for VTE prophylaxis, respectively (Table 3) [42, 43]. Many of the recommendations found in the best practices document are not as scenario-specific as those in evidence-based medicine guidelines documents but instead provide a practical framework for managing critically ill TBI patients.

Methodology and Classification of Evidence

Brain Trauma Foundation

Classification of evidence for the BTF's 4th edition TBI Guidelines was based on the stringent requirements set by the IOM criteria for the development of guidelines. The BTF performed a systematic evidence review and synthesis and then followed the methods for the development of recommendations detailed below. The literature search (Ovid/MEDLINE) from 2006 to November 2013 resulted in a large number of studies. (For the topic of cerebrospinal fluid drainage, the literature was searched from 1980 to November 2013, and decompressive craniectomy literature was searched from 2001 to November 2013.) Two members of the Methods team were assigned to each topic and reviewed titles and abstracts. The reviewers read the abstracts and eliminated citations using predetermined inclusion/exclusion criteria (Table 4). Full

Table 4 Inclusion and exclusion criteria for classification of evidence for the Brain Trauma Foundation's Guidelines for the Management of Severe TBI, 4th edition

Inclusion criteria	Exclusion criteria
Population (note: population criteria may be relaxed, and studies used as indirect evidence if no direct evidence is available)	
Human subjects	Animal or mechanical simulations; not human subjects
85% of population must be	**If more than 15% are**
Adults	Children
Traumatic brain injury, non-penetrating	Brain injury not from trauma (e.g., stroke) or penetrating injury (gunshot, foreign object) or mixed pathology without separation of outcomes
In-hospital	Prehospital or outpatient treatment
GCS 3–8, or results presented for subgroup with this GCS	GCS ≥ 9 with no results presented by GCS subgroups
N ≥ 25	N < 25
Interventions	
Decompressive craniectomy	Studies of type of bone flap replacement
Prophylactic hypothermia	
Hyperosmolar therapy	
Cerebrospinal fluid drainage	
Ventilation therapy	Hyperbaric O_2
Anesthetics, analgesics, and sedatives	
Steroids	

Table 4 (continued)

Inclusion criteria	Exclusion criteria
Nutrition	
Infection prophylaxis	
Deep vein thrombosis	
Antiseizure prophylaxis	
ICP monitoring	
CPP monitoring	
Advanced cerebral monitoring	
Blood pressure thresholds	
ICP thresholds	
CPP thresholds	
Advanced cerebral monitoring thresholds	
Comparator/study designs	
Two or more groups defined by differences in intervention (or monitoring or thresholds) and compared on an included outcome	Purely prognostic studies (nontreatment factors that affect outcome) that are not thresholds
Randomized controlled trials, cohort studies, case-control studies	Descriptive studies (e.g., natural history or characteristics of injury or of course of treatment)
Cohort studies, retrospective or prospective	Case studies, case series
Case-control studies	Assessment of technologies (differences, cost, feasibility of use)
	Studies that assess the psychometrics of a measure (validity, reliability, etc.)
	New drug or device efficacy trials
Outcomes	
Mortality (inpatient or post-discharge)	Physiologic measure without a link to an included outcome
Morbidity/harms (e.g., pneumonia, bleeding, infection, ischemia, reoperation, etc.)	
Function (GOS other functional measure)	
Health services use (length of stay in hospital, in ICU, etc.)	
Change in ICP (for treatments explicitly aimed at lowering ICP)	
Publication	
English	Not English
Publication date: 2000 or later (for updated topics)	Studies published prior to 2000
Research study	Editorial, comments, letters

GCS Glasgow Coma Score, *ICP* intracranial pressure, *CCP* cerebral perfusion pressure, *GOS* Glasgow Outcome Scale, *ICU* intensive care unit

texts of articles were reviewed if one of the reviewers considered the article relevant. Further discrepancies were discussed and resolved through consensus or with the use of a third reviewer. Full-text publications were then reviewed by one or more clinical investigators who took the lead on the topic. The clinical investigators read the papers critically and determined whether the selected texts met the inclusion criteria. The Methods team then abstracted data from each publication, and another member evaluated the texts for errors. Information was recorded about the study population, design, and results. For topics where meta-analysis publications were considered, the study characteristics and results were independently abstracted by two people and verified by a third member. Two reviewers independently evaluated each study and rated the study as Class 1, 2, or 3 evidence based on a combination of study design and quality rating. Class 1 is the highest class and is limited to good-quality randomized trials. Class 2 includes moderate-quality randomized control trials and good-quality cohort or case-control studies. Class 3 is the lowest class and is given to low-quality randomized control trials, moderate to low-quality cohort or case-control studies, case series, and other noncomparative designs. After the classification, the studies were assessed for quality based on four domains: (1) the aggregate quality of the studies, (2) the consistency of the results, (3) whether the evidence provided was direct or indirect, and (4) the precision of the evidence. Applicability is the extent to which the research finding was useful in informing recommendations for a broader population and more specifically the population of interest. For applicability, consideration was made to include geographic location and type of hospital.

Level of recommendation was designated as Level I, Level IIA, Level IIB, or Level III. Recommendation was based on the classification of evidence, quality of the body of evidence, and consideration of applicability. Level I recommendation was based on a high-quality body of evidence. Level IIA recommendation was based on a moderate-quality body of evidence. Level II B and III recommendations were based on a low-quality body of evidence. A Level IIB recommendation was based on Class 2 body of evidence with direct evidence but of low quality, whereas a Level III recommendation was based on Class 3 studies or on Class 2 studies with only indirect evidence. The 4th edition was finalized with a peer review. The peer review committee consisted of topic-specific TBI clinicians, methodologists, representatives of specialty societies, and related stakeholders. Additionally, a comprehensive review was conducted by the members of the AANS/CNS Joint Guideline Committee in collaboration with the clinical investigators and Methods team.

Guidelines for the Management of Penetrating Brain Injury

A group of experts in the treatment of patients with PBI from varying fields including neurosurgery, neurology, neuropsychology, and clinical epidemiology assembled to produce the PBI guidelines. A MEDLINE search was performed to identify articles published from January 1966 to January 2000 using key search words pertaining to penetrating head injury. The search was limited to papers in English with human subjects. Two independent reviewers then read the abstracts and rejected or approved them based on appropriateness of the subject material. Full articles were then evaluated, the evidence was classified into Class 1, 2, or 3, and recommendations were derived. The methodology used in the production of the guidelines is evidence based and follows the recommendations of the IOM; however, the treatment recommendations specific to PBI were limited because of the paucity of research in that targeted subject. Additionally, the literature evaluated for the guidelines included prognostic indicators to define features that correlated to poor outcomes to aid with communicating with families of victims of PBI.

Table 5 Categories of evidence of therapeutic effectiveness

Class 1	Based on evidence from 1 or more high-quality, well-designed randomized controlled trials
Class 2	Based on evidence from 1 or more trials such as nonrandomized trials, cohort studies, or case-control studies
Class 3	Based on evidence from case series, case reports, comparative studies, and expert opinion

Surgical Management of Traumatic Brain Injury

The literature search was performed using the National Library of Medicine database. The search covered the era from 1975 to 2006 and was limited to studies written in the English language involving humans with TBI and their surgical management. The articles were evaluated with a critical assessment of the methodology as well as clinical questions addressed and the type of study conducted. Additionally, the quality of the studies was assessed as it related to errors in design execution or conclusions reached. All articles were then cross reviewed, and consensus was reached on disagreements among the panel. The literature was then classified into three categories of evidence ranging from Class 1 to Class 3 evidence (Table 5). All of the recommendations were considered at the option level because of the quality of articles, which were classified into Class 3 evidence.

Neurocritical Care Society

Experts in the fields of neurosurgery, neurocritical care, neurology, critical care, neuroanesthesia, nursing, pharmacy, internal medicine, infectious disease, and informatics convened. The committee generated several clinical questions regarding several areas of TBI management specifying the patient group of interest, intervention, comparators, and outcomes of interest. Two

experts were assigned to each clinical question of interest. With the assistance of a medical librarian, the committee performed a critical literature search and review of available evidence. The abstracts were reviewed by committee members, and the quality of the data was assessed, and recommendations were developed using the GRADE system (Grades of Recommendation Assessment, Development, and Evaluation) ranging from high to very low. The GRADE system classifies recommendations as strong (recommended) or weak (suggested) based on the balance between benefits, risks, cost, and burden and according to the quality of evidence. Recommendations were also based on trade-offs, taking into account the estimated size of the effect for the main outcomes, the confidence limits around those estimates, and relative value placed on each outcome. Consideration was also placed on translation of the evidence into practice in a specific setting while adjusting for important factors that could be expected to modify the size of the expected effects.

A meeting was held with the full committee where the evidence and summaries were presented and, after discussion by the entire panel, approval of the document was finalized. The final consensus statement was submitted for a final review by experts within NCS and reviewers from other stakeholder societies.

American College of Surgeons

The ACS statement noted that data from well-designed, controlled studies on acute management of traumatic brain injury are sparse. The Committee on Trauma compiled an evidence-based guideline but with the disclaimer that the scarcity of high-quality studies limits the strength and scope of their recommendations. The recommendations were based on the best available evidence or lack thereof and based overall on the consensus opinion of the expert panel. Multiple consensus-driven clinical research trial protocols from prior TBI studies were consulted (including

COBRIT [44, 45], PRoTECT III [42], and SYNAPSE [46]). The members of the expert panel were listed and comprised neurosurgeons, surgeons, emergency physicians, neurologist, and critical care specialists. The ACS TQIP does acknowledge the participation of members of the AANS/CNS Joint Section of Neurotrauma and Critical Care, the NCS, and the American College of Emergency Medicine but explicitly stated that the content is solely the responsibility of the authors and does not represent the views of the supporting entities.

Protocols Versus Individualized Therapy

Patient outcomes are improved by the delivery of evidence-based protocols, which can standardize treatments and reduce variability of clinical care. A protocol-based guideline can educate clinicians and help guide medical personnel to provide interventions and manage the natural course related to TBI by standardizing practice. As a result, studies have demonstrated improved neurological outcomes with the use of center-specific TBI protocols [47–49]. This success led to translation of the BTF guidelines into more than 15 languages with copies available worldwide.

A concern with protocols and guidelines is the perceived contribution to loss of physician autonomy in decision-making. Additionally, the early implementation of protocols can hinder the development of clinical expertise and impede the ability to develop clinical reasoning skills, which might be necessary in individual cases. A protocol-driven approach also results in lack of consideration of pathophysiological variation among patients and their varying severity of injuries. Clearly, patients from a heterogeneous population have differing physiologic requirements. As such, there are areas where individualized therapy is needed. With the gradual development of neurocritical care, the understanding of disease pathophysiology and its complexity has also evolved. Recent advances and introduction of neuromonitoring devices that measure cerebrovascular autoregulation, brain tissue oxygen-

ation, and perfusion increased the complexity of the management of TBI. Thus, implementation of personalized care to account for patient variability in a team-based approach to neurocritical care is an avenue that can potentially lead to improved outcomes.

Limitations of Guidelines

Lack of High-Quality Evidence

Guideline recommendations are based on the most up-to-date evidence available supporting the use or practice of specific therapies; however, limitations do exist with their use. As already noted, a key limitation to TBI guidelines is the lack of high-quality evidence to back recommendations, which may result in not recommending proven therapies for lack of evidence. Recommendations based on inaccurate or poor evidence can lead to suboptimal or harmful practices. Furthermore, persistent gaps in the evidence knowledge base are reflected in the guidelines. Despite the addition of publications over time, some recommendations still lack strong evidence. For example, BTF describes the use of hyperosmolar therapy and hypertonic saline as important therapies in the armamentarium of practitioners for the management of elevated ICP in patients with traumatic intracranial injuries; however, the use of which agent at which times, the optimal route of administration, optimal combinations, and the precise mechanisms of action are yet to be determined. The use of mannitol is recommended without high-quality evidence to support its use based upon decades of clinical experience. Mannitol is believed to reduce ICP by inducing osmotic fluid shifts out of brain tissue into the bloodstream but also by reducing blood viscosity, which leads to improved microcirculatory flow of blood and decreased cerebral blood volume and thus decreased ICP. Despite the fact that it is clearly evident through clinical use that mannitol and hyperosmolar therapy are highly effective in treating elevated ICP, the guidelines have insufficient evidence about the effects on clinical outcomes to support the use of any specific hyperosmolar agent or usage pattern for patients with severe TBI. Moreover, as the field of neurosurgery evolves, the recommendations provided currently will become outdated with time. Different methodological considerations will yield differences in levels of recommendations and confidence in the evidence. The BTF 3rd edition guidelines gave Level II and III recommendations about the use of mannitol and hyperosmolar therapy, but these recommendations were not carried over to the 4th edition because they were derived from studies that did not meet Class 3 criteria. Additionally, hypertonic saline is used as an alternative agent to hyperosmolar agent but lacks sufficient evidence from comparative studies to support a formal recommendation. However, because the potential need for hyperosmolar therapy to reduce ICP is still recognized, the 4th edition restated the 3rd edition recommendations and made no new additions. Another example is with the surgical evacuation of epidural hematomas. Patients with acute epidural hematomas and a GCS < 8 with evidence of a "blown pupil" benefit from early intervention and achieve better outcomes. Although there is lack of evidence to endorse such recommendation, no neurosurgeon would allow these symptoms to go unaddressed without surgical intervention, especially in patients who have a good chance at recovery [23], because of ethical considerations and proven clinical efficacy outside of trial scenarios.

Lack of Protocols

The lack of treatment protocols is an additional limitation of the current TBI guidelines. Treatment protocols would provide best practices, guidance, and suggestions; however, they were not discussed in the guidelines. The BTF prides itself that its TBI guidelines are a product of stringent review of the literature evaluating the current evidence and deriving recommendations based on available studies. Thus, the currently available guidelines are limited to areas where the evidence base was established according to stringent criteria. Treatment protocols that are critical in guiding practitioners are often not described in the guidelines. As a result, the ACS TQIP Best Practices document was developed, and the BTF is in the process of developing an updated protocol that dissects the treatment of elevated ICP into three tiers based on risk and efficacy. This approach is the framework adopted by recent studies such as COBRIT, PRoTECT III, SYNAPSE, and TRACK-TBI. Additional protocols are currently still in the development phase.

Need for Individualized Care

Clinical guidelines recommendations usually are focused around providing a universal approach to neurophysiologic management of TBI. However, a one-size-fits-all approach does not account for individual pathophysiological variation and a wide range of severity of injuries in TBI patients. Multimodal neuromonitoring strategies allow clinicians to provide individualized treatment tailored to the patient's pathophysiology based on the use of continuous ICP transduction, assessment of autoregulation using the pressure reactivity index, monitoring of partial pressure of oxygen, continuous electroencephalography, and cerebral microdialysis. Implementation of multimodal neuromonitoring can allow clinicians to treat TBI using personalized management within the context of protocol-driven care. However, recommendations to utilize multimodal neuromonitoring lack stringent evidence-based backing and also steer away from standardization of care. Further investigation is currently required to further understand and determine how to integrate personalized medicine into clinical guidelines.

Expert Opinion

Prior to the advent of evidence-based guidelines, clinical guidelines were based on consensus developed through expert opinion. The opinions of experts were based on personal clinical experience and knowledge, new information attained from attending conferences and symposiums, and practice styles of other experts in the field [50]. However, expert opinion is prone to personal bias and limited by human errors. The IOM criteria for developing guidelines designate the use of expert opinion as Class 3 evidence, although expert opinion can play a key role in guidelines especially with developing recommendations for practice. Additionally, expert recommendations are used to assess and evaluate the literature when formulating evidence-based guidelines [23, 26]. The BTF guidelines are rigorous and based on evidence evaluated based on the highest standard available, whereas the NCS, ACS, Guidelines for Surgical Management of TBI, and Guidelines for PBI recommendations take into consideration some component of expert opinion, which can introduce bias and at times be the source of wrong treatments. The BTF does not include expert opinions that are not based on current evidence standards. Rather, the guidelines are intended to enable the derivation of institutional protocols while considering all aspects of the care of patients with severe TBI that rely partially on some expert opinions. However, the limitations of this approach include a lack of actionable recommendations on which to formulate the basis for care. All types of analyses should be taken together when developing clinical approaches to care.

Conclusions

Using the Evidence to Inform Clinical Research Questions

Despite having guidelines that are based on the most current evidence-based research, there are still gaps in the evidence base for severe TBI management. The BTF added 102 new studies to its library of evidence between the transitions from the 3rd edition to the 4th edition, but even these new studies generally lack the design of meaningful and effective research. Just as there is a need to have processes for the development of guidelines, there is a need to design and establish a systematic

process for developing a research agenda that starts with conversation about the scope, topics, management, and research methods. Most neurotraumatologists agree that the process should include identification and refinement of topics for studies that could serve to fill critical gaps in guidelines, improve study design, and incorporate state-of-the-art methods for synthesizing the literature and assessing the evidence.

References

1. Lugtenberg M, Burgers JS, Westert GP. Effects of evidence-based clinical practice guidelines on quality of care: a systematic review. Qual Saf Health Care. 2009;18(5):385–92.
2. Jacoby I. Evidence and consensus. JAMA. 1988;259(20):3039.
3. White LJ, Ball JR. The Clinical Efficacy Assessment Project of the American College of Physicians. Int J Technol Assess Health Care. 1985;1(1):69–74.
4. Eddy DM. Clinical decision making: from theory to practice. Practice policies—guidelines for methods. JAMA. 1990;263(13):1839–41.
5. Eddy DM. Clinical decision making: from theory to practice. Guidelines for policy statements: the explicit approach. JAMA. 1990;263(16):2239–2240, 2243.
6. Institute of Medicine. Clinical Practice Guidelines: Directions for a New Program. The National Academies Press: Washington, DC; 1990.
7. Institute of Medicine. Guidelines for Clinical Practice: From Development to Use. The National Academies Press: Washington, DC; 1992.
8. Institute of Medicine. Clinical Practice Guidelines We Can Trust. The National Academies Press: Washington, DC; 2011.
9. Coronado VG, McGuire LC, Sarmiento K, Bell J, Lionbarger MR, Jones CD, et al. Trends in traumatic brain injury in the U.S. and the public health response: 1995-2009. J Saf Res. 2012;43(4):299–307.
10. Myburgh JA, Cooper DJ, Finfer SR, Venkatesh B, Jones D, Higgins A, et al. Epidemiology and 12-month outcomes from traumatic brain injury in Australia and New Zealand. J Trauma. 2008;64(4):854–62.
11. Bruns J Jr, Hauser WA. The epidemiology of traumatic brain injury: a review. Epilepsia. 2003;44(Suppl 10):2–10.
12. Bullock R, Chesnut RM, Clifton G, Ghajar J, Marion DW, Narayan RK, et al. Guidelines for the management of severe head injury. Brain Trauma Foundation. Eur J Emerg Med. 1996;3(2):109–27.
13. Bullock R, Chesnut R, Clifton G, Ghajar J, Marion D, Narayan R, et al. Guidelines for the management

of severe traumatic brain injury. J Neurotrauma. 2000;17(6–7):449–554.

14. Brain Trauma Foundation, American Association of Neurological Surgeons, Congress of Neurological Surgeons. Guidelines for the management of severe traumatic brain injury. J Neurotrauma. 2007;24(Suppl 1):S1–106.

15. Carney N, Totten AM, O'Reilly C, Ullman JS, Hawryluk GW, Bell MJ, et al. Guidelines for the management of severe traumatic brain injury, fourth edition. Neurosurgery. 2017;80(1):6–15.

16. Badjatia N, Carney N, Crocco TJ, Fallat ME, Hennes HM, Jagoda AS, et al. Guidelines for prehospital management of traumatic brain injury 2nd edition. Prehosp Emerg Care. 2008;12(Suppl 1):S1–52.

17. Chestnut R, Ghajar J, Maas A, Marion D, Servadei F, Teasdale G, et al. Management and prognosis of severe traumatic brain injury. Part 2: early indicators of prognosis in severe traumatic brain injury. J Neurotrauma. 2000;17:557–627.

18. Kochanek PM, Carney N, Adelson PD, Ashwal S, Bell MJ, Bratton S, et al. Guidelines for the acute medical management of severe traumatic brain injury in infants, children, and adolescents—second edition. Pediatr Crit Care Med. 2012;13(Suppl 1):S1–82.

19. Knuth T, Letarte P, Ling G, Moores L, Rhee P, Tauber D, et al. Guidelines for the field management of combat-related head trauma. New York: Brain Trauma Foundation; 2005.

20. Hutchinson PJ, Kolias AG, Timofeev IS, Corteen EA, Czosnyka M, Timothy J, et al. Trial of decompressive craniectomy for traumatic intracranial hypertension. N Engl J Med. 2016;375(12):1119–30.

21. Gabriel EJ, Ghajar J, Jagoda A, Pons PT, Scalea T, Walters BC, et al. Guidelines for prehospital management of traumatic brain injury. J Neurotrauma. 2002;19(1):111–74.

22. Carney NA, Chesnut R, Kochanek PM, American Association for Surgery of Trauma, Child Neurology Society, International Society for Pediatric Neurosurgery, et al. Guidelines for the acute medical management of severe traumatic brain injury in infants, children, and adolescents. Pediatr Crit Care Med. 2003;4(3 Suppl):S1.

23. Anonymous. Part 1: Guidelines for the management of penetrating brain injury. Introduction and methodology. J Trauma. 2001;51(2 Suppl):S3–6.

24. Anonymous. Part 2: Prognosis in penetrating brain injury. J Trauma. 2001;51(2 Suppl):S44–86.

25. Thurman D, Guerrero J. Trends in hospitalization associated with traumatic brain injury. JAMA. 1999;282(10):954–7.

26. Bullock MR, Chesnut R, Ghajar J, Gordon D, Hartl R, Newell DW, et al. Surgical management of acute subdural hematomas. Neurosurgery. 2006;58(3 Suppl):S16–24; discussion Si–iv.

27. Souter MJ, Blissitt PA, Blosser S, Bonomo J, Greer D, Jichici D, et al. Recommendations for the critical care management of devastating brain injury: prog-

nostication, psychosocial, and ethical management: a position statement for healthcare professionals from the Neurocritical Care Society. Neurocrit Care. 2015;23(1):4–13.

28. Le Roux P, Menon DK, Citerio G, Vespa P, Bader MK, Brophy GM, et al. Consensus summary statement of the International Multidisciplinary Consensus Conference on Multimodality Monitoring in Neurocritical Care: a statement for healthcare professionals from the Neurocritical Care Society and the European Society of Intensive Care Medicine. Intensive Care Med. 2014;40(9):1189–209.

29. Fried HI, Nathan BR, Rowe AS, Zabramski JM, Andaluz N, Bhimraj A, et al. The insertion and management of external ventricular drains: an evidence-based consensus statement: a statement for healthcare professionals from the Neurocritical Care Society. Neurocrit Care. 2016;24(1):61–81.

30. Frontera JA, Lewin JJ 3rd, Rabinstein AA, Aisiku IP, Alexandrov AW, Cook AM, et al. Guideline for reversal of antithrombotics in intracranial hemorrhage: executive summary. A statement for healthcare professionals from the Neurocritical Care Society and the Society of Critical Care Medicine. Crit Care Med. 2016;44(12):2251–7.

31. Nyquist P, Bautista C, Jichici D, Burns J, Chhangani S, DeFilippis M, et al. Prophylaxis of venous thrombosis in neurocritical care patients: an evidence-based guideline: a statement for healthcare professionals from the Neurocritical Care Society. Neurocrit Care. 2016;24(1):47–60.

32. Diringer MN, Bleck TP, Hemphill JC 3rd, Menon D, Shutter L, Vespa P, et al. Critical care management of patients following aneurysmal subarachnoid hemorrhage: recommendations from the Neurocritical Care Society's Multidisciplinary Consensus Conference. Neurocrit Care. 2011;15(2):211–40.

33. Brophy GM, Bell R, Claassen J, Alldredge B, Bleck TP, Glauser T, et al. Guidelines for the evaluation and management of status epilepticus. Neurocrit Care. 2012;17(1):3–23.

34. Torbey MT, Bosel J, Rhoney DH, Rincon F, Staykov D, Amar AP, et al. Evidence-based guidelines for the management of large hemispheric infarction: a statement for health care professionals from the Neurocritical Care Society and the German Society for Neuro-intensive Care and Emergency Medicine. Neurocrit Care. 2015;22(1):146–64.

35. Sharma OP, Oswanski MF, Joseph RJ, Tonui P, Westrick L, Raj SS, et al. Venous thromboembolism in trauma patients. Am Surg. 2007;73(11):1173–80.

36. Rogers FB, Cipolle MD, Velmahos G, Rozycki G, Luchette FA. Practice management guidelines for the prevention of venous thromboembolism in trauma patients: the EAST practice management guidelines work group. J Trauma. 2002;53(1):142–64.

37. Geerts WH, Bergqvist D, Pineo GF, Heit JA, Samama CM, Lassen MR, et al. Prevention of venous thromboembolism: American College of Chest Physicians

evidence-based clinical practice guidelines (8th edition). Chest. 2008;133(6 Suppl):381S–453S.

38. American College of Surgeons Committee on Trauma. ACS TQIP geriatric trauma management guidelines. https://www.facs.org/~/media/files/quality%20programs/trauma/tqip/geriatric%20guide%20tqip.ashx: American College of Surgeons.

39. American College of Surgeons Committee on Trauma. ACS TQIP massive transfusion in trauma guidelines. https://www.facs.org/~/media/files/quality%20programs/trauma/tqip/massive%20transfusion%20in%20trauma%20guildelines.ashx: American College of Surgeons.

40. American College of Surgeons Committee on Trauma. ACS TQIP best practices in the management of orthopaedic trauma. https://www.facs.org/~/media/files/quality%20programs/trauma/tqip/tqip%20bpgs%20in%20the%20management%20of%20orthopaedic%20traumafinal.ashx: American College of Surgeons.

41. American College of Surgeons Committee on Trauma. ACS TQIP best practices in the management of traumatic brain injury. https://www.facs.org/~/media/files/quality%20programs/trauma/tqip/traumatic%20brain%20injury%20guidelines.ashx: American College of Surgeons.

42. Wright DW, Yeatts SD, Silbergleit R, Palesch YY, Hertzberg VS, Frankel M, et al. Very early administration of progesterone for acute traumatic brain injury. N Engl J Med. 2014;371(26):2457–66.

43. Pastorek RA, Cripps MW, Bernstein IH, Scott WW, Madden CJ, Rickert KL, et al. The Parkland Protocol's modified Berne-Norwood criteria predict two tiers of risk for traumatic brain injury progression. J Neurotrauma. 2014;31(20):1737–43.

44. Zafonte R, Friedewald WT, Lee SM, Levin B, Diaz-Arrastia R, Ansel B, et al. The citicoline brain injury treatment (COBRIT) trial: design and methods. J Neurotrauma. 2009;26(12):2207–16.

45. Zafonte RD, Bagiella E, Ansel BM, Novack TA, Friedewald WT, Hesdorffer DC, et al. Effect of citicoline on functional and cognitive status among patients with traumatic brain injury: Citicoline brain injury treatment trial (COBRIT). JAMA. 2012;308(19):1993–2000.

46. Skolnick BE, Maas AI, Narayan RK, van der Hoop RG, MacAllister T, Ward JD, et al. A clinical trial of progesterone for severe traumatic brain injury. N Engl J Med. 2014;371(26):2467–76.

47. Palmer S, Bader MK, Qureshi A, Palmer J, Shaver T, Borzatta M, et al. The impact on outcomes in a community hospital setting of using the AANS traumatic brain injury guidelines. J Trauma. 2001;50(4):657–64.

48. Patel HC, Menon DK, Tebbs S, Hawker R, Hutchinson PJ, Kirkpatrick PJ. Specialist neurocritical care and outcome from head injury. Intensive Care Med. 2002;28(5):547–53.

49. Vukic M, Negovetic L, Kovac D, Ghajar J, Glavic Z, Gopcevic A. The effect of implementation of guidelines for the management of severe head injury on patient treatment and outcome. Acta Neurochir. 1999;141(11):1203–8.

50. Eibling D, Fried M, Blitzer A, Postma G. Commentary on the role of expert opinion in developing evidence-based guidelines. Laryngoscope. 2014;124(2):355–7.

Functional Neurosurgery for Sequelae of Traumatic Brain Injury

William R. Y. Carlton Jr. and Gregory J. A. Murad

Abbreviations

ABR	Auditory brainstem responses
BDNF	Brain-derived neurotrophic factor
CM	Centromedian thalamus
DBS	Deep brain stimulation
EEG	Electroencephalogram
ET	Essential tremor
GPi	Globus pallidus internal nucleus
ITP	Interthalamic peduncle
LTP	Long-term potentiation
MCS	Minimally conscious state
NAcc	Nucleus accumbens
NGF	Nerve growth factor
RMNS	Right median nerve electrical stimulation
SCC	Subgenual cingulate cortex
SCS	Spinal cord stimulation
SSEP	Somatosensory evoked potentials
STN	Subthalamic nucleus
TBI	Traumatic brain injury
tDCS	Transcranial direct-current stimulation
TMS	Transcranial magnetic stimulation
VC/VS	Ventral capsule/ventral striatum
VIM	Ventral intermediate nucleus
VOA	Ventral oral anterior nucleus
VOP	Ventral oral posterior nucleus
VPL	Ventroposterolateral nucleus
VS	Vegetative state

W. R. Y. Carlton Jr., MD · G. J. A. Murad,
MD, FAANS (✉)
Department of Neurosurgery, Shands Hospital of the
University of Florida, Gainesville, FL, USA
e-mail: William.carlton@neurosurgery.ufl.edu;
murad@neurosurgery.ufl.edu

Introduction

Traumatic brain injury (TBI) accounted for about 2.5 million visits to the emergency department (ED) in 2010, with more than 280,000 hospitalizations, more than 52,000 deaths, and $60 billion in medical costs and lost productivity [1–3]. It is estimated that between 3.2 and 5.3 million Americans are living with sequelae from moderate to severe TBI—greater than 1% of the general population [4]. TBI leads to an inflammatory cascade that causes significant damage to brain parenchyma, both locally due to mechanical injury and globally due to ischemia, shear injury, oxidative stress, and excitotoxicity. Differing injury mechanisms lead to differing cellular damage patterns, including receptor-mediated damage, oxidative damage, mitochondrial dysfunction, apoptosis, and calcium-mediated damage [5–7]. The end result of this damage is neurological dysfunction in both motor and cognitive domains. Motor deficits include paresis, tremor, dystonia, and ballismus. Cognitive deficits include impairments in consciousness, attention, information processing, problem-solving, and memory. Recovery from TBI is variable due to this widespread damage. Multiple new and exciting

© Springer International Publishing AG, part of Springer Nature 2018
S. D. Timmons (ed.), *Controversies in Severe Traumatic Brain Injury Management*,
https://doi.org/10.1007/978-3-319-89477-5_18

technologies are available to aid in this recovery and will be reviewed and described in this chapter.

Multiple therapies exist for limiting neurological disabilities in TBI patients, including occupational, physical, and cognitive rehabilitation, but there remains critical need for more effective therapies, including pharmacological or surgical treatments. Despite nearly 100 years of effort, and hundreds of millions of dollars of investment, no successful phase III clinical trial investigating a pharmacological intervention to mitigate the effects of TBI has been completed, with the Protect III and Synapse Trials the most recent to fail [8]. Recent advances in the understanding of brain circuitry and technical advances in neurostimulation technologies have created enthusiasm for the possibility of electrical stimulation of the nervous system to promote functional recovery in patients with acquired brain disorders. In 2013, the Defense Advanced Research Projects Agency (DARPA) also moved funding into these areas, including the RAM (restoring active memory) and RAM replay initiatives, with a stated goal "to develop and test a wireless, fully implantable neural interface medical device for human clinical use. The device would facilitate the formation of new memories and the retrieval of existing ones in individuals who have lost these capacities as a result of traumatic brain injury or neurological disease" [9]. In 2014, the BRAIN Initiative of the National Institutes of Health (NIH) and National Institute of Neurological Disorders and Stroke (NINDS) has begun to aggressively fund research into these areas as well to further understand the potential technologies, targets, and biomarkers that may allow for significant improvements in recovery of function after TBI.

Functional Techniques for Motor Disorders

Functional techniques for recovery after brain injury (including those extrapolated from the literature for stroke) involve the application of electrical or magnetic current to alter or modify brain circuitry. This can be peripheral, transcranial, or via implanted electrodes, either over the cerebral cortex or subcortical stimulation through deep brain electrodes. Noninvasive stimulation carries the advantage of safety, but the trade-off in efficacy involves a lack of spatial accuracy and speed of effect (Fig. 1).

Noninvasive Treatments for Motor Disorders

Transcranial stimulation can be achieved using either magnetic current induction or direct-current application. Transcranial magnetic stimulation (TMS) involves using a magnetic field to induce electric current within the brain. In this technology, electrical current is passed through a coil overlying the skull, which in turn induces a magnetic field that penetrates the skull, inducing electric current within the cortex, causing neuronal depolarization [10]. Transcranial direct-current stimulation (tDCS) involves the application of direct current to alter resting membrane potentials. In this technology, two or more electrodes are placed over the scalp, and direct current flows through the skull into the cortex. The current enters through the anode, exits via cathode, and depolarizes or hyperpolarizes underlying neurons based on the polarity of the stimulation [11, 12]. TMS can be used to decrease hyperexcitability in normal cortex or increase excitability in damaged cortex. High-frequency TMS (10–20 Hz) enhances cortical excitability. Presumably this is due to changes in neural excitability and modulation of long-term potentiation. It may also reduce excess GABAergic inhibition, promote compensatory plasticity, and inhibit maladaptive plasticity [13, 14]. Low-frequency (<1 Hz) TMS can reduce cortical excitability. This is presumed to have similar effects on long-term potentiation and also decreases glutamatergic excitotoxicity while improving plasticity [15, 16]. As a direct-current application, tDCS can involve either anodal or cathodal stimulation. Anodal stimulation (1–2 mA) enhances cortical excitability. This depolarizes neuronal resting membranes, changes NMDA receptors, and modulates long-

Spectra of Brain Stimulation

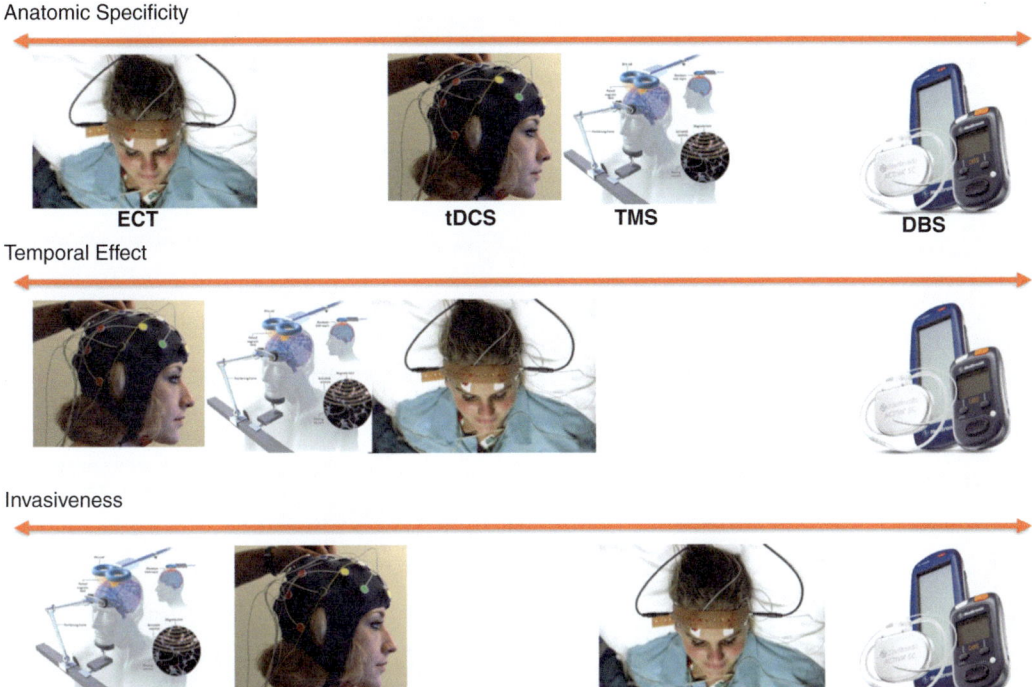

Anatomic Specificity

ECT   tDCS   TMS   DBS

Temporal Effect

Invasiveness

Fig. 1 Examples of brain stimulation techniques, placed in order of degree, moving from the left of each row to the right; with the left of the figure the least, and the right of the figure the most. *ECT* electroconvulsive therapy, *tDCS* transcranial direct-current stimulation, *TMS* transcranial magnetic stimulation, *DBS* deep brain stimulation

term potentiation. Similar to high-frequency TMS, GABAergic inhibition may be reduced, and compensatory plasticity may be improved [17]. Alternatively, cathodal stimulation (1–2 mA) reduces cortical excitability [18]. It also depolarizes neuronal resting membranes and changes N-methyl-D-aspartate (NMDA) receptor activation, improving long-term potentiation (LTP). Similar to low-frequency TMS, it also may decrease glutamatergic excitotoxicity and promote neuroplasticity. In studies of stroke patients, underlying normal cortex may become hyperexcitable due to loss of contralateral inhibition, and TMS may help reduce this issue [19–22]. Although the literature is small in TBI, early results have shown some promise.

Both of these technologies, however, while relatively safe are limited, as mentioned earlier. The penetration of the cortex is variable and may be inhibited by damaged cortex, or physical changes of the skull and brain due to surgery [23, 24]. Also, deep brain structures cannot be accessed for modulation [25]. Knowledge about circuitry from direct recording of electrophysiologic data is limited by these same factors. Finally, these technologies are noncontinuous and episodic, which limits their effectiveness in nonclinical settings, rather than an implant, which can provide continuous or on-demand stimulation.

The timing of the use of these technologies also varies depending on the stage of the injury. The specific brain injury response will vary with time according to the stimulatory technology used [26]. Overall, these technologies have been used widely for anecdotal success, but the data supporting their use derives from limited numbers of case reports (Table 1) [14, 27–40].

Table 1 Transcranial magnetic stimulation (TMS) and transcranial direct-current stimulation (tDCS) in traumatic brain injury (TBI)

Author	Stimulation method	Type of TBI	Study type	Stimulation location	Results
Louise-Bender Pape et al., 2009 [14]	TMS	Chronic severe	Case report (1)	DLPFC	Transient behavioral improvement
Cosentino et al., 2010 [27]	TMS	Chronic TBI	Case report (1)	Right temporal cortex	Significant improvement in auditory hallucinations
Kang et al., 2012 [28]	tDCS	Chronic TBI w/ attentional problems	Double-blind crossover (9)	Anodal, left DLPFC	Improved reaction time
Bonni et al., 2013 [29]	TMS	Chronic severe	Case report (1)	Left parietal cortex	Improved cognition
Kreuzer et al., 2013 [30]	TMS	Chronic severe with tinnitus	Case report (1)	Left primary auditory cortex	Improved tinnitus
Pistoia, et al., 2013 [31]	TMS	Chronic, vegetative state	Cross sectional (6)	Nondominant cortical motor hand area	Improved coma recovery score and ADLs in 3/6
Lesniak, et al., 2014 [32]	tDCS	Chronic severe	Randomized controlled (23)	Anodal, left DLPFC	No difference in cognitive outcome measurements
Angelakis et al., 2014 [33]	tDCS	Chronic severe	Case series (10)	Anodal, left DLPFC	4/10 with significant cognitive improvement
Thibaut et al., 2014 [34]	tDCS	25 severe TBI, 30 nontraumatic injury	Double-blind crossover (55)	Anodal, left DLPFC	Transient improvement in consciousness, nonsignificant
Middleton et al., 2014 [35]	tDCS	Chronic severe TBI, or stroke	Open label (8)	Bihemispheric	Mild motor improvement
Nielson et al., 2015 [36]	TMS	Chronic severe	Case report (1)	Right DLPFC	Improvement in depression and ADLs
Koski et al., 2015 [37]	TMS	Chronic mild	Open label (15)	Left DLPFC	Improvement in symptom severity
Ulam et al., 2015 [38]	tDCS	Subacute TBI	Randomized controlled (26)	Anodal, left DLPFC	Neuropsychiatric test improvement in treated group
Naro et al., 2015 [39]	tDCS	Chronic severe	Crossover (25)	Anodal, orbitofrontal cortex	Increased M1 excitability and short-term cortical excitability in treated patients
Fecteau et al., 2015 [40]	TMS	Subacute moderate to severe	Case control (20 TBI, 20 normal controls)	Left M1 cortex	Increased M1 excitability in TBI patients vs. healthy controls posttreatment

TBI traumatic brain injury, *TMS* transcranial magnetic stimulation, *tDCS* transcranial direct-current stimulation, *DLPFC* dorsolateral prefrontal cortex, *ADLs* activities of daily living

Invasive Treatment for Motor Disorders

Invasive stimulation for motor disorders has involved direct cortical stimulation, which has been applied in animal models of TBI [41, 42] and more widely in animal models of stroke. This involves low-frequency stimulation via implanted cortical electrodes to aid in recovery after injury [41–44]. Molecular mechanisms of successful stimulation show increased dendritic growth in the areas of stimulation, with a concomitant decrease in local astrogliosis [45, 46]. Animal studies led to phase I [47] and II trials [47–49], which demonstrated safety and efficacy, and eventually culminated in the phase III Everest trial for rehabilitation in poststroke patients [50]. In this trial, cortical electrodes were implanted epidurally over intact motor cortex in the ipsilesional hemisphere in a predetermined area based on functional magnetic resonance imaging (fMRI). The epidural electrodes were then attached to an implanted pulse generator, which could be externally programmed. Of the 152 patients randomized, 58 were in the control arm and 94 in the implant arm. These groups subsequently went through either regular rehabilitation or stimulated rehabilitation for 6 weeks, followed by multiple blinded assessments at time points up to 24 weeks after trial entry. Assessments involved the use of UEFM (Upper-Extremity Fugl-Meyer scale) and AMAT (Arm Motor Ability Test) scores. UEFM is an assessment of neurological and motor function, while AMAT is a qualitative and quantitative assessment of upper limb function in daily activities. Overall, patients in the investigational group showed no statistical difference at 4 and 12 weeks, but statistically significant improvements were seen in both scores at 24 weeks. For the subset of patients who showed motor movements at low stimulation thresholds, improvement was even greater, with 69% of patients meeting the primary endpoint vs.

29% in the control group. Complications in the trial were minimal, in keeping with the small morbidity associated with implantation of other stimulation devices. Overall, this trial showed the promise for epidural direct cortical stimulation and may be translatable to TBI as well.

Direct cortical stimulation has also been used in central pain syndromes as well as trigeminal neuralgia [51–55]. However, these technologies have had limited effects. Fontaine et al. [55] performed a meta-analysis of the literature and reported on 210 patients, of whom 45% had sustained improvement at 1 year, with a mean improvement of 57% on visual analog scales. Further study in this area is also ongoing, with DBS for pain disorders also being explored [56, 57].

The other method of stimulation that is widely used for movement and motor disorders is subcortical deep brain stimulation. Since its approval by the US Food and Drug Administration (FDA) in 2002, DBS has become the gold standard for motor manifestations of parkinsonism [58–60] and is well studied for essential tremor (ET) and dystonia [61]. Animal models of TBI have also been studied with response to DBS. Tabansky et al. [62] examined an animal model of TBI with subsequent DBS of the central thalamus, which showed significant improvement in motor coordination as well as initiation of movement compared to control animals. As tremor, dystonia, and parkinsonism are also sequelae of TBI, DBS may have efficacy in treating patients with these symptoms (Table 2) [63–78].

Post-TBI kinetic tremor is a well-described long-term motor sequela and may occur in as little as a few weeks out to 2 or more years postinjury [79, 80]. Multiple studies of patients after severe TBI have shown that 19–45% of subjects will develop kinetic tremor at some time point in their recovery [76]. Treatment for refractory tremor includes similar targets as those used for ET as well as novel targets. Multiple case reports exist of stimulation of the ventral intermediate

Table 2 Deep brain stimulation (DBS) for motor sequelae of traumatic brain injury (TBI)

Author	Study type (number of patients)	Type of TBI	Stimulation location	Results
Broggi et al., 1993 [63]	Case report (1)	Chronic TBI, right-sided tremor	Left VIM	Improved function and tremor
Nguyen and Degos, 1993 [64]	Case report (1)	Chronic TBI, postural and UE tremor	VIM	Improved tremor and functional limb use
Sellal et al., 1993 [65]	Case report (1)	Chronic TBI	Left VPL	Improvement in dystonia and right UE function
Loher et al., 2000 [66]	Case report (1)	Chronic TBI	GPi	Improved pain and dystonia
Umemura et al., 2004 [67]	Case report (1)	Chronic TBI with tremor	Left VIM	Improved function and ADLs
Green and Aziz, 2005 [68]	Case report (1)	Chronic TBI with left UE tremor and ballismus	Right VOP/zona incerta (ZI)	Increased functional use of arm with some loss of fine motor control
Capelle et al., 2006 [69]	Case report (1)	Chronic TBI, dystonia	Right VPL and GPi	No change
Foote et al., 2006 [70]	Case reports (4)	Chronic TBI tremor (3) and MS tremor (1)	Two leads, VIM/VOP border, and VOA/VOP border	Improved function, significant placebo effect
Broggi et al., 2006 [71]	Case reports (3)	Chronic TBI, tremor	ZI and VOA/VOP	All regained ability to perform self-feeding and personal care
Kuhn et al., 2008 [72]	Case report (1)	Chronic TBI	Posterior hypothalamus	Eliminated self-mutilation behavior in study period
Franzini et al., 2011 [73]	Case series (9)	Chronic TBI with unilateral (6) or bilateral (3) tremor	VIM	>50% tremor improvement in all cases, three patients with worsened speech function after bilateral DBS
Reese et al., 2011 [74]	Case report (1)	Chronic severe TBI	VIM, STN	Decreased tremor and rigidity
Kim et al., 2012 [75]	Case reports (4)	Chronic severe TBI with dystonia	GPi	Improvement in dystonia rating scale scores and QOL
Issar et al., 2013 [76]	Case series (5)	Chronic severe TBI	Bilateral VIM, GPi	Reduction of tremor
Carvalho et al., 2014 [77]	Case report (1)	Chronic severe TBI	Right GPi	Improved tremor
Follett et al., 2014 [78]	Case report (1)	Chronic severe TBI	Staged (6 months) bilateral VIM	Improved UE and voice tremor, stable dystonia, and leg tremor

TBI traumatic brain injury, *VIM* ventral intermediate nucleus, *VPL* ventroposterolateral nucleus, *UE* upper extremity, *GPi* globus pallidus internal nucleus, *VOP* ventral oral posterior nucleus, *VOA* ventral oral anterior nucleus, *STN* subthalamic nucleus, *QOL* quality of life

nucleus (VIM) [74, 76, 78] (similar to ET). Foote et al. showed dual-lead stimulation of VIM/ventral oral anterior nucleus (VOA)/ventral oral posterior nucleus (VOP) [70, 81] (Fig. 2). Others have shown globus pallidus internal nucleus (GPi) stimulation to help in this area [76].

Post-TBI dystonia and parkinsonism have also been treated with DBS. Dystonia can occur early or in a much delayed fashion (>5 years) after TBI [75, 82, 83] and appears more likely after thalamic or basal ganglia injury [84–86]. Case reports of ventroposterolateral nucleus (VPL) [65], GPi [66], and unilateral [87, 88] or bilateral [89] VOA stimulation have all shown efficacy for dystonia from TBI as well as anoxic brain injury. A case series of four patients treated by Kim

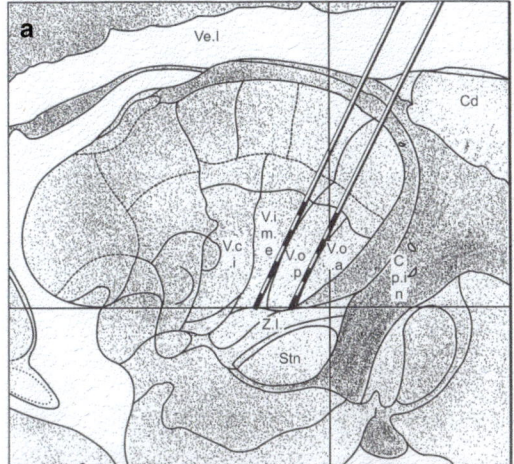

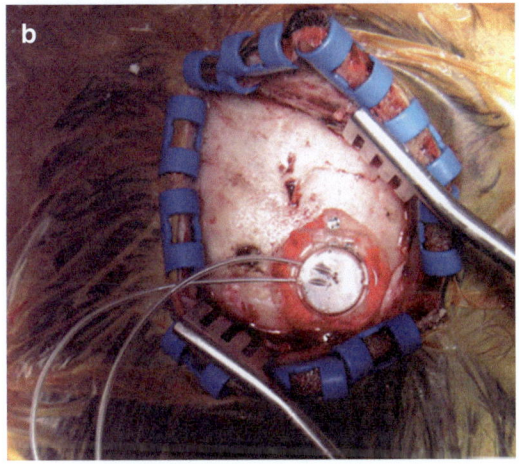

Fig. 2 Dual-lead deep brain stimulation (DBS) implantation in a patient with post-traumatic tremor. (**a**) Reconstruction of the two leads implanted for post-traumatic tremor. *V.c.i* ventralis caudalis, *V.im* ventralis intermedius, *V.o.p* ventralis oralis posterior, *V.o.a* ventralis oralis anterior, *Cp.i* internal capsule, *Z.i.* zona incerta, *Stn* subthalamic nucleus, *Cd* caudate nucleus, *Ve.l* lateral ventricle. Reprinted with permission from Michael S. Okun, Kelly D. Foote, inventors; University of Florida Research Foundation Inc., assignee. Multiple lead method for deep brain stimulation. US patent 8295935 B2. Oct 23, 2012. (**b**) Intraoperative photo of dual-lead implantation coming through single burr hole cover

et al. [75] with unilateral GPi DBS showed significant improvements in all four patients in the Burke-Fahn-Marsden Dystonia Rating Scale movement and disability scores.

Post-traumatic parkinsonism is characterized by similar motor manifestations as de novo Parkinson disease (PD), including resting tremor, bradykinesia, and rigidity. The pathologic and electrophysiologic mechanisms of post-traumatic parkinsonism have yet to be elucidated [90], but the similarity in phenotype [91] suggests that DBS may be a beneficial strategy. Although no large-scale reports exist, post-traumatic parkinsonism is likely to respond to DBS with similar targets as de novo parkinsonism.

Functional Treatments for Cognitive Disorders

Perhaps the most exciting areas of functional treatments for TBI include cognitive disorders. These include depression, disorders of consciousness, post-traumatic epilepsy, and disorders of learning and memory. Again, stimulation for treatment of these disorders can be noninvasive or surgical/invasive.

Noninvasive Treatments for Cognitive Disorders

Noninvasive stimulation paradigms again include tDCS and TMS. TMS has been shown to enhance cognitive function and improve aphasia [92, 93] in case reports of chronic stroke. This is through reducing hyperexcitability in normal cortex, as well as increased excitability in damaged cortex [94, 95]. Similar efficacy has been shown with tDCS for ipsilateral left frontotemporal stimulation [96], as well as in homologous areas of the contralateral nondamaged hemisphere. Dorsolateral prefrontal stimulation for depression in TBI has been marginally successful (Table 1) [28, 97].

Another exciting area of noninvasive stimulation for TBI has been peripheral right median nerve stimulation. Multiple proposed physiologic mechanisms of stimulation exist. These include activation of the ascending reticular activating system and dopaminergic pathways after prolonged stimulation, increased central brain-derived neurotrophic factor (BDNF) and nerve growth factor (NGF) facilitating neuroplasticity, increased cerebral perfusion and neurotransmitter metabolism, or activation of central thalamocortical projections important in arousal [98–100]. Various studies starting in the 1980s showed promise for this technique to improve arousal in patients after severe TBI [98, 99, 101]. More recently, Lei et al. published on a cohort of 437 comatose patients after severe TBI who were randomized to 2 weeks of RMNS vs. control [100]. Patients in the RMNS group showed a trend toward increased Glasgow Coma Scale (GCS) scores (8.43 vs. 7.47, $P = 0.053$) at 2 weeks, and significantly more patients returned to consciousness at 6 months (59.8% vs. 46.2%). In the subset of those who regained consciousness, functional independence measurement (FIM) score was also significantly higher. The treatment had no observable complications and thus represents a safe and easy technique with the potential to improve long-term arousal and recovery in comatose patients.

Invasive Treatments for Cognitive Disorders

Regarding surgical treatments for cognitive improvement in TBI, DBS has had a significant amount of investigation, mainly in animal models, but more recently in human trials, for memory function in Alzheimer's disease as well as epilepsy, depression (not necessarily TBI-related), and minimally conscious states (Table 3) [102–107].

Post-traumatic seizures are another common late effect of TBI [108, 109]. Long-term risks of seizure are up to 16% in severe TBI patients, and the prevalence of seizure in TBI ranges from 4 to 20%. TBI patients are up to 30 times more likely to develop epilepsy than age-matched controls [110, 111]. DBS has been studied for treatment refractory epilepsy, as Fisher et al. [111] reported in the SANTE (Stimulation of the Anterior Nucleus of the Thalamus) trial, a double-blinded study that demonstrated significant benefits in terms of seizure reduction. Another novel treatment paradigm introduced in epilepsy, but possibly with broader implications, is that of closed-loop stimulation. The responsive neurostimulation system (RNS) (NeuroPace, Inc.) was approved for use in the USA by the FDA in 2013 and involves implanted recording electrodes in up to two seizure foci, with separate stimulation electrodes to arrest seizure propagation [112]. Single-electrode systems to both detect and stim-

Table 3 Deep brain stimulation (DBS) for cognitive sequelae of traumatic brain injury (TBI)

Author	Study type (number of patients)	Type of TBI	Stimulation location	Results
Hassler et al., 1969 [102]	Case report (3)	Chronic TBI, MCS	Central thalamus	Improved consciousness
Tsubokawa et al., 1990 [103]	Case series (8)	Chronic TBI, VS	Mesencephalic RF, thalamus	Three patients regained communication
Yamamoto and Katayama, 2005 [104]	Case series (26, 12 were TBI)	Chronic VS (9/21) MCS (3/5)	Thalamic CM parafascicular complex (VS and MCS) Mesencephalic RF (2/21 VS)	8/21 patients improved from VS but remained total care, 4/5 MCS patients improved to live at home
Schiff et al., 2007 [105]	Case report (1)	Chronic severe TBI, MCS	Bilateral CM thalamus	Improved coma recovery score and function
Giacino et al., 2012 [106]	Case report (1)	Chronic severe TBI, MCS	CM thalamus	Improved communication, feeding, motor function
Rezai et al., 2016 [107]	Prospective open label (4)	Chronic severe TBI	Bilateral NAcc and anterior limb IC	3/4 met a priori improvement criteria in Mayo-Portland adaptability inventory-4

MCS minimally conscious state, *VS* vegetative state, *CM* centromedian, *NAcc* nucleus accumbens, *RF* reticular formation

ulate through the same electrode are also in development and may make responsive or closed-loop DBS a possibility [113].

DBS has been studied widely in depression, and as depression represents the most common sequelae of TBI, seen in up to 80% of patients [114], DBS may be a potential treatment for medically refractory cases [115, 116]. In TBI, subgenual cingulate cortex (SCC) overactivity appears to correlate with symptoms and thus represents a target for neuromodulation. Other targets for stimulation include ventral capsule/ventral striatum (VC/VS), nucleus accumbens (NAcc), subthalamic nucleus (STN), and inter-thalamic peduncle (ITP) [117–119]. Although multiple case reports exist with response rates of 45–92% and remission rates as high as 35%, these have not been undertaken specifically for TBI-related depression.

Disorders of consciousness have also been explored for invasive treatments, including DBS and spinal cord stimulation (SCS). Stimulation of the upper cervical cord, C2–4, has been shown to increase cerebral blood flow, arousal, and upper extremity motor function in patients in minimally conscious state (MCS) from a variety of insults, including TBI [120–122]. Kanno et al. [123] employed SCS for a nonrandomized, observation group of 214 patients with vegetative state (VS) or MCS from stroke, anoxia, and TBI (106 patients) over a 20-year period (1986–2005). Patients underwent C2–4 implantation with stimulation in alternating 15-min periods during waking hours. Using the author's self-designed non-validated outcome measures, 54% achieved excellent or good outcome with regard to arousal and self-awareness, with 64% of those in the TBI group achieving this outcome. The study was limited by its nonrandomized, nonblinded design, as well as early implementation, which meant that spontaneous recovery may have contributed significantly to the outcomes. However, it does suggest the need for further investigation in this area.

DBS was initially tried in animal models with VS and MCS and in a few case reports starting in the late 1960s [102] extending into the early 2000s [103, 124–126]. Renewed interest in this area occurred with the 2007 publication by Schiff

et al. [105] of bilateral central thalamic stimulation for a 38-year-old patient who remained in a minimally conscious state more than 6 years following a severe TBI. The central thalamus is believed to have diffuse cortical connections that allow for arousal. Stimulation of this area may lead to depolarization of cortical and striatal neurons, release of thalamocortical transmissions by inhibition of pallidothalamic projections, facilitation of cortico-cortical connections, or facilitation of central and cortical synaptic plasticity [106, 127–130]. In Schiff's elegant study [105], after a preintervention washout period involving structured rehabilitation, and immediate postoperative testing and threshold stimulation, they performed a double-blind alternating crossover study. Stimulation was alternated with the DBS being turned on or off for 30-day intervals out to 180 days. Rehabilitation with speech, physical, occupational, and cognitive therapy began prior to surgery and was continued during the stimulation period. Blinded assessments using the JFK Coma Recovery Scale-Revised (CRS-R) were performed by the rehabilitation staff during the on and off periods. Overall, CRS-R subscales for arousal, limb control, and oral feeding all showed statistical improvements, and all other subscales showed nonsignificant improvement. This publication thrusts the ethical concerns of deep brain stimulation into the forefront and has resulted in numerous commentaries [131–133] on the delicate nature of offering hope to patients in minimally conscious states and selecting the correct patients for intervention [127]. The ethical questions regarding the correct diagnosis of patients in minimally conscious states (MCS) or vegetative states (VS), and the difficulty in explaining these conditions and their expected course to family members, remain challenging. The sensitivity, specificity, and costs of different diagnostic tests also remain to be elucidated. Efforts to identify radiographic [132] and electrophysiologic biomarkers to identify those patients who will most likely benefit from these treatments are ongoing. Yamamoto et al. [121] attempted to answer this question in another group of patients using electrophysiologic measurements to aid in patient selection for intervention. In a cohort of

128 patients with TBI, anoxia, and stroke (107 with VS), the authors performed auditory brainstem responses (ABR), somatosensory evoked potentials (SSEP), pain-related P250 [134], and continuous electroencephalogram (EEG) spectral analysis. (Pain-related P250 [pain-related potential] is a positive potential appearing at a latency of 200–300 ms by giving a stimulus such that the subject feels pain. It is believed that it is not a response due to a simple sensation of pain but rather subsequent information processing of the stimulus, and thus representative of higher cortical function.) After initial evaluation of nonresponders to DBS and SCS therapy, they set four electrophysiologic inclusion criteria: recordable Vth wave of the ABR, recordable N20 of the SSEP, desynchronization or slight desynchronization pattern of EEG, and pain-related P250 with an amplitude over 7 microvolts. In total, 21 patients were treated with DBS (19 centromedian/parafascicular thalamus, 2 mesencephalic reticular formation) for VS, 10 of whom met criteria, with 8 of these showing improved arousal and emergence from VS, although all remained bedbound. Five MCS patients met criteria and had DBS implantation, all of whom improved to meet criteria for functional interaction and no longer remained in MCS. SCS was performed on ten patients, eight of whom met criteria, and seven of these improved to no longer be in MCS. Comparisons of cerebral blood flow and cerebral metabolic rate of oxygen between prestimulation and on-stimulation patients in both the DBS and SCS groups showed significant improvements. Although this was a nonblinded nonrandomized study, the findings continue to spark interest in the area. Most recently, Rezai et al. [107] showed efficacy in four long-term severe TBI patients with disabling frontal lobe dysfunction with bilateral stimulator implants into the anterior limb of the internal capsule and the NAcc, targets that have been used previously for the treatment of depression. Three of the four patients met a priori criteria for improvement on the Mayo-Portland Adaptability Inventory-4, and all four showed improvement vs. baseline. Ongoing trials for minimally conscious patients

currently are being funded by the Brain Initiative, with centromedian (CM) thalamus again as the target.

DBS is also being investigated for memory and cognitive enhancement in organic brain disease. Recently, trials in early Alzheimer's disease have shown safety in DBS implantation in the fornix with some efficacy in improving working and visuospatial memory [135, 136]. Similarly, research involving stimulating implanted depth electrodes in the entorhinal cortex of epilepsy patients resulted in marked improvement in memory, whereas hippocampal stimulation did not [137]. A wide variety of targets for either cognitive/memory restoration or augmentation are also currently being explored, including pedunculopontine nuclei, nucleus basalis of Meynert, and the anterior nucleus of the thalamus [138].

Conclusions

Future Developments

Future developments in the treatment of TBI-related functional disorders look promising. In the 15 years since DBS was first approved in the USA for the treatment of Parkinson's disease, a wide variety of targets and pathologies have become areas of investigation for therapeutic benefit [138–141]. The most promising of these areas is electrophysiologic biomarkers, which will allow for more targeted treatment. In the recent past, multiple decoupled circuits have been discovered including β(beta)-band neuronal synchronization of the basal ganglia [142] and increased cortical phase-amplitude coupling [143] in patients with Parkinson's disease, pathological high-frequency oscillations in patients with focal epilepsy [144], and decreased phase-amplitude coupling in Tourette's syndrome [145]. Although the initial insult in TBI is different than de novo movement disorders, the pathologic disruptions of function likely overlap in terms of their electrophysiologic signatures. Using these biomarkers as targets, more targeted therapies and stimulation paradigms can be designed, and more direct compari-

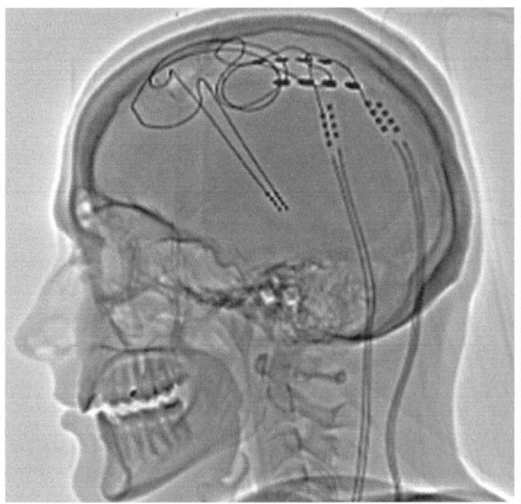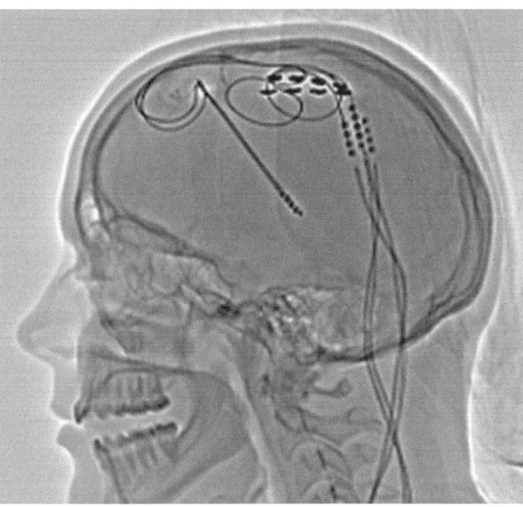

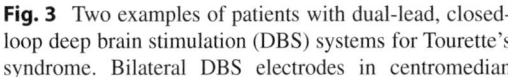

Fig. 3 Two examples of patients with dual-lead, closed-loop deep brain stimulation (DBS) systems for Tourette's syndrome. Bilateral DBS electrodes in centromedian (CM-Pf) thalamus with bilateral subdural strip electrodes overhead motor cortex connected to Medtronic Activa PC+S sensing and stimulating devices

sons of effectiveness can be made. Similarly, identifying pathologic alterations of circuits will make responsive DBS rather than continuous technologies a reality. This closed-loop stimulation is already a target for extratemporal epilepsy [112] using the RNS system as mentioned previously and is currently being studied in Parkinson's disease animal models [146] as well as in human trials for patients with Tourette's syndrome (Fig. 3) [145, 147]. In the future, on-demand stimulation, including both cortical and/or subcortical targets, will greatly improve therapeutic responses, side effect profiles, and battery life for patients undergoing DBS procedures.

An enormous amount of study has gone into the exploration of functional treatments for neurologic disability, both de novo and acquired. TBI represents an ever-growing population of patients who may benefit from these investigations. Both noninvasive and invasive technologies have shown early promise in the treatment of post-traumatic disorders of the brain, and as greater understanding of neural circuitry and its dysfunctions is achieved, functional neurosurgeons will have the ability to provide an increasing number of treatment options with improving efficacy.

References

1. Thurman DJ, Alverson C, Dunn KA, Guerrero J, Sniezek JE. Traumatic brain injury in the United States: a public health perspective. J Head Trauma Rehabil. 1999;14(6):602–15.
2. Guerrero JL, Thurman DJ, Sniezek JE. Emergency department visits associated with traumatic brain injury: United States, 1995–1996. Brain Inj 2000;14(2):181–6.
3. Corso P, Finkelstein E, Miller T, Fiebelkorn I, Zaloshnja E. Incidence and lifetime costs of injuries in the United States. Inj Prev. 2006;12(4):212–8.
4. Anonymous. Report to congress on traumatic brain injury in the United States: epidemiology and rehabilitation. Atlanta, GA: Centers for Disease Control and Prevention, Prevention NCfIPaCDoUI.
5. Bramlett HM, Dietrich WD. Pathophysiology of cerebral ischemia and brain trauma: similarities and differences. J Cereb Blood Flow Metab. 2004;24(2):133–50.
6. Kristian T, Siesjo BK. Calcium in ischemic cell death. Stroke. 1998;29(3):705–18.
7. Syntichaki P, Tavernarakis N. The biochemistry of neuronal necrosis: rogue biology? Nat Rev Neurosci. 2003;4(8):672–84.
8. Skolnick BE, Maas AI, Narayan RK, van der Hoop RG, MacAllister T, Ward JD, et al. A clinical trial of progesterone for severe traumatic brain injury. N Engl J Med. 2014;371(26):2467–76.
9. Anonymous. http://www.darpa.mil/program/our-research/darpa-and-the-brain-initiative.

10. Kobayashi M, Pascual-Leone A. Transcranial magnetic stimulation in neurology. Lancet Neurol. 2003;2(3):145–56.

11. Shah PP, Szaflarski JP, Allendorfer J, Hamilton RH. Induction of neuroplasticity and recovery in post-stroke aphasia by non-invasive brain stimulation. Front Hum Neurosci. 2013;7:888.

12. Nitsche MA, Cohen LG, Wassermann EM, Priori A, Lang N, Antal A, et al. Transcranial direct current stimulation: state of the art 2008. Brain Stimul. 2008;1(3):206–23.

13. Khedr EM, Ahmed MA, Fathy N, Rothwell JC. Therapeutic trial of repetitive transcranial magnetic stimulation after acute ischemic stroke. Neurology. 2005;65(3):466–8.

14. Louise-Bender Pape T, Rosenow J, Lewis G, Ahmed G, Walker M, Guernon A, et al. Repetitive transcranial magnetic stimulation-associated neurobehavioral gains during coma recovery. Brain Stimul. 2009;2(1):22–35.

15. Mansur CG, Fregni F, Boggio PS, Riberto M, Gallucci-Neto J, Santos CM, et al. A sham stimulation-controlled trial of rTMS of the unaffected hemisphere in stroke patients. Neurology. 2005;64(10):1802–4.

16. Fregni F, Boggio PS, Valle AC, Rocha RR, Duarte J, Ferreira MJ, et al. A sham-controlled trial of a 5-day course of repetitive transcranial magnetic stimulation of the unaffected hemisphere in stroke patients. Stroke. 2006;37(8):2115–22.

17. Tohyama T, Fujiwara T, Matsumoto J, Honaga K, Ushiba J, Tsuji T, et al. Modulation of event-related desynchronization during motor imagery with transcranial direct current stimulation in a patient with severe hemiparetic stroke: a case report. Keio J Med. 2011;60(4):114–8.

18. Vines BW, Cerruti C, Schlaug G. Dual-hemisphere tDCS facilitates greater improvements for healthy subjects' non-dominant hand compared to uni-hemisphere stimulation. BMC Neurosci. 2008;9:103.

19. Boroojerdi B, Diefenbach K, Ferbert A. Transcallosal inhibition in cortical and subcortical cerebral vascular lesions. J Neurol Sci. 1996;144(1–2):160–70.

20. Murase N, Duque J, Mazzocchio R, Cohen LG. Influence of interhemispheric interactions on motor function in chronic stroke. Ann Neurol. 2004;55(3):400–9.

21. Classen J, Schnitzler A, Binkofski F, Werhahn KJ, Kim YS, Kessler KR, et al. The motor syndrome associated with exaggerated inhibition within the primary motor cortex of patients with hemiparetic. Brain. 1997;120(Pt 4):605–19.

22. Fregni F, Pascual-Leone A. Hand motor recovery after stroke: tuning the orchestra to improve hand motor function. Cogn Behav Neurol. 2006;19(1):21–33.

23. Wassermann EM, Zimmermann T. Transcranial magnetic brain stimulation: therapeutic promises and scientific gaps. Pharmacol Ther. 2012;133(1):98–107.

24. Datta A, Bikson M, Fregni F. Transcranial direct current stimulation in patients with skull defects and skull plates: high-resolution computational fem study of factors altering cortical current flow. NeuroImage. 2010;52(4):1268–78.

25. Tofts PS. The distribution of induced currents in magnetic stimulation of the nervous system. Phys Med Biol. 1990;35(8):1119–28.

26. Demirtas-Tatlidede A, Vahabzadeh-Hagh AM, Bernabeu M, Tormos JM, Pascual-Leone A. Noninvasive brain stimulation in traumatic brain injury. J Head Trauma Rehabil. 2012;27(4):274–92.

27. Cosentino G, Giglia G, Palermo A, Panetta ML, Lo Baido R, Brighina F, et al. A case of post-traumatic complex auditory hallucinosis treated with rTMS. Neurocase. 2010;16(3):267–72.

28. Kang EK, Kim DY, Paik NJ. Transcranial direct current stimulation of the left prefrontal cortex improves attention in patients with traumatic brain injury: a pilot study. J Rehabil Med. 2012;44(4):346–50.

29. Bonni S, Mastropasqua C, Bozzali M, Caltagirone C, Koch G. Theta burst stimulation improves visuospatial attention in a patient with traumatic brain injury. Neurol Sci. 2013;34(11):2053–6.

30. Kreuzer PM, Landgrebe M, Frank E, Langguth B. Repetitive transcranial magnetic stimulation for the treatment of chronic tinnitus after traumatic brain injury: a case study. J Head Trauma Rehabil. 2013;28(5):386–9.

31. Pistoia F, Sacco S, Carolei A, Sara M. Corticomotor facilitation in vegetative state: results of a pilot study. Arch Phys Med Rehabil. 2013;94(8):1599–606.

32. Lesniak M, Polanowska K, Seniow J, Czlonkowska A. Effects of repeated anodal tDCS coupled with cognitive training for patients with severe traumatic brain injury: a pilot randomized controlled trial. J Head Trauma Rehabil. 2014;29(3):E20–9.

33. Angelakis E, Liouta E, Andreadis N, Korfias S, Ktonas P, Stranjalis G, et al. Transcranial direct current stimulation effects in disorders of consciousness. Arch Phys Med Rehabil. 2014;95(2):283–9.

34. Thibaut A, Bruno MA, Ledoux D, Demertzi A, Laureys S. tDCS in patients with disorders of consciousness: sham-controlled randomized double-blind study. Neurology. 2014;82(13):1112–8.

35. Middleton A, Fritz SL, Liuzzo DM, Newman-Norlund R, Herter TM. Using clinical and robotic assessment tools to examine the feasibility of pairing tDCS with upper extremity physical therapy in patients with stroke and TBI: a consideration-of-concept pilot study. NeuroRehabilitation. 2014;35(4):741–54.

36. Nielson DM, McKnight CA, Patel RN, Kalnin AJ, Mysiw WJ. Preliminary guidelines for safe and effective use of repetitive transcranial magnetic stimulation in moderate to severe traumatic brain injury. Arch Phys Med Rehabil. 2015;96(4 Suppl):S138–44.

37. Koski L, Kolivakis T, Yu C, Chen JK, Delancy S, Ptito A. Noninvasive brain stimulation for persistent

postconcussion symptoms in mild traumatic brain injury. J Neurotrauma. 2015;32(1):38–44.

38. Ulam F, Shelton C, Richards L, Davis L, Hunter B, Fregni F, et al. Cumulative effects of transcranial direct current stimulation on EEG oscillations and attention/working memory during subacute neurorehabilitation of traumatic brain injury. Clin Neurophysiol. 2015;126(3):486–96.

39. Naro A, Calabro RS, Russo M, Leo A, Pollicino P, Quartarone A, et al. Can transcranial direct current stimulation be useful in differentiating unresponsive wakefulness syndrome from minimally conscious state patients? Restor Neurol Neurosci. 2015;33(2):159–76.

40. Fecteau S, Dickler M, Pelayo R, Kumru H, Bernabeu M, Opisso Salleras E, et al. Cortical excitability during passive action observation in hospitalized adults with subacute moderate to severe traumatic brain injury: a preliminary TMS study. Neurorehabil Neural Repair. 2015;29(6):548–56.

41. Plautz EJ, Barbay S, Frost SB, Friel KM, Dancause N, Zoubina EV, et al. Post-infarct cortical plasticity and behavioral recovery using concurrent cortical stimulation and rehabilitative training: a feasibility study in primates. Neurol Res. 2003;25(8):801–10.

42. Yoon YS, Yu KP, Kim H, Kim HI, Kwak SH, Kim BO. The effect of electric cortical stimulation after focal traumatic brain injury in rats. Ann Rehabil Med. 2012;36(5):596–608.

43. Kleim JA, Bruneau R, VandenBerg P, MacDonald E, Mulrooney R, Pocock D. Motor cortex stimulation enhances motor recovery and reduces peri-infarct dysfunction following ischemic insult. Neurol Res. 2003;25(8):789–93.

44. Teskey GC, Flynn C, Goertzen CD, Monfils MH, Young NA. Cortical stimulation improves skilled forelimb use following a focal ischemic infarct in the rat. Neurol Res. 2003;25(8):794–800.

45. Zheng J, Liu L, Xue X, Li H, Wang S, Cao Y, et al. Cortical electrical stimulation promotes neuronal plasticity in the peri-ischemic cortex and contralesional anterior horn of cervical spinal cord in a rat model of focal cerebral ischemia. Brain Res. 2013;1504:25–34.

46. Adkins-Muir DL, Jones TA. Cortical electrical stimulation combined with rehabilitative training: enhanced functional recovery and dendritic plasticity following focal cortical ischemia in rats. Neurol Res. 2003;25(8):780–8.

47. Brown JA, Lutsep HL, Weinand M, Cramer SC. Motor cortex stimulation for the enhancement of recovery from stroke: a prospective, multicenter safety study. Neurosurgery. 2006;58(3):464–73.

48. Levy R, Ruland S, Weinand M, Lowry D, Dafer R, Bakay R. Cortical stimulation for the rehabilitation of patients with hemiparetic stroke: a multicenter feasibility study of safety and efficacy. J Neurosurg. 2008;108(4):707–14.

49. Huang M, Harvey RL, Stoykov ME, Ruland S, Weinand M, Lowry D, et al. Cortical stimulation for upper limb recovery following ischemic stroke: a small phase ii pilot study of a fully implanted stimulator. Top Stroke Rehabil. 2008;15(2):160–72.

50. Levy RM, Harvey RL, Kissela BM, Winstein CJ, Lutsep HL, Parrish TB, et al. Epidural electrical stimulation for stroke rehabilitation: results of the prospective, multicenter, randomized, single-blinded Everest trial. Neurorehabil Neural Repair. 2016;30(2):107–19.

51. Katayama Y, Tsubokawa T, Yamamoto T. Chronic motor cortex stimulation for central deafferentation pain: experience with bulbar pain secondary to Wallenberg syndrome. Stereotact Funct Neurosurg. 1994;62(1–4):295–9.

52. Meyerson BA, Lindblom U, Linderoth B, Lind G, Herregodts P. Motor cortex stimulation as treatment of trigeminal neuropathic pain. Acta Neurochir Suppl (Wien). 1993;58:150–3.

53. Nguyen JP, Keravel Y, Feve A, Uchiyama T, Cesaro P, Le Guerinel C, et al. Treatment of deafferentation pain by chronic stimulation of the motor cortex: report of a series of 20 cases. Acta Neurochir Suppl. 1997;68:54–60.

54. Tsubokawa T, Katayama Y, Yamamoto T, Hirayama T, Koyama S. Chronic motor cortex stimulation in patients with thalamic pain. J Neurosurg. 1993;78(3):393–401.

55. Fontaine D, Hamani C, Lozano A. Efficacy and safety of motor cortex stimulation for chronic neuropathic pain: critical review of the literature. J Neurosurg. 2009;110(2):251–6.

56. Nardone R, Holler Y, Leis S, Holler P, Thon N, Thomschewski A, et al. Invasive and non-invasive brain stimulation for treatment of neuropathic pain in patients with spinal cord injury: a review. J Spinal Cord Med. 2014;37(1):19–31.

57. Bittar RG, Kar-Purkayastha I, Owen SL, Bear RE, Green A, Wang SY, et al. Deep brain stimulation for pain relief: a meta-analysis. J Clin Neurosci. 2005;12(5):515–9.

58. Weaver FM, Follett K, Stern M, Hur K, Harris C, Marks WJ Jr, et al. Bilateral deep brain stimulation vs. best medical therapy for patients with advanced Parkinson disease: a randomized controlled trial. JAMA. 2009;301(1):63–73.

59. Schuepbach WM, Rau J, Knudsen K, Volkmann J, Krack P, Timmermann L, et al. Neurostimulation for Parkinson's disease with early motor complications. N Engl J Med. 2013;368(7):610–22.

60. Deep-Brain Stimulation for Parkinson's Disease Study G, Obeso JA, Olanow CW, Rodriguez-Oroz MC, Krack P, Kumar R, et al. Deep-brain stimulation of the subthalamic nucleus or the pars interna of the globus pallidus in Parkinson's disease. N Engl J Med. 2001;345(13):956–63.

61. Vidailhet M, Vercueil L, Houeto JL, Krystkowiak P, Benabid AL, Cornu P, et al. Bilateral deep-brain stimulation of the globus pallidus in primary generalized dystonia. N Engl J Med. 2005;352(5):459–67.

62. Tabansky I, Quinkert AW, Rahman N, Muller SZ, Lofgren J, Rudling J, et al. Temporally-patterned deep brain stimulation in a mouse model of multiple traumatic brain injury. Behav Brain Res. 2014;273:123–32.

63. Broggi G, Brock S, Franzini A, Geminiani G. A case of posttraumatic tremor treated by chronic stimulation of the thalamus. Mov Disord. 1993;8(2):206–8.

64. Nguyen JP, Degos JD. Thalamic stimulation and proximal tremor. A specific target in the nucleus ventrointermedius thalami. Arch Neurol. 1993;50(5):498–500.

65. Sellal F, Hirsch E, Barth P, Blond S, Marescaux C. A case of symptomatic hemidystonia improved by ventroposterolateral thalamic electrostimulation. Mov Disord. 1993;8(4):515–8.

66. Loher TJ, Hasdemir MG, Burgunder JM, Krauss JK. Long-term follow-up study of chronic globus pallidus internus stimulation for posttraumatic hemidystonia. J Neurosurg. 2000;92(3):457–60.

67. Umemura A, Samadani U, Jaggi JL, Hurtig HI, Baltuch GH. Thalamic deep brain stimulation for posttraumatic action tremor. Clin Neurol Neurosurg. 2004;106(4):280–3.

68. Green AAT. Deep brain stimulation for post traumatic tremor. ACNR. 2005;5(1):38.

69. Capelle HH, Grips E, Weigel R, Blahak C, Hansjorg B, Wohrle JC, et al. Posttraumatic peripherally-induced dystonia and multifocal deep brain stimulation: case report. Neurosurgery. 2006;59(3):E702; discussion E702.

70. Foote KD, Seignourel P, Fernandez HH, Romrell J, Whidden E, Jacobson C, et al. Dual electrode thalamic deep brain stimulation for the treatment of posttraumatic and multiple sclerosis tremor. Neurosurgery. 2006;58(4 Suppl 2):ONS-280-285; discussion ONS-285-286.

71. Broggi GFA, Tringali G, Ferroli P, Marras C, et al. Deep brain stimulation as a functional scalpel. In: Chang JWKY, Yamamoto T, editors. Advances in functional and reparative neurosurgery. Vienna: Springer; 2006. p. 9–13.

72. Kuhn J, Lenartz D, Mai JK, Huff W, Klosterkoetter J, Sturm V. Disappearance of self-aggressive behavior in a brain-injured patient after deep brain stimulation of the hypothalamus: technical case report. Neurosurgery. 2008;62(5):E1182; discussion E1182.

73. Franzini A, Cordella R, Messina G, Marras CE, Romito LM, Carella F, et al. Deep brain stimulation for movement disorders. Considerations on 276 consecutive patients. J Neural Transm (Vienna). 2011;118(10):1497–510.

74. Reese R, Herzog J, Falk D, Lutzen U, Pinsker MO, Mehdorn HM, et al. Successful deep brain stimulation in a case of posttraumatic tremor and hemiparkinsonism. Mov Disord. 2011;26(10):1954–5.

75. Kim JP, Chang WS, Chang JW. The long-term surgical outcomes of secondary hemidystonia associated with post-traumatic brain injury. Acta Neurochir. 2012;154(5):823–30.

76. Issar NM, Hedera P, Phibbs FT, Konrad PE, Neimat JS. Treating post-traumatic tremor with deep brain stimulation: report of five cases. Parkinsonism Relat Disord. 2013;19(12):1100–5.

77. Carvalho KS, Sukul VV, Bookland MJ, Koch SA, Connolly PJ. Deep brain stimulation of the globus pallidus suppresses post-traumatic dystonic tremor. J Clin Neurosci. 2014;21(1):153–5.

78. Follett MA, Torres-Russotto D, Follett KA. Bilateral deep brain stimulation of the ventral intermediate nucleus of the thalamus for posttraumatic midbrain tremor. Neuromodulation. 2014;17(3):289–91.

79. Louis ED, Lynch T, Ford B, Greene P, Bressman SB, Fahn S. Delayed-onset cerebellar syndrome. Arch Neurol. 1996;53(5):450–4.

80. Krauss JK, Jankovic J. Head injury and post-traumatic movement disorders. Neurosurgery. 2002;50(5):927–939; discussion 939-940.

81. Foote KD, Okun MS. Ventralis intermedius plus ventralis oralis anterior and posterior deep brain stimulation for posttraumatic holmes tremor: two leads may be better than one: technical note. Neurosurgery. 2005;56(2 Suppl):E445; discussion E445.

82. Krauss JK, Mohadjer M, Braus DF, Wakhloo AK, Nobbe F, Mundinger F. Dystonia following head trauma: a report of nine patients and review of the literature. Mov Disord. 1992;7(3):263–72.

83. Silver JK, Lux WE. Early onset dystonia following traumatic brain injury. Arch Phys Med Rehabil. 1994;75(8):885–8.

84. Chuang C, Fahn S, Frucht SJ. The natural history and treatment of acquired hemidystonia: report of 33 cases and review of the literature. J Neurol Neurosurg Psychiatry. 2002;72(1):59–67.

85. Krauss JK, Trankle R, Raabe A. Tremor and dystonia after penetrating diencephalic-mesencephalic trauma. Parkinsonism Relat Disord. 1997;3(2):117–9.

86. King RB, Fuller C, Collins GH. Delayed onset of hemidystonia and hemiballismus following head injury: a clinicopathological correlation. Case report. J Neurosurg. 2001;94(2):309–14.

87. Constantoyannis C, Kagadis GC, Ellul J, Kefalopoulou Z, Chroni E. Nucleus ventralis oralis deep brain stimulation in postanoxic dystonia. Mov Disord. 2009;24(2):306–8.

88. Katsakiori PF, Kefalopoulou Z, Markaki E, Paschali A, Ellul J, Kagadis GC, et al. Deep brain stimulation for secondary dystonia: results in 8 patients. Acta Neurochir. 2009;151(5):473–8; discussion 478.

89. Ghika J, Villemure JG, Miklossy J, Temperli P, Pralong E, Christen-Zaech S, et al. Postanoxic generalized dystonia improved by bilateral VOA thalamic deep brain stimulation. Neurology. 2002;58(2):311–3.

90. Peran P, Catani S, Falletta Caravasso C, Nemmi F, Sabatini U, Formisano R. Supplementary motor area activation is impaired in severe traumatic brain injury parkinsonism. J Neurotrauma. 2014;31(7):642–8.

91. Wong JC, Hazrati LN. Parkinson's disease, parkinsonism, and traumatic brain injury. Crit Rev Clin Lab Sci. 2013;50(4–5):103–6.

92. Medina J, Norise C, Faseyitan O, Coslett HB, Turkeltaub PE, Hamilton RH. Finding the right words: transcranial magnetic stimulation improves discourse productivity in non-fluent aphasia after stroke. Aphasiology. 2012;26(9):1153–68.

93. Naeser MA, Martin PI, Nicholas M, Baker EH, Seekins H, Kobayashi M, et al. Improved picture naming in chronic aphasia after TMS to part of right Broca's area: an open-protocol study. Brain Lang. 2005;93(1):95–105.

94. Fitzgerald PB, Fountain S, Daskalakis ZJ. A comprehensive review of the effects of rTMS on motor cortical excitability and inhibition. Clin Neurophysiol. 2006;117(12):2584–96.

95. Ohyama M, Senda M, Kitamura S, Ishii K, Mishina M, Terashi A. Role of the nondominant hemisphere and undamaged area during word repetition in poststroke aphasics. A pet activation study. Stroke. 1996;27(5):897–903.

96. Jo JM, Kim YH, Ko MH, Ohn SH, Joen B, Lee KH. Enhancing the working memory of stroke patients using tDCS. Am J Phys Med Rehabil. 2009;88(5):404–9.

97. Fitzgerald PB, Hoy KE, Maller JJ, Herring S, Segrave R, McQueen S, et al. Transcranial magnetic stimulation for depression after a traumatic brain injury: a case study. J ECT. 2011;27(1):38–40.

98. Cooper EB, Cooper JB. Electrical treatment of coma via the median nerve. Acta Neurochir Suppl. 2003;87:7–10.

99. Cooper JB, Jane JA, Alves WM, Cooper EB. Right median nerve electrical stimulation to hasten awakening from coma. Brain Inj. 1999;13(4):261–7.

100. Lei J, Wang L, Gao G, Cooper E, Jiang J. Right median nerve electrical stimulation for acute traumatic coma patients. J Neurotrauma. 2015;32(20):1584–9.

101. Peri CV, Shaffrey ME, Farace E, Cooper E, Alves WM, Cooper JB, et al. Pilot study of electrical stimulation on median nerve in comatose severe brain injured patients: 3-month outcome. Brain Inj. 2001;15(10):903–10.

102. Hassler R, Ore GD, Bricolo A, Dieckmann G, Dolce G. EEG and clinical arousal induced by bilateral long-term stimulation of pallidal systems in traumatic vigil coma. Electroencephalogr Clin Neurophysiol. 1969;27(7):689–90.

103. Tsubokawa T, Yamamoto T, Katayama Y, Hirayama T, Maejima S, Moriya T. Deep-brain stimulation in a persistent vegetative state: follow-up results and criteria for selection of candidates. Brain Inj. 1990;4(4):315–27.

104. Yamamoto T, Kobayashi K, Kasai M, Oshima H, Fukaya C, Katayama Y. DBS therapy for the vegetative state and minimally conscious state. Acta Neurochir Suppl. 2005;93:101–4.

105. Schiff ND, Giacino JT, Kalmar K, Victor JD, Baker K, Gerber M, et al. Behavioural improvements with thalamic stimulation after severe traumatic brain injury. Nature. 2007;448(7153):600–3.

106. Giacino J, Fins JJ, Machado A, Schiff ND. Central thalamic deep brain stimulation to promote recovery from chronic posttraumatic minimally conscious state: challenges and opportunities. Neuromodulation. 2012;15(4):339–49.

107. Rezai AR, Sederberg PB, Bogner J, Nielson DM, Zhang J, Mysiw WJ, et al. Improved function after deep brain stimulation for chronic, severe traumatic brain injury. Neurosurgery. 2016;79(2):204–11.

108. Ritter AC, Wagner AK, Fabio A, Pugh MJ, Walker WC, Szaflarski JP, et al. Incidence and risk factors of posttraumatic seizures following traumatic brain injury: a traumatic brain injury model systems study. Epilepsia. 2016;57(12):1968–77.

109. Annegers JF, Hauser WA, Coan SP, Rocca WA. A population-based study of seizures after traumatic brain injuries. N Engl J Med. 1998;338(1):20–4.

110. Larkin M, Meyer RM, Szuflita NS, Severson MA, Levine ZT. Post-traumatic, drug-resistant epilepsy and review of seizure control outcomes from blinded, randomized controlled trials of brain stimulation treatments for drug-resistant epilepsy. Cureus. 2016;8(8):e744.

111. Fisher R, Salanova V, Witt T, Worth R, Henry T, Gross R, et al. Electrical stimulation of the anterior nucleus of thalamus for treatment of refractory epilepsy. Epilepsia. 2010;51(5):899–908.

112. Morrell MJ, Group RNSSiES. Responsive cortical stimulation for the treatment of medically intractable partial epilepsy. Neurology. 2011;77(13):1295–304.

113. Stypulkowski PH, Stanslaski SR, Denison TJ, Giftakis JE. Chronic evaluation of a clinical system for deep brain stimulation and recording of neural network activity. Stereotact Funct Neurosurg. 2013;91(4):220–32.

114. Jorge RE, Robinson RG, Moser D, Tateno A, Crespo-Facorro B, Arndt S. Major depression following traumatic brain injury. Arch Gen Psychiatry. 2004;61(1):42–50.

115. Mayberg HS, Lozano AM, Voon V, McNeely HE, Seminowicz D, Hamani C, et al. Deep brain stimulation for treatment-resistant depression. Neuron. 2005;45(5):651–60.

116. Hamani C, Diwan M, Macedo CE, Brandao ML, Shumake J, Gonzalez-Lima F, et al. Antidepressant-like effects of medial prefrontal cortex deep brain stimulation in rats. Biol Psychiatry. 2010;67(2):117–24.

117. Kubu CS, Malone DA, Chelune G, Malloy P, Rezai AR, Frazier T, et al. Neuropsychological outcome after deep brain stimulation in the ventral capsule/ventral striatum for highly refractory obsessive-compulsive disorder or major depression. Stereotact Funct Neurosurg. 2013;91(6):374–8.

118. Taghva AS, Malone DA, Rezai AR. Deep brain stimulation for treatment-resistant depression. World Neurosurg. 2013;80(3–4):S27 e17–24.

119. Lozano AM, Mayberg HS, Giacobbe P, Hamani C, Craddock RC, Kennedy SH. Subcallosal cingulate gyrus deep brain stimulation for treatment-resistant depression. Biol Psychiatry. 2008;64(6):461–7.

120. Yamamoto T, Katayama Y, Obuchi T, Kobayashi K, Oshima H, Fukaya C. Spinal cord stimulation for treatment of patients in the minimally conscious state. Neurol Med Chir (Tokyo). 2012;52(7):475–81.

121. Yamamoto T, Katayama Y, Obuchi T, Kobayashi K, Oshima H, Fukaya C. Deep brain stimulation and spinal cord stimulation for vegetative state and minimally conscious state. World Neurosurg. 2013;80(3–4):S30 e31–9.

122. Matsui T, Asano T, Takakura K, Yamada R, Hosobuchi Y. Beneficial effects of cervical spinal cord stimulation (cscs) on patients with impaired consciousness: a preliminary report. Pacing Clin Electrophysiol. 1989;12(4 Pt 2):718–25.

123. Kanno T, Morita I, Yamaguchi S, Yokoyama T, Kamei Y, Anil SM, et al. Dorsal column stimulation in persistent vegetative state. Neuromodulation. 2009;12(1):33–8.

124. Yamamoto T, Katayama Y. Deep brain stimulation therapy for the vegetative state. Neuropsychol Rehabil. 2005;15(3–4):406–13.

125. Yamamoto T, Katayama Y, Kobayashi K, Kasai M, Oshima H, Fukaya C. DBS therapy for a persistent vegetative state: ten years follow-up results. Acta Neurochir Suppl. 2003;87:15–8.

126. Yamamoto T, Katayama Y, Oshima H, Fukaya C, Kawamata T, Tsubokawa T. Deep brain stimulation therapy for a persistent vegetative state. Acta Neurochir Suppl. 2002;79:79–82.

127. Shah SA, Schiff ND. Central thalamic deep brain stimulation for cognitive neuromodulation—a review of proposed mechanisms and investigational studies. Eur J Neurosci. 2010;32(7):1135–44.

128. Schiff ND. Moving toward a generalizable application of central thalamic deep brain stimulation for support of forebrain arousal regulation in the severely injured brain. Ann N Y Acad Sci. 2012;1265:56–68.

129. Schiff ND. Central thalamic contributions to arousal regulation and neurological disorders of consciousness. Ann N Y Acad Sci. 2008;1129:105–18.

130. Shirvalkar P, Seth M, Schiff ND, Herrera DG. Cognitive enhancement with central thalamic electrical stimulation. Proc Natl Acad Sci U S A. 2006;103(45):17007–12.

131. Phan TG. Disorders of consciousness: are we ready for a paradigm shift? Lancet Neurol. 2013;12(2):131–2.

132. Jox RJ, Bernat JL, Laureys S, Racine E. Disorders of consciousness: responding to requests for novel diagnostic and therapeutic interventions. Lancet Neurol. 2012;11(8):732–8.

133. Jox RJ, Bernat JL, Laureys S, Racine E. Disorders of consciousness: are we ready for a paradigm shift?—authors' reply. Lancet Neurol. 2013;12(2):132.

134. Katayama Y, Tsubokawa T, Harano S, Tsukiyama T. Dissociation of subjective pain report and pain-related late positive components of cerebral evoked potentials in subjects with brain lesions. Brain Res Bull. 1985;14(5):423–6.

135. Laxton AW, Tang-Wai DF, McAndrews MP, Zumsteg D, Wennberg R, Keren R, et al. A phase i trial of deep brain stimulation of memory circuits in Alzheimer's disease. Ann Neurol. 2010;68(4):521–34.

136. Lozano AM, Fosdick L, Chakravarty MM, Leoutsakos JM, Munro C, Oh E, et al. A phase ii study of fornix deep brain stimulation in mild Alzheimer's disease. J Alzheimers Dis. 2016;54(2):777–87.

137. Suthana N, Haneef Z, Stern J, Mukamel R, Behnke E, Knowlton B, et al. Memory enhancement and deep-brain stimulation of the entorhinal area. N Engl J Med. 2012;366(6):502–10.

138. Bick SK, Eskandar EN. Neuromodulation for restoring memory. Neurosurg Focus. 2016;40(5):E5.

139. Shin SS, Dixon CE, Okonkwo DO, Richardson RM. Neurostimulation for traumatic brain injury. J Neurosurg. 2014;121(5):1219–31.

140. Roy HA, Green AL, Aziz TZ. State of the art: novel applications for deep brain stimulation. Neuromodulation. 2017;21(2):126–34.

141. Li S, Zaninotto AL, Neville IS, Paiva WS, Nunn D, Fregni F. Clinical utility of brain stimulation modalities following traumatic brain injury: current evidence. Neuropsychiatr Dis Treat. 2015;11: 1573–86.

142. Hammond C, Bergman H, Brown P. Pathological synchronization in Parkinson's disease: networks, models and treatments. Trends Neurosci. 2007;30(7):357–64.

143. de Hemptinne C, Ryapolova-Webb ES, Air EL, Garcia PA, Miller KJ, Ojemann JG, et al. Exaggerated phase-amplitude coupling in the primary motor cortex in Parkinson disease. Proc Natl Acad Sci U S A. 2013;110(12):4780–5.

144. Zijlmans M, Jiruska P, Zelmann R, Leijten FS, Jefferys JG, Gotman J. High-frequency oscillations as a new biomarker in epilepsy. Ann Neurol. 2012;71(2):169–78.

145. Rossi PJ, Opri E, Shute JB, Molina R, Bowers D, Ward H, et al. Scheduled, intermittent stimulation of the thalamus reduces tics in Tourette syndrome. Parkinsonism Relat Disord. 2016;29:35–41.

146. Rosin B, Slovik M, Mitelman R, Rivlin-Etzion M, Haber SN, Israel Z, et al. Closed-loop deep brain stimulation is superior in ameliorating parkinsonism. Neuron. 2011;72(2):370–84.

147. Okun MS, Foote KD, Wu SS, Ward HE, Bowers D, Rodriguez RL, et al. A trial of scheduled deep brain stimulation for Tourette syndrome: moving away from continuous deep brain stimulation paradigms. JAMA Neurol. 2013;70(1):85–94.

The Future of Clinical Trials in Traumatic Brain Injury

David S. Hersh, Beth M. Ansel, and Howard M. Eisenberg

Clinical Trials in Traumatic Brain Injury: Learning from the Past

Over the past three decades, dozens of clinical trials have examined therapeutic strategies and neuroprotective agents for the treatment of traumatic brain injury (TBI). Extensive preclinical and clinical work has produced a better understanding of the pathophysiology that underlies TBI and has facilitated the development of evidence-based guidelines with regard to nutrition, oxygenation, intracranial pressure (ICP) monitoring, and surgical intervention [1]. Recent attention has focused on a number of pharmacological agents evaluated in experimental TBI models that target one or more of the events that cause neurological dysfunction. The search for a neuroprotective agent that will improve clinical outcomes, particularly for patients with moderate or severe TBI, however, remains elusive [2, 3]. In a recent state of the science overview, Bragge et al. [4] identified 207 randomized controlled trials that investi-gated acute interventions for moderate or severe TBI. The authors highlighted the failure of the numerous randomized clinical trials that have studied pharmacological interventions, noting that of 13 "robust" trials involving nine individual neuroprotective agents, none yielded consistently positive results [4].

One of the most recent examples of this phenomenon occurred in 2014, when the *New England Journal of Medicine* published the results of two large Phase III trials targeting early neuroprotection with progesterone. Both failed to demonstrate the efficacy of progesterone as a neuroprotective agent following moderate or severe TBI [5, 6]. The disappointing results were surprising, given that more than 300 preclinical studies in a variety of animal models had demonstrated the ability of progesterone, when given early, to reduce inflammation, edema, and cell death and improve functional outcomes following injury [7].

Data resulting from two Phase II trials also provided promising results. ProTECT II (Progesterone for the Treatment of TBI—Experimental Clinical Treatment trial) was a randomized, double-blinded, placebo-controlled Phase II trial involving 100 patients with moderate or severe TBI at a level 1 trauma center [8]. Treatment resulted in significantly lower 30-day mortality rates for patients with severe TBI and higher outcome scores for patients with moderate TBI. Concurrently, a Phase II trial in Hangzhou,

D. S. Hersh, MD · H. M. Eisenberg, MD (✉)
Department of Neurosurgery, University of Maryland, Baltimore, MD, USA
e-mail: dhersh@som.umaryland.edu; heisenberg@som.umaryland.edu

B. M. Ansel, PhD, CCC-SLP
The Eunice Kennedy Shriver National Institute of Child Health and Human Development, The National Institutes of Health, Spencerville, MD, USA

© Springer International Publishing AG, part of Springer Nature 2018
S. D. Timmons (ed.), *Controversies in Severe Traumatic Brain Injury Management*,
https://doi.org/10.1007/978-3-319-89477-5_19

China, randomized 159 patients with severe TBI [9]. Treatment resulted in significantly lower mortality rates and better outcome scores at 3 and 6 months post-injury.

The encouraging Phase II results led to two double-blinded, randomized, two-arm, multi-center Phase III trials. ProTECT III, sponsored by the National Institute of Neurological Disorders and Stroke (NINDS) involved 49 centers and was designed to enroll 1200 patients with a Glasgow Coma Scale (GCS) score of 4–12 [6]. The trial was stopped after 882 patients were enrolled when an interim analysis revealed no significant differences in mortality or functional outcomes 6 months after injury. A simultaneous Phase III study, SYNAPSE (Study of a Neuroprotective Agent, Progesterone, in Severe Traumatic Brain Injury), sponsored by BHR Pharma, enrolled 1195 patients with a GCS score of 3–8 across 180 centers in 21 countries. This study also found no significant differences in functional outcomes at 3 or 6 months post-injury [5].

The addition of progesterone to the expanding list of clinical trial failures has prompted many TBI researchers to call for a critical reappraisal of the design, conduct, and analysis of TBI trials. Some have argued that key limitations in preclinical research continue to hinder the translation of bench science to the clinical world. Others have focused on the details of the clinical trials themselves, arguing that the heterogeneous nature of TBI calls for unique considerations with regard to trial design, sample size, subject recruitment, outcome measurement, and statistical analysis [4, 7]. Some take a more global view, believing that TBI treatments that target a single pathophysiological mechanism with a single pharmacological agent are unlikely to succeed: the inherent complexity of TBI instead requires a systems biology approach to address multiple interacting variables in a more sophisticated manner [10]. It will be essential to consider each of these approaches to shape a more successful future for clinical trials in TBI.

Bridging the Gap: From Preclinical and Early Clinical Data to Phase III Trial Design

Translating preclinical animal studies to clinical trials remains an ongoing challenge. Preclinical TBI research has been criticized for not representing the clinical realities of treatment. To date, many experimental models of TBI have involved small rodents with lissencephalic brains. Some investigators suggest larger, gyrencephalic mammals would more closely predict human responses to treatment [10]. Regardless of the model system studied, one of the inherent issues in TBI research is the clinically complex and variable phenomenon of TBI. Traumatic brain injury occurs through a number of different mechanisms, including falls, motor vehicle accidents, and penetrating injuries. Injuries may be focal or diffuse in nature and exist across a spectrum of severity. TBI may occur in isolation, or patients may be affected by polytrauma involving multiple organ systems. Conversely, preclinical models of TBI involve standardized, predictable, reproducible injuries. As a result, the preclinical findings of any given experiment may be relevant to only a particular subset of TBI patients [10].

Despite these limitations, preclinical studies have provided important information to help delineate the pathophysiology that underlies various forms of TBI. Preclinical work targeting glutamate excitotoxicity established that this pathophysiological process plays an important role in patients with contusions or traumatic subarachnoid hemorrhage, as opposed to patients with diffuse injuries [11]. Preclinical data also provided valuable information to guide the dosing, treatment schedule, and route of administration in Phase I and Phase II trials [7, 12]. For example, preclinical work involving tirilazad, a potentially neuroprotective aminosteroid, revealed that sex-based differences in metabolism result in subtherapeutic levels in females [11]. Additionally, preclinical data suggested that progesterone has an inverted U-shaped dose-response curve and that doses above a certain threshold may have diminished efficacy—information that potentially contributed to the failure of the Phase III trials [7, 12].

The challenge is how to translate preclinical animal studies to the clinical setting. In the experimental environment of preclinical studies, investigators have the ability to control factors such as dosing, pretreatment, or the treatment window following injury. This is not possible in the clinical setting, where injuries are unpredictable, rendering pretreatment impossible and rapid treatment challenging at best [10]. As a result, a recently completed Phase III trial (EPO-TBI) randomized patients with moderate or severe TBI to erythropoietin versus placebo within 24 h of injury, despite preclinical work that suggested a shorter therapeutic window [13, 14]. In addition, TBI often occurs within a complex of other injuries and medical issues that compromise the controlled treatment paradigm. Decisions regarding the appropriate dosing and treatment schedule can therefore be complicated by safety concerns that may not be relevant in preclinical experiments. In the EPO-TBI trial, for example, the theoretical risk of thrombotic complications prevented many subjects from receiving a full course of erythropoietin [13]. Therefore, while preclinical data may preliminarily guide early clinical studies, Phase I and II trials will also continue to play a pivotal role in refining the dosing and scheduling of the therapeutic agent under investigation.

The Impact of Patient Heterogeneity on Trial Design, Inclusion Criteria, and Sample Size

Patient heterogeneity not only complicates the translation of preclinical data to clinical research but also influences the design, execution, and analysis of the clinical trial. Including heterogeneous patients with variable prognoses decreases statistical power, since patients with a good prognosis might do well even without the intervention, while patients with a poor prognosis might have a bad outcome even with the intervention, making it difficult to detect a true treatment effect. Three approaches have been advocated to address the inherent patient heterogeneity in TBI research: (1) identifying and studying more homogeneous patient populations, (2) broadening the inclusion criteria and increasing the sample size in order to meet the power requirements of the study as well as make trials more generalizable, or (3) conducting large observational studies and applying the principles of comparative effectiveness research.

The first approach offers the most direct solution to patient heterogeneity by attempting to eliminate it entirely. Although TBI patients may be characterized by various mechanisms of injury, pathophysiologic processes, radiographic patterns, and levels of severity, clinical trials can be designed with strict inclusion criteria in an effort to study a more homogeneous population [4, 15, 16]. Although minimizing heterogeneity will increase statistical power, there are several factors to consider with this approach. First, rigid inclusion criteria will reduce the number of patients who are screened for study eligibility. As a result, recruitment rates will decline, and it will take longer to complete the study enrollment. This limitation has been demonstrated in several recently published clinical trials, including the DECRA (DEcompressive CRAniectomy) trial, which began enrollment in 2002 and was published in 2011, and the more recent RESCUEicp trial, which began enrollment in 2006 and was published in 2016 [17–19]. A second issue is that despite recent advances in imaging and efforts to improve the classification of TBI, it remains difficult to identify truly homogeneous patient populations. Reliance on the GCS score as a means of categorizing subjects in a clinical trial ignores the enormous variability that exists among individuals with a particular GCS. Investigators are recognizing the scientific and pragmatic implications of relying on the GCS score alone. The COBRIT (Citicoline Brain Injury Treatment) trial, for example, included neuroimaging findings as part of the inclusion criteria [20, 21]. Future clinical trials will benefit from incorporating genomics, biomarkers, and emerging imaging modalities, in order to characterize patients more effectively. Developing more accurate and specific patient profiles will enable the enrollment of patients who are more likely to respond similarly to an intervention, thereby increasing the likelihood of identifying a treatment effect [15].

A second strategy takes the opposite approach, arguing that instead of incorporating strict inclusion criteria, studies should broaden their enrollment and increase their sample size. Proponents of this approach believe that larger numbers of subjects will decrease the risk of significant differences between the study groups while simultaneously increasing the generalizability of the study results. This approach embraces patient heterogeneity but recognizes that including more heterogeneous patients, in particular those with an extreme prognosis, reduces the statistical power of the study and increases the required sample size [22]. In their state of the science overview, Bragge et al. [4] revealed that the majority of the randomized clinical trials that they identified were single-center studies that enrolled fewer than 100 patients. Only 14 of the 191 completed trials enrolled more than 500 patients. The small, single-center studies were more likely to find a positive treatment effect when compared with large multicenter studies, likely due to an overestimation of the effect size. Recognizing this issue, investigators have begun to design and execute TBI "mega trials" involving thousands of patients. The first TBI mega trial was the CRASH (Corticosteroid Randomization After Significant Head injury) trial, which studied the effect of a 48-h infusion of methylprednisolone in patients with moderate or severe TBI [23]. The trial was stopped after 10,008 patients were enrolled (of the 20,000 planned) after an interim analysis demonstrated a higher mortality rate at 14 days in the treatment group. The CRASH trial used broad inclusion criteria to enroll large numbers of patients and employed the minimization method [24] of allocating patients to ensure that the baseline characteristics of the patients in each study group remained well balanced [22, 25].

The third approach abandons the concept of a randomized clinical trial entirely and instead proposes that TBI research can be performed in the context of large observational studies. Randomized trials test the efficacy of a treatment under prespecified, controlled conditions. Large observational studies monitor the impact of the intervention under the "messy" conditions of the real world, thereby making the results more generalizable [22]. Proponents of this approach embrace the heterogeneity that exists between centers, rather than between patients, and suggest that large observational studies will capture the differences in treatment that are provided across a variety of prehospital, hospital, and post-discharge settings [19, 26]. This intrinsic variability across different centers and countries can be used to identify "best practices" through the process of comparative effectiveness research [10]. These analyses are achieved by capturing high-quality data, developing robust risk-adjustment models that allow researchers to adjust for baseline characteristics that affect prognosis, and using statistical models (e.g., random effects models) that enable differences between centers to be rigorously analyzed [15].

Developing More Sophisticated Outcome Measures: Moving Beyond the Glasgow Outcome Scale

Choosing appropriate outcome measures represents another critical step in clinical trial design that will become increasingly important in future TBI trials. The National Institute of Child Health and Human Development (NICHD) TBI Clinical Trials (TBI-CT) Network was specifically designed to address the need for more precise multidimensional TBI classification, meaningful outcome measures and design features, and to implement rigorous clinical trials within the acute and rehabilitation phases. A series of primary and secondary outcome measures were designed to reflect the global status of the patient and capture a broad perspective of functional and cognitive parameters that are important post-TBI [27]. A complementary approach is the goal of the ongoing TBI Endpoints Development (TED) Initiative.

The NICHD TBI-CT Network and the TED Initiative recognize that the complex impact of TBI on multiple components of a patient's life post-injury makes it difficult to quantify the effect of an intervention with a single outcome measure [28]. Bragge et al. [4] reported that among the 207 randomized clinical trials that have evaluated acute interventions for moderate to severe TBI, the most frequently measured outcomes have included early mortality, late mortality, ICP, and the Glasgow Outcome Scale (GOS) at 6 months. Only 23% of the trials identified a superior effect of the intervention being studied, with clinical outcome measures such as the GOS or mortality being less likely to demonstrate an effect as compared to surrogate endpoints such as the ICP or length of stay.

This raises two questions. First, are the appropriate timepoints being examined? It is possible that 6–12 months post-injury is not enough time to capture the full recovery from a moderate or severe TBI. Conversely, if studies try to incorporate later timepoints, patients (and in particular, TBI patients) are more likely to be lost to follow-up [29]. Additional confounders are also likely to play a role as the duration of follow-up increases, and those patients who do return for follow-up are more likely to represent a selected subset of patients. Nevertheless, time should be considered as one of the dimensions of TBI outcome, with more continuity between acute and post-acute research [10].

Secondly, are the outcome measures themselves appropriate? Early and late mortality, although commonly measured primary outcomes, have been criticized for failing to capture quality of life (QOL) components that are of key importance to patients. For example, the RESCUEicp trial concluded that in TBI patients with refractory intracranial hypertension, decompressive craniectomy improves survival but that many of the patients who survive are in a vegetative or severely disabled state [18]. Similarly, the EPO-TBI trial found that in a subset of patients without intracranial mass lesions, erythropoietin improves survival but without a concomitant increase in dichotomized extended GOS (GOS-E) scores [13, 14]. Therefore, it is critical to examine functional outcome measures in addition to survival. The GOS, or alternatively the more detailed GOS-E, has been most commonly used. The GOS-E is an 8-point ordinal rating scale that is determined by surveying patients and/or their caregivers face to face or by phone. However, the nuances of the different points on the scale are often lost in clinical trials due to dichotomization of the GOS-E into "favorable" or "unfavorable" outcomes [22]. This oversimplification ignores the multidimensional nature of outcome following TBI, which can be characterized by physical limitations, cognitive deficits, poor executive function, and, as a result, difficulty with employment and socialization [10]. Furthermore, the assignment of "upper severe disability" (when dividing severe disability into upper and lower categories) has been variably assigned to either good or poor outcomes on the dichotomized GOS-E, with valid arguments for doing so on both sides.

Recently, increased emphasis has been placed on the need to incorporate a cognitive endpoint into TBI research, given that cognitive deficits are hallmarks of TBI patients across severity. A cognitive endpoint would add a level of detail not captured by the GOS or GOS-E and would enable researchers to distinguish between patients who scored at the upper end of the outcome scale. Additionally, since cognition is affected by multiple TBI processes, a cognitive endpoint would measure the overall effect of an intervention, rather than its impact on a specific pathophysiologic process [30]. One option for measuring cognitive outcome is to incorporate a battery of tests that explore various cognitive domains, including attention, memory, processing speed, and executive functioning. An alternative option is to use a cognition composite score, which would provide a single endpoint. This is the approach that was taken by the COBRIT trial [20, 21] and would be useful in validation studies, discussions with the Food and Drug Administration (FDA), meta-analyses, and discussions with families [30]. However, composite outcome measurements should *not* be used if the treatment effect is not equal across all of the components of the composite score [28].

In addition to long-term cognitive endpoints, future clinical trials will benefit from incorporating early mechanistic targeting using short-term surrogate endpoints in order to obtain early verification that the intervention is having the expected effect on individual pathophysiological processes. For example, in a recently completed Phase II trial evaluating the use of glibenclamide (RP-1127) as a neuroprotective agent following TBI (NCT01454154), the primary outcomes were changes in the degree of edema and hemorrhage at 72 h post-injury relative to baseline imaging rather than long-term survival or functional outcomes. Further advances in neuroimaging and TBI biomarkers will facilitate early mechanistic targeting by allowing specific pathophysiological processes to be tracked and early responses to treatment to be determined. This will allow more precise targeting of the particular mechanisms that are involved in that patient's injury. Innovative monitoring modalities, including microdialysis and brain tissue oximetry, may also play a role in differentiating between individual pathophysiologies, enabling the application of "precision medicine" by targeting treatments to individual patients. This would allow patients to serve as their own controls by tracking their responses over time, enabling the early confirmation of a treatment effect [10, 22].

Innovative Techniques for the Statistical Analysis of Clinical Trial Data

While the design issues described earlier will be critical when planning future clinical trials in TBI, the proper analysis of trial data is also integral. Two analytical methods that have attracted much attention are (1) covariate adjustment and (2) ordinal analysis. Covariate adjustment has been advocated as a method for handling patient heterogeneity, since including patients with different prognoses (particularly those with extremely good or extremely poor prognoses) decreases the statistical power of the study. While

one approach is to perform "prognostic targeting" by including only those patients with an intermediate prognostic risk, the resultant decrease in the recruitment rate would extend the duration of the study. Covariate adjustment, on the other hand, allows for broad enrollment criteria but adjusts the estimate of the treatment effect for predictors of outcome, thereby accounting for unbalanced prognostic factors [22, 26].

In order to accurately apply the principle of covariate adjustment, it is necessary to first know which variables are predictors of patient outcome. Much of this information has been derived from the International Mission on Prognosis and Clinical Trial (IMPACT) Design in TBI study group, an international multidisciplinary study group that was initiated in 2003 in order to improve the design and analysis of TBI clinical trials. The IMPACT investigators had several goals, one of which was to develop and validate sophisticated prognostic models using the data from numerous randomized clinical trials and observational studies. Their work resulted in (1) a core model that utilizes demographic and injury severity variables including age, GCS motor score, and pupillary reactivity; (2) an extended model that incorporates radiographic information and secondary insults such as hypoxia and hypotension; and (3) a laboratory model based on data such as glucose and hemoglobin levels [11, 31, 32]. These models allow the prognostic risk estimate to be calculated and reported for the treatment and the placebo groups separately, thereby obtaining a less biased estimate of the treatment effect [11, 22].

Ordinal analysis has also become increasingly recognized as an important element of clinical trial analysis (Fig. 1). The GOS or the GOS-E, which is among the most commonly utilized outcome measures in TBI studies, is often dichotomized into "favorable" or "unfavorable" outcomes. However, even within each group of outcomes, differences in the GOS can reflect clinically meaningful differences. Therefore, dichotomization does not fully utilize the ordinal scale, which characterizes the GOS [22, 26]. One alternative is the sliding dichotomy approach, which adjusts the threshold for "favorable" vs.

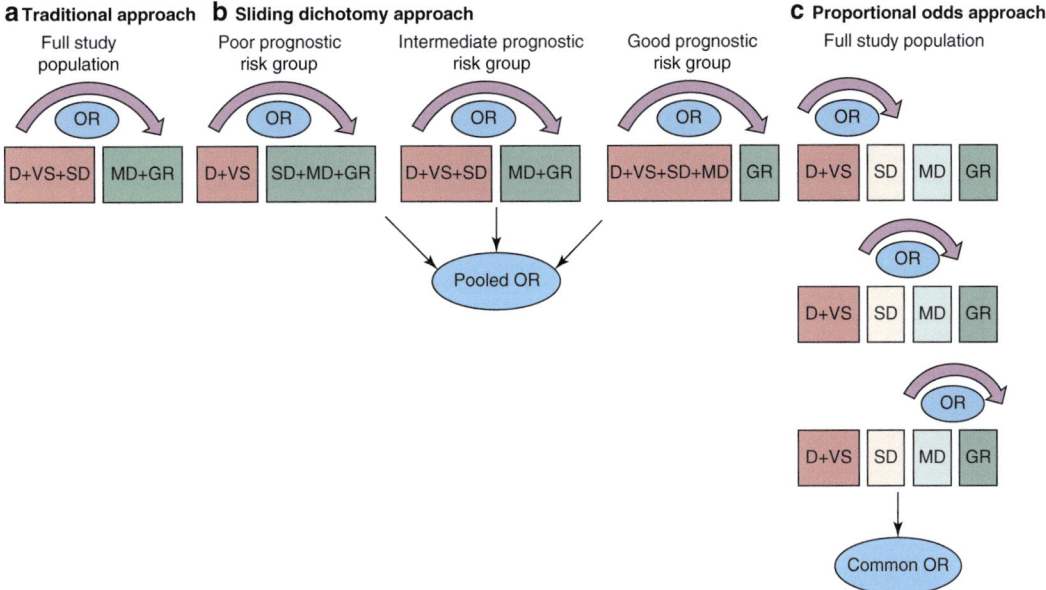

Fig. 1 Approaches to analyze the Glasgow Outcome Scale as the primary outcome measure in randomized controlled trials of traumatic brain injury. The traditional approach (**a**) to efficacy analysis is to dichotomize the Glasgow Outcome Scale into unfavorable outcomes (dead [D], vegetative state [VS], or severe disability [SD]) versus favorable outcomes (moderate disability [MD] or good recovery [GR]). The proportions of patients with an unfavorable outcome in the treatment and placebo groups are compared by calculating an odds ratio (OR) with logistic regression analysis. With the sliding dichotomy approach (**b**), the study population is first subdivided in (e.g., three) equally large prognostic risk groups. For each of the risk groups, the point of the dichotomy of the Glasgow Outcome Scale is based on the baseline prognostic risk (e.g., for patients in the good prognostic risk group, only good recovery is judged a favorable outcome). A pooled odds ratio is calculated, which can be interpreted as the summary measure for having a better outcome than expected. With the proportional odds approach (**c**), the population is not subdivided. The proportional odds model considers every possible way the Glasgow Outcome Scale can be dichotomized, assuming that the odds ratio for a better versus a worse outcome is similar wherever the scale is dichotomized (the proportional odds assumption). The common odds ratio can be interpreted as a summary measure for the shift in outcome across the full scale. Reprinted with permission from Maas AI, Murray GD, Roozenbeek B, Lingsma HF, Butcher I, McHugh GS, et al.; International Mission on Prognosis Analysis of Clinical Trials in Traumatic Brain Injury (IMPACT) Study Group, Advancing care for traumatic brain injury: findings from the IMPACT studies and perspectives on future research. Lancet Neurol. 2013 Dec;12(12):1200–10

"unfavorable" according to the baseline prognostic risk. Patients with a very poor prognosis may consider survival to be a favorable outcome, whereas those with a very good prognosis will have higher expectations for their functional status. Another alternative involves proportional odds regression, an analytical method that measures an "overall effect" (i.e., the common odds ratio) by taking into account every possible point where the ordinal scale can be dichotomized. This strategy relies on the assumption that the odds ratio is identical wherever the scale is dichotomized and measures the overall shift across the GOS [26]; however, this assumption may not be a valid one.

The IMPACT database allowed simulations to be conducted using each of these analytical approaches. The investigators found that the incorporation of ordinal analysis, whether via a sliding dichotomy approach or using proportional odds analysis, increased the statistical power and reduced the sample size requirements by 23–30%. Combining ordinal analysis with covariate adjustment increased the statistical power even further, reducing the sample size requirements by up to 50%. These findings were validated by applying the two approaches to the data that were obtained during the CRASH trial [26]. Although covariate adjustment has been used in less than one-quarter of the randomized clinical trials that have been performed to date, and ordinal analysis has been used even less frequently, both approaches should be considered in future clinical trials in TBI [4].

Looking to the Future: International and Multidisciplinary Collaboration

In order to overcome the current limitations of TBI research, a fundamental change in the way clinical trials are perceived is underway. Multidisciplinary working groups have come to realize that single-center randomized trials are insufficient and are instead advocating the systematic collection of large-scale data via patient registries so that observational studies can be performed and systems biology-based approaches can be applied [19]. Large-scale data collection across multiple sites in various countries requires careful classification and organization and has culminated in the development of formal common data elements (CDEs) [33]. The International Initiative on TBI Research (InTBIR) was founded for this purpose in 2011 (Table 1). InTBIR, which is a col-

Table 1 Studies funded in the context of the International Initiative for Traumatic Brain Injury Research (InTBIR) (Reprinted with permission from Maas AI, Murray GD, Roozenbeek B, Lingsma HF, Butcher I, McHugh GS, et al.; International Mission on Prognosis Analysis of Clinical Trials in Traumatic Brain Injury (IMPACT) Study Group, Advancing care for traumatic brain injury: findings from the IMPACT studies and perspectives on future research. Lancet Neurol. 2013 Dec;12(12):1200–10)

	Institution and Principal Investigator	Project
European Commission		
CENTER-TBI	Antwerp University Hospital (A Maas) University of Cambridge (D Menon)	Collaborative European NeuroTrauma Effectiveness Research in TBI
CREACTIVE	IRCCS—Istituto di Ricerche Farmacologiche Mario Negri Milano (G Bertolini)	Collaborative Research on Acute Traumatic Brain Injury in Intensive Care Medicine in Europe
US National Institutes of Health		
ADAPT	Children's Hospital of Pittsburgh (M Bell)	Approaches and Decisions for Acute Pediatric TBI
TRACK-TBI	University of California (G Manley)	Transforming Research and Clinical Knowledge in Traumatic Brain Injury
Canadian Institutes of Health Research[a]		
Safe to Play	Hotchkiss Brain Institute, University of Calgary (C Emery)	A longitudinal research program to establish best practice in the prevention, early diagnosis, and management of sport-related concussion in youth ice hockey players
Innovation Through the Use of Common Data	McGill University (I Gagnon)	Generating innovation through the use of common data: improving the diagnosis and treatment of pediatric and adolescent mild traumatic brain injury in Canada
Play Game	University of Calgary (K Barlow)	Postconcussion syndrome Affecting Youth: GABAergic effects of Melatonin
Postconcussion Problems in Pediatric TBI	Children's Hospital of Eastern Ontario, University of Ottawa (R Zemek)	Predicting Persistent Postconcussive Problems in Pediatrics (SP)
"NeuroCare" as Innovation in Intervention	University of Toronto (M Keightley)	A Neurophysiological Approach to Determine Readiness for Return to Activity

[a]Also 15 catalyst grants (1-year duration) and 3 new postdoctoral awards; co-funding partners for the team grants are Fonds de recherche du Québec Santé, Hotchkiss Brain Institute, Ontario Brain Institute, and Ontario Neurotrauma Foundation

laboration between the European Commission, the US NINDS, and the Canadian Institute of Health Research, undertakes projects whose focus is standardized data collection, in order to facilitate comparative effectiveness research (15). By encouraging international, multidisciplinary data collection, InTBIR will increase the generalizability of TBI research [26].

One of the key projects within InTBIR, the Collaborative European NeuroTrauma Effectiveness Research in TBI (CENTER-TBI) study, will involve the collection of prospective, nonrandomized, observational core data from up to 80 sites in 22 countries over 18 months. The goal is to produce a registry containing enough data to perform comprehensive comparative effectiveness research and identify best practices [15]. Similarly, the Transforming Research and Clinical Knowledge in TBI (TRACK-TBI) study is a large, multicenter, prospective observational study whose goal is to design a platform for collecting and analyzing clinical, biomarker, and imaging data [33].

These projects reflect a growing trend toward increased international and multidisciplinary cooperation within the TBI research community. As the complexity and heterogeneity of TBI become better appreciated, enthusiasm for single-center randomized trials involving a single neuroprotective agent continues to wane. Innovative approaches involving the collection of high-quality large-scale data, novel trial design, inclusion criteria and sample sizes that account for patient heterogeneity, more sophisticated outcome measurements, and rigorous statistical analysis will shape the future of clinical trials in TBI for many years to come.

Acknowledgments and Disclosures This work was supported in part by the Department of Defense PTSD/TBI Clinical Consortium (HME). Dr. Eisenberg is an unpaid consultant for InSightec Ltd. and is an independent neurotrauma consultant to the National Football League.

References

1. Carney N, Totten AM, O'Reilly C, Ullman JS, Hawryluk GW, Bell MJ, et al. Guidelines for the management of severe traumatic brain injury, fourth edition. Neurosurgery. 2016;80(1):6–15.

2. Maas AI, Roozenbeek B, Manley GT. Clinical trials in traumatic brain injury: past experience and current developments. Neurotherapeutics. 2010;7(1):115–26.

3. Maas AI, Steyerberg EW, Murray GD, Bullock R, Baethmann A, Marshall LF, et al. Why have recent trials of neuroprotective agents in head injury failed to show convincing efficacy? A pragmatic analysis and theoretical considerations. Neurosurgery. 1999;44(6):1286–98.

4. Bragge P, Synnot A, Maas AI, Menon DK, Cooper DJ, Rosenfeld JV, et al. A state-of-the-science overview of randomized controlled trials evaluating acute management of moderate-to-severe traumatic brain injury. J Neurotrauma. 2016;33(16):1461–78.

5. Skolnick BE, Maas AI, Narayan RK, van der Hoop RG, MacAllister T, Ward JD, et al. A clinical trial of progesterone for severe traumatic brain injury. N Engl J Med. 2014;371(26):2467–76.

6. Wright DW, Yeatts SD, Silbergleit R, Palesch YY, Hertzberg VS, Frankel M, et al. Very early administration of progesterone for acute traumatic brain injury. N Engl J Med. 2014;371(26):2457–66.

7. Stein DG. Embracing failure: what the Phase III progesterone studies can teach about TBI clinical trials. Brain Inj. 2015;29(11):1259–72.

8. Wright DW, Kellermann AL, Hertzberg VS, Clark PL, Frankel M, Goldstein FC, et al. Protect: a randomized clinical trial of progesterone for acute traumatic brain injury. Ann Emerg Med. 2007;49(4):391–402, 402 e391–392.

9. Xiao G, Wei J, Yan W, Wang W, Lu Z. Improved outcomes from the administration of progesterone for patients with acute severe traumatic brain injury: a randomized controlled trial. Crit Care. 2008;12(2):R61.

10. Maas AI, Menon DK, Lingsma HF, Pineda JA, Sandel ME, Manley GT. Re-orientation of clinical research in traumatic brain injury: report of an International Workshop on Comparative Effectiveness Research. J Neurotrauma. 2012;29(1):32–46.

11. Maas AI, Steyerberg EW, Marmarou A, McHugh GS, Lingsma HF, Butcher I, et al. Impact recommendations for improving the design and analysis of clinical trials in moderate to severe traumatic brain injury. Neurotherapeutics. 2010;7(1):127–34.

12. Schumacher M, Denier C, Oudinet JP, Adams D, Guennoun R. Progesterone neuroprotection: the background of clinical trial failure. J Steroid Biochem Mol Biol. 2016;160:53–66.

13. Menon DK, Maas AI. EPO in traumatic brain injury: two strikes...but not out? Lancet. 2015;386(10012):2452–4.

14. Nichol A, French C, Little L, Haddad S, Presneill J, Arabi Y, et al. Erythropoietin in traumatic brain injury (EPO-TBI): a double-blind randomised controlled trial. Lancet. 2015;386(10012):2499–506.

15. Maas AI, Menon DK, Steyerberg EW, Citerio G, Lecky F, Manley GT, et al. Collaborative European Neurotrauma Effectiveness Research in Traumatic Brain Injury (CENTER-TBI): a prospective longitudinal observational study. Neurosurgery. 2015;76(1):67–80.

16. Menon DK, Maas AI. Traumatic brain injury in 2014. Progress, failures and new approaches for TBI research. Nat Rev Neurol. 2015;11(2):71–2.

17. Cooper DJ, Rosenfeld JV, Murray L, Arabi YM, Davies AR, D'Urso P, et al. Decompressive craniectomy in diffuse traumatic brain injury. N Engl J Med. 2011;364(16):1493–502.

18. Hutchinson PJ, Kolias AG, Timofeev IS, Corteen EA, Czosnyka M, Timothy J, et al. Trial of decompressive craniectomy for traumatic intracranial hypertension. N Engl J Med. 2016;375(12):1119–30.

19. Timmons SD, Toms SA. Comparative effectiveness research in neurotrauma. Neurosurg Focus. 2012;33(1):E3.

20. Zafonte RD, Bagiella E, Ansel BM, Novack TA, Friedewald WT, Hesdorffer DC, et al. Effect of citicoline on functional and cognitive status among patients with traumatic brain injury: Citicoline Brain Injury Treatment Trial (COBRIT). JAMA. 2012;308(19):1993–2000.

21. Zafonte R, Friedewald WT, Lee SM, Levin B, Diaz-Arrastia R, Ansel B, et al. The Citicoline Brain Injury Treatment (COBRIT) trial: design and methods. J Neurotrauma. 2009;26(12):2207–16.

22. Roozenbeek B, Lingsma HF, Maas AI. New considerations in the design of clinical trials for traumatic brain injury. Clin Investig (Lond). 2012;2(2):153–62.

23. Edwards P, Arango M, Balica L, Cottingham R, El-Sayed H, Farrell B, et al. Final results of MRC CRASH, a randomised placebo-controlled trial of intravenous corticosteroid in adults with head injury-outcomes at 6 months. Lancet. 2005;365(9475):1957–9.

24. White SJ, Freedman LS. Allocation of patients to treatment groups in a controlled clinical study. Br J Cancer. 1978;37(5):849–57.

25. Edwards P, Farrell B, Lomas G, Mashru R, Ritchie N, Roberts I, et al. The MRC CRASH trial: study design, baseline data, and outcome in 1000 randomised patients in the pilot phase. Emerg Med J. 2002;19(6):510–4.

26. Maas AI, Murray GD, Roozenbeek B, Lingsma HF, Butcher I, McHugh GS, et al. Advancing care for traumatic brain injury: findings from the impact studies and perspectives on future research. Lancet Neurol. 2013;12(12):1200–10.

27. Bagiella E, Novack TA, Ansel B, Diaz-Arrastia R, Dikmen S, Hart T, et al. Measuring outcome in traumatic brain injury treatment trials: recommendations from the traumatic brain injury clinical trials network. J Head Trauma Rehabil. 2010;25(5):375–82.

28. Alali AS, Vavrek D, Barber J, Dikmen S, Nathens AB, Temkin NR. Comparative study of outcome measures and analysis methods for traumatic brain injury trials. J Neurotrauma. 2015;32(8):581–9.

29. Zelnick LR, Morrison LJ, Devlin SM, Bulger EM, Brasel KJ, Sheehan K, et al. Addressing the challenges of obtaining functional outcomes in traumatic brain injury research: missing data patterns, timing of follow-up, and three prognostic models. J Neurotrauma. 2014;31(11):1029–38.

30. Silverberg ND, Crane PK, Dams-O'Connor K, Holdnack J, Ivins BJ, Lange RT, et al. Developing a cognition endpoint for traumatic brain injury clinical trials. J Neurotrauma. 2017;34(2):363–71.

31. Roozenbeek B, Lingsma HF, Lecky FE, Lu J, Weir J, Butcher I, et al. Prediction of outcome after moderate and severe traumatic brain injury: external validation of the International Mission on Prognosis and Analysis of Clinical Trials (IMPACT) and Corticoid Randomisation After Significant Head injury (CRASH) prognostic models. Crit Care Med. 2012;40(5):1609–17.

32. Sun H, Lingsma HF, Steyerberg EW, Maas AI. External validation of the international mission for prognosis and analysis of clinical trials in traumatic brain injury: prognostic models for traumatic brain injury on the study of the neuroprotective activity of progesterone in severe traumatic brain injuries trial. J Neurotrauma. 2016;33(16):1535–43.

33. Yue JK, Vassar MJ, Lingsma HF, Cooper SR, Okonkwo DO, Valadka AB, et al. Transforming research and clinical knowledge in traumatic brain injury pilot: multicenter implementation of the common data elements for traumatic brain injury. J Neurotrauma. 2013;30(22):1831–44.

34. Wright DWYS, Silbergleit R, Palesch YY, Hertzberg VS, Frankel M, Goldstein FC, Caveney AF, Howlett-Smith H, Bengelink EM, Manley GT, Merck LH, Janis LS, Barsan WG, Investigators NETT. Very early administration of progesterone for acute traumatic brain injury. N Engl J Med. 2014;371(26):2457–66.

Who's My Doctor? Team-Based Management

James Leiphart and James Ecklund

Introduction

The unexpected happens: There is a motor vehicle crash, a fall from scaffolding at a construction site, a gunshot, and a resulting traumatic brain injury (TBI). The EMTs arrive, stabilize the injured patients, and take them to the hospital for care. Then the care becomes complicated. The patient is evaluated by the emergency department medical team and may be admitted to that hospital or may be transferred to a higher-level trauma care hospital. Hospital admission may be to a trauma intensive care unit (ICU), a neuro ICU, or even a medical ICU. There may be in-house ICU coverage 24 h a day, 7 days a week by an ICU team, or one physician may be responsible for ICU care during the entire ICU stay—covering from home at night and on weekends. There could be trauma doctors providing care and almost certainly a neurosurgeon as well, but the delineation of who is in charge of what part of the care may not be clear. The involvement of residents, fellows, and medical students may add

additional complexities to care, especially with work hour restrictions for residents and frequent sign outs. A new doctor or team of doctors may care for the patient once out of the ICU but still in the hospital, and a completely different doctor or team of doctors will be responsible for rehabilitation.

This complexity coupled with a higher standard of care for head trauma than in the past creates new challenges. Decades ago, much less was known about head trauma, and fewer treatments were available. Standard of care was stabilizing vital signs and nursing the injured patient in a quiet environment with little stimulation. Many hospitals were able to provide this level of care, and usually only one doctor was necessary for managing the care. Increased knowledge about brain injury, better care for the injured, and increased concern about the impact of doctor fatigue on patient care have led to our environment of transfers of care, collaboration, and team approaches. The care is decidedly better, but the new approach sometimes leaves the patient and the patient's family wondering, "Who's my doctor?" In this chapter we will explore the evidence, or lack thereof, that has led to this multitude of caregivers and discuss the positive and negative impacts resulting from this type of care.

J. Leiphart, MD, PhD, FACS
J. Ecklund, MD, FACS (✉)
Inova Neuroscience and Spine Institute,
Falls Church, VA, USA
e-mail: James.Leiphart@inova.org;
James.Ecklund@inova.org

Specialized Trauma Centers and the Trauma Team

Improvements in traumatic brain injury outcomes have occurred over time but appear to be grouped around specific time periods in which there have been significant changes in the way patients are cared for. A recent comprehensive review of the traumatic brain injury literature over the past 150 years has elucidated the periodic nature of the improvements in outcome and has attempted to establish the causes of the improvements [1]. The authors report a nearly 50% decrease in mortality over a 150-year period, but the improvements in outcomes came in specific epochs. They report a gradual improvement in mortality from traumatic brain injury over the period of 1885–1930. There was subsequently no improvement in survivability until the period between 1970 and 1990 when traumatic brain injury mortality again decreased significantly. The authors express some surprise that there were no improvements between 1930 and 1970 because this period saw significant advances in resuscitation techniques and greater availability of neurosurgeons. However, they note that this period also saw a great increase in severe traumatic brain injury from high-speed motor vehicle collisions. They attribute the reductions in mortality between 1970 and 1990 to the introduction of computed tomography (CT) scanning and intracranial pressure (ICP) monitoring. Although this study found no improvement in TBI mortality from 1990 onward, another study of TBI outcomes in New York State from 2001 to 2009 did find a decrease in TBI patient mortality from 22 to 13% with the implementation of the Trauma Foundation Guidelines for the Management of Severe Traumatic Brain Injury [2]. This agrees with the results from a single trauma center that implemented the same guidelines in 1995 and found a 4.5% reduction in mortality among TBI patients from 18.2 to 13.7% comparing the period before guidelines (1991–1996) to the period after implementing the guidelines (1997–2000) [3]. Another trauma center saw a decrease in mortality from TBI from 27.8 to 18.8% comparing their pre-guidelines period (1999–2000) to the guide-lines period (2001–2006) [4], and a third trauma center found a decrease in overall TBI-related mortality from 19.95 to 13.5% comparing the period before implementing standardized care guidelines (1992–1996) to the period in which multiple consensus guidelines were used (1997–2000) [5]. Protocol-driven TBI therapy led to improved outcomes in severe TBI patients being treated in the neuroscience ICU [6]. These results would suggest that higher-level trauma centers that are able to perform ICP monitoring and have traumatic brain injury protocols in place would have better overall outcomes in TBI.

Several studies evaluating TBI outcomes in relation to the trauma center providing care have supported this conclusion. Three studies have shown decreased mortality rates for TBI in high-volume trauma centers compared to lower-volume trauma centers [7–9], but no volume-mortality relationship was found for TBI patients in another study [10]. This agrees with the finding of lower mortality among all ICU patients in high-volume hospitals compared to lower-volume hospitals [11]. Lower mortality in all patients in level 1 trauma centers compared to non-trauma centers has been reported [12]. Significant variability in outcomes of TBI between various medical centers has also been found [13]. One study reported an 8% increase in mortality among TBI patients treated at non-neurosurgical centers compared to those treated at neurosurgical centers [14]. However, the transfer of patients also seems to be associated with risks to patients with traumatic brain injury. Two studies have demonstrated higher mortality among TBI patients transferred to higher-level trauma centers from other medical centers compared to TBI patients who were brought directly to the same higher-level trauma centers following their injuries [15, 16]. Should all traumatic brain injury patients be brought directly to high-volume level 1 trauma centers with neurosurgical services available to improve their care? Although there is evidence that it would improve outcomes, the challenge remains that this approach would rely on triage at the level of the first responder who lacks the additional information the emergency department physicians and CT scan may provide; therefore the resultant low threshold for transport of potentially head-injured patients to high-volume level 1 medical centers could overwhelm those medical centers' resources. The literature does support the transfer of the severe TBI patient to the high-volume medical center as is currently a common practice. A multicenter study of moderate to severe TBI patients indicates that currently 86% of TBI patients are directly transported to the participating level 1 trauma center [17].

The survival outcome advantage for TBI appears to be due to access to neurosurgical care and the use of TBI guidelines. Given the complexity of TBI and the treatment modalities necessary for effective care of severe TBI, effective treatment requires a multidisciplinary approach with close collaboration between the neurosurgeon and the trauma surgery service [18]. The role of the trauma surgeon over time has changed, threatening the availability of this key partner in the care of the TBI patient. Subspecialization and technological advances have reduced the number of surgical procedures performed by the trauma surgeon. One study found that only 11% of patients on the trauma service at a single level 1 trauma center were operated on by a trauma surgeon [19]. This means that the majority of care delivered by the trauma surgeon is nonsurgical, which could lead to dissatisfaction among trauma surgeons and difficulty filling trauma surgery positions in the future. One effort to combat this trend is the movement to add acute care surgery to the trauma surgery service, which adds elective surgery procedures to the care they deliver [20]. This approach has the potential to increase interest in trauma surgery subspecialization among general surgeons, a key component to modern TBI treatment strategies, but it also necessitates rotation in and out of the acute trauma care service leading to an increased number of physicians being primarily responsible for the patient's care over time.

Intensive Care Unit

Intensive care unit (ICU) care is a critical component of the care of all severe TBI and many moderate TBI patients [21]. ICU care is necessary for maintaining oxygenation and perfusion, providing nutrition with appropriate glycemic control, controlling temperature and seizures, monitoring and treating ICP, and managing ventilation and the necessary concomitant sedation required, all of which can have a significant impact on the outcome for the TBI patient. A multicenter study of moderate and severe TBI patients showed that 70% were admitted to the ICU (83% of severe TBI patients) [17]. Ninety-six percent of these patients required mechanical ventilation, and 38% of the severe and 8% of the moderate TBI patients admitted to the ICU required ICP monitoring. Reductions in mortality over the history of TBI treatment have been partially attributed to ICU care [1, 22]. Protocol-driven ICU care is associated with improved TBI patient outcomes [2–6]. The volume of TBI patients seen in the ICU does not seem to make a difference in mortality [10]. ICU care is a necessity for many TBI patients, but there is significant variability in how ICU care is delivered, from single practitioner coverage to a team approach with 24-h, 7-day-a-week in-house coverage with rotating physicians in charge.

The vast majority of moderate to severe TBI patients are cared for at level 1 trauma centers, which have 24-h in-house critical care provided by the trauma surgery service, so patterns of ICU physician coverage in TBI have not been explicitly studied. However, for those non-level 1 trauma centers that manage the care of mild-to-moderate TBI patients, ICU coverage by intensivists may make a difference in patient outcomes. The only guidance in this area comes from studies of intensivist coverage of general ICU critical care patients. This literature is mixed in its findings. Some studies have found better patient outcomes in ICUs that have intensivist-led teams [23, 24], but this finding is not universal [25], and in-house overnight intensivist coverage for general ICU patients produced no measureable benefit in patient outcomes [26]. It is difficult to believe that these findings, especially those that did not demonstrate benefit of intensivist-led care and overnight in-house intensivist coverage, can be generalized to the care of the moderate to severe TBI patient population—one of the most complex patient populations cared for in the ICU. Protocol-driven care, which has demonstrated benefits in TBI patient outcomes, requires an intensity of management that could not be delivered without 24-h in-house intensivist care, so one could reasonably conclude that better outcomes among the TBI population do require 24-h in-house coverage by an intensivist, which includes the trauma surgeons in their critical care capacity.

Even though there is a benefit outcome of ICU care for the TBI patient, negative effects of the ICU environment have been documented. The constant high ICU noise level has a negative impact on patient sleep [27, 28]. Only about half of the patients in ICU surveys felt that the environment was not too noisy [29, 30]. ICU patients sleep nearly 8 h in a 24-h sleep cycle, but the sleep is highly fragmented, and the majority of the sleep is in stage 1 or stage 2 [31]. The authors of the study demonstrating this disrupted sleep point out that disrupted sleep is associated with immune dysfunction and may impede successful recovery. Noise reduction strategies can be helpful, improving patient sleep by 10–68% [28]. The psychological impact of being in the ICU can be significant as well. Prolonged ICU care can lead to posttraumatic stress disorder, both in patients and in their family members, delirium, hallucinations, delusions, confusion, agitation, depression, anxiety, and bizarre dreams or nightmares [32]. Although some patients report remembering everything about their ICU stay [33], most patients have unclear recollections [30], and many recall dreams that were sometimes confused with reality [30, 32, 34]. The most important desire of patients and their families in the ICU is to feel safe [32], but in one study, 55% of patients reported being frightened the majority of the time [29]. It is known that stress inhibits the immune response in ICU patients [35], so stress reduction by the patient care team is not only a patient quality of life issue but also critical to patients' abilities to fight disease and have optimum outcomes.

How do we mitigate the stress innate to the ICU experience for so many patients? One important step is to understand each patient's concerns and needs. A study of patient's reported concerns compared to nurses impressions of patient concerns showed important differences [36]. The number 1 and 2 concerns for patients in the ICU were tubes in the nose and mouth and being stuck by needles, neither of which were rated highly as perceived concerns by nurses. Nurses reported not being in control of yourself and being tied down highly as concerns of the patients, whereas these were not within the top five concerns of the patients. There was clear concordance between patients' concerns and nurses' impressions of their concerns when it came to being in pain and being unable to sleep, but the study suggested that better understanding of patient needs could help in addressing them and reducing ICU stress.

The following exchange was reported in a paper on patients' experiences in the ICU [33]:

> "Ann is a 65-year-old woman who spent two months in the intensive care unit (ICU), most of that time in critical condition. Years later she looked terrific. I described her as an 'ICU success story.' She started to cry, explaining that her experience in ICU had taken away her dignity. She remembered being washed in bed, lying naked, while staff joked about their social lives. She told me that without dignity she would rather be dead. Every day for the past 3 years she has wished that she was dead."

Clearly, misunderstanding of a patient's emotional and psychological needs can be devastating to the effort of optimizing her or his emotional state and improving her or his ability to fight disease.

Another clear strategy for reducing stress is improving communication. Poor communication has been identified as a major source of stress among ICU patients [29, 33]. In the care of TBI patients, the necessity for transfers to higher level of care, collaboration between neurosurgical and trauma surgery clinicians, and changes in primary physician caregivers innate to 24-h in-house ICU coverage all have the potential to lead to fragmented and ineffective communication, which could increase patient and family stress.

The following is another example of a family's experience during their daughter's ICU stay [33]:

"(It was) said in front of me that Kathy was not going to be all right and that we may as well pull the plug... (The nurse) was talking to another nurse at the foot of the bed and I was sitting beside Kathy. I could hear him clearly," patient's mother. "The two years that Kathy had been sick, we were always told exactly what was going on. We were used to being talked to as if we knew what was being talked about... This was the approach we were used to—honest communication. We found this a great help. Kathy especially needs to know what is going on. To have some uppity (expletive)-wik like that (in the ICU)—it's pretty upsetting," patient's father.

This illustrates both how helpful effective communication can be and the potential detrimental effect of even a single episode of poor communication. This is not limited to nurse interaction but could come from any member of the patient care team. Every patient interaction has the potential to help or to harm, whether it be the primary physician, the consultant, the resident, the physician's assistant, the medical student, the nurse, the tech, or even the person delivering the food tray or cleaning the room. All are important in creating the environment of good communication. Regular and effective communication between all of the caregivers for each patient is essential in producing effective, consistent communication with patients and families.

The nursing staff is an important resource that must be effectively leveraged in creating effective communication in the ICU and producing a lower-stress environment. Patients have reported the positive experience of feeling safe and secure from having a nurse close to them [29]. Nurses have by far the greatest amount of time interacting with the patients and their families. Frequently, nurses will be assigned to the same patients day after day, so nurses have the potential to have the greatest impact on reducing patient stress. A key component to optimizing the positive impact of the nurses in the ICU is communication between the physicians and the nurses. This communication is not always optimal [37]. Another component is effective nurse-patient communication. A study found that the majority of nurse-patient communications were effective, but patients felt that 40% of the communications with nurses were somewhat to

extremely difficult [38]. Of importance in the care of TBI patients, ICU nurses find it more difficult to communicate with unconscious patients and patients who cannot effectively communicate back, creating barriers to the potential benefit provided by nurse-patient interactions [39]. Another clear component in optimizing the positive impact of nurses on patient communication and care is the nurse-to-patient ratio. A nurse-to-patient ratio of 1:1.5 was found to be associated with lower risk of inpatient death [40]. Whether this is from more communication and positive effects of emotional well-being on the patients' ability to fight disease or a more direct ability to deliver patient care more effectively when dealing with fewer patients, the effect cannot be ignored and should be considered in trying to achieve the best possible care for TBI patients.

ICU care is necessary for many TBI patients, but it is an artificial environment with negative influences as well as positive. For this reason we must continue to evaluate where we can improve patient care and make the improvements necessary.

Impact of Night and Weekend Shifts: Transfers of Care

The increased number of physicians involved in the care of the TBI patient leads to increased transfers of care between clinicians and more frequent sign outs. Sign outs and transfers of care have risks of their own that require study and adaptation to reduce the potential harm. One study that looked at 88 house staff sign-out sessions, including the sign outs of 503 patients, found that 5 patients had delays in diagnosis related to sign out, 1 of which resulted in an ICU transfer, and 4 patients had near misses [41]. This approximately 1% risk of error and similar risk of near miss is not terribly high but does present an opportunity for improvement in the pursuit of 100% patient safety. Another study of house staff sign outs found inconsistencies between the first and second sign outs in 22% of cases in which a second sign out was performed during the same day [42]. The factors that were found to be associated with better sign out were patient familiarity, feeling responsible for the patient, single sign out per day, senior resident presence at sign out, and a comprehensive written sign out. This is a very clear demonstration that the risks increase with the increased number of sign outs. It also provides techniques by which sign outs can be made more effective beyond the obvious reduction in the number of sign outs. Another study of 26 interns caring for 82 patients over 2 call nights found a self-reported rate of 25 incidents resulting from communication error [43]. In resident surveys about sign outs, 31% reported that an event occurred for which they were inadequately prepared because of ineffective sign out [44]. This occurred in an equal rate among residents within the regular care team as residents cross covering at night, and half of these incidents were with patients whom the resident had cared for in the past.

There are many opportunities for improvement in the removal of identified barriers to effective sign out [45]. The physical setting should be private and quiet. The social setting should be facilitating to the open exchange of all information with a lack of hierarchical structure. Language barriers among physicians should be recognized and may require repeating back information to verify correct communication. Direct communication between clinicians in a face-to-face interaction is always superior to electronic communication and to written-only sign out. Time constraints can diminish the effectiveness of sign out, so adequate time should be allocated for sign out. And standard education concerning sign out methods, commonly neglected as a tool, could improve reliability and accuracy of sign outs. A limited association between resident handoff training and patient outcomes has been reported [46]. A study of postsurgical handoffs at a single institution showed that some type of distraction was present in almost every handoff, with three or more distractions in 70% of handoffs and six or more distractions in 35% of handoffs [47]. Eliminating such distractions will be important in improving patient safety, especially in the current environment of increasing transfers of patient care.

A number of different handover tools have been developed in an attempt to improve patient care [48–56]. These handover tools were developed in the British National Medical System with the implementation of the European Working Time Directive that limits physicians to a 13-h shift [55]. The Royal College of Physicians recognized that handovers of care are a time when errors are more likely to occur, which prompted a number of the medical centers and clinical services within those medical centers to implement or standardize handover tools and put in place policies that would encourage their use. The majority of these tools are electronic, but some protocols involved placing a printed copy with the patient's chart and required signatures from the physician initiating the transfer of care and the physician receiving the transfer of care. Although some of the studies focused on shift-change handover tools [50, 54, 56], mostly on surgical services [50, 54], the majority of the handover tools were developed for more effective handover on the weekends [48, 49, 51–53, 55]. This is because of a study within the English National Health System that found a higher 30-day mortality rate for patients admitted to the hospital over the weekend [57]. One theory is that the increased mortality is at least partially from inadequate patient handover to the weekend covering physicians [48]. All of these studies succeeded in their measured end point of increasing utilization of their handover tool, but none attempted to measure patient outcome improvements from the handover tools—a shortcoming of the studies. Standardized handover is thought to improve patient care, but there remains a lack of objective evidence.

Anesthesiologists perform regular handovers of patients that are frequently ill and always have acute physiological issues. Following anesthesia best practices in patient handover may help improve TBI patient handover in our current environment of increased transfers of care. A recent systematic review of the anesthesia handover literature resulted in the following recommendations for patient handover that encapsulate many of the ideas already discussed and may be a good template in designing standardized patient handover protocols for TBI patients [58]. The recommendations from this article are as follows:

1. Prepare monitor, alarms, equipment, and fluids before patient arrival.
2. Complete urgent care tasks before the verbal handover.
3. Set aside time for handover communication. Avoid performing other tasks during this time and, conversely, limit conversation while performing tasks.
4. Use the "sterile cockpit"—only patient-specific conversation or urgent clinical interruptions can occur during the handover.
5. All relevant members of the operating room and postoperative receiving teams should be present during the handover.
6. Only one care provider should speak at a time, with minimal distractions and interruptions.
7. Provide an opportunity to ask questions and voice concerns.
8. Document the handover.
9. Use supporting documentation, e.g., lab test results and anesthesia chart.
10. Use structured checklists to guide communication and ensure completeness of information. Use forms or reference cards as reminders.
11. Use protocols to standardize processes.
12. Provide formal team or handover training.

These recommendations could be taken in part or in whole and adapted to the TBI patient care scenario. The most important concept to take away from the discussion of handovers is the necessity of developing a standardized approach and eliminating or minimizing distractions to optimize patient safety in this error-prone but necessary reality of patient care.

Resident Duty Hour Restrictions and Impact on Patient Ownership

Postgraduate medical education has changed greatly over the past two decades, especially in the area of regulations surrounding work hours for resident physicians and interns. The origin of the resident physician or "house officer," another common term for the postgraduate trainee, is just

how the title describes: a physician who is in "house," the hospital, at all times. The original house officers would study under the supervision of one or more physicians and would be given a room in the hospital to sleep. The expectation was that this individual would be in the hospital at all times until the end of training. The time period of training was left up to the physician or physicians providing the training and could be as short as 1 or 2 years, depending on the development of the physician in training. The concept was that of immersion in the care of the patient so that the entire course of the disease process would be appreciated and the resident physician would understand the commitment to complete ownership of each patient under his care. Long before resident physician work hours came under scrutiny following the tragic incident involving Libby Zion in 1984 and work hour restrictions for resident physicians were implemented nationally by the Accreditation Council for Graduate Medical Education (ACGME) in 2003, this pattern of having a "house officer" essentially living in the hospital had been replaced. Residencies were more regimented, with set periods of time necessary to complete training and published call schedules to clarify the rotation of duty necessary for the service to be covered 24 h a day. However, work hours remained long, commonly reaching 100–120 h per week or possibly more.

Resident duty hours, physician fatigue, and supervision of physicians in training came under scrutiny following the highly publicized unexpected death of Libby Zion and the resulting grand jury investigation [59]. One of the recommendations of the grand jury was for the Department of Health to regulate the working hours of resident physicians and interns in training. This episode and the grand jury's findings gained national attention and prompted calls for federal regulation. To stave off the introduction of federal legislation and to keep the regulation of the physician training process with physicians, the ACGME implemented its own regulations for resident work hour restrictions. The initial regulations in 2003 limited all physicians in internship or residency to a maximum of 24 h of continuous duty, a minimum of 10 h off between shifts, and a maximum of 80 h of clinical care activities per week. The updated regulations that went into effect in 2011 further limited the intern work hours to a maximum of 16 h per shift [60]. Several justifications for long resident and intern working hours have been put forward [59]. The most compelling of these are arguments that work hour restrictions will impact patient care, both for current and future patients. The arguments for current patient care impacts go both ways. Some clinicians believe that limiting resident work hours will decrease physician fatigue and improve patient safety, while others believe that limited hours will require more patient care handoffs, which are prone to errors and omissions, and will unnecessarily place patients under the care of physicians who do not know their clinical case the best. The argument for patient care in the future is that future patients will be jeopardized by the training of physicians who do not take ownership of their patients and the care of their illnesses but who rather see themselves as part of an assembly line of care in which they do their limited portion and send the patient down the line to the next station. Because of the significant potential impact on patient care, the evidence for or against these impressions should be examined, and any detrimental effects should be mitigated.

We will start by discussing impressions of the work hour restrictions by the different groups involved and then discuss if any of their issues have been addressed by studies. Less than half of program directors responding to a survey gave overall approval to the 2011 resident guidelines, only 48% approved of restricting senior residents to 24-h shifts, and 71.6% disagreed with limiting the interns to 16-h shifts [60]. The biggest concerns for the program directors were the negative effect on resident education, the negative effects on preparedness for senior roles, the negative impact on patient "ownership," the loss of continuity of care, and the increased number of handoffs. There is also the concern among physician educators that by putting so much focus on the duty hours and wellness of physicians in training, the focus on patient service as the driving principle of the profession will be reduced [61].

Clinicians understand the importance of the family caregiver needing to care for himself or herself to be able to care for his or her loved one. Physicians routinely advise family members of critically ill patients with traumatic brain injury to get some rest when they have been at the bedside for 24 h or longer. Physicians understand that many decisions will need to be made as the family member directs the care of her or his loved one and the need to rest to make the most appropriate decisions. Although physicians are quick to advise patient family members to seek rest, they are sometimes reluctant to seek rest themselves.

Resident and intern perceptions of the work hour restrictions vary. A survey of resident perceptions conducted in 2004, shortly after implementation of the first round of work hour restrictions in 2003, showed varied impressions of the impact on resident training and patient care, the majority of which were negative [62]. The residents discussed the intended consequences of the work hour restrictions including improved well-being and less time in the hospital and the unintended consequences of the work hour restrictions including more discontinuity and work hour rules as a goal. The surveyed residents felt that only improved well-being had a positive effect on decreasing patient care mistakes, with all three other consequences leading to increased patient care errors. Resident surveys were performed prior to the increased limit in resident work hours implemented in 2011 [63, 64]. While 51% of the residents felt that the work hour restrictions would have a positive effect on resident quality of life, 44% of residents felt that the effect on patient care would be negative, with only 33% feeling the impact would be positive. The majority felt the impact on resident education would be negative, with 54% responding that the effect on their fund of knowledge would be negative and 63% responding that there would be a negative effect on their preparedness for assuming more senior roles [63]. Of surveyed surgical residents, 80.3% felt that the duty hour restrictions would decrease continuity of care, 57.6% felt they would decrease coordination of care, 48% felt they would impede their ability to acquire medical knowledge, 67.4% felt they would decrease their time in the operating room, 52.8% felt they would decrease their time with patients, and 52.8% felt they would decrease their educational experience. On a positive note, the majority felt the work hour restrictions would increase or not change the majority of ACGME core competencies (66.5–74.7%), and 61.5% of interns thought that they would decrease resident fatigue [64]. A resident survey following implementation of the new 2011 ACGME guidelines found that the majority felt that supervision was unchanged (73.8%), there was an increase in transfers of care (72.0%), the quality of life of the interns increased while the quality of life of the senior residents decreased, and their amount of rest (50.1% of respondents) and number of hours they worked (58.9% of respondents) remained unchanged [65].

Opinions among patients and the general public vary considerably from the perception of program directors and residents. The framework from which patients form their perceptions is significantly different because patients are for the most part unaware of the hours residents spend on duty and have grossly underestimated the average shift and work week lengths for residents [66, 67], similar to the underestimation by the general public [68]. Surveyed patients were much more concerned about resident fatigue than transfers of care [66, 67, 69], likely because they would have personal experience being fatigued, but patient care transfers would be an unfamiliar concept. Approximately half of the patients surveyed supported work hour restrictions for residents [66, 69]. Given these perceptions it is surprising that in two of three surveys, slightly more patients reported that they would rather have a physician familiar with their care even if the physician was fatigued [66] or not in compliance with work hour restrictions [69]. In the third survey, 57.1% of patients reported that they would select a well-rested physician who was unfamiliar with their care over a doctor who knew them but was fatigued [67]. In a survey of the public, the average of responses on the maximum amount of time a resident should work per shift was 10.9 h, and the maximum time a resi-

dent should work in a week was 50 h [68]. Only 1% of respondents felt that it was acceptable for residents to work more than 24 consecutive hours.

These opinions, both for and against the resident work hour restrictions, are based on opinions concerning benefit of the restrictions. But the important question in determining the significance to TBI patients is the data concerning impacts on patient care. Several studies have demonstrated improved patient outcomes associated with changes in line with the new work hour restrictions. Studies of ICU care before and after changes in intern schedules that limited working shifts to 16 h or less [70] and that eliminated 24-h work shifts in favor of separate day and night shifts [71] showed fewer attentional failures and fewer serious medical errors, respectively, during the hour restriction schedule period. Fewer order entry errors in the ICU have also been reported with resident work hour restrictions [72].

A study of surgical patients demonstrated a 28% greater chance of death before resident work hour restrictions compared to when the restrictions were in place, but this was not statistically significant, and a difference in morbidity was not found [73]. A study of trauma patient outcomes found a decrease in mortality rate with the 80-h resident work week restrictions compared to the pre-restriction period, which was statistically significant [74].

Other analyses have found a negative effect of the work hour restrictions. One group found an increased rate of accidental puncture or laceration and postoperative pulmonary embolus or deep vein thrombosis following implementation of work hour restrictions [75]. In a randomized intensive care unit study, there was no significant difference in complication rate after implementation of work hour restrictions compared to before, but seven of eight complications considered preventable occurred during the work hour restriction period, and no difference for residents in Stanford Sleepiness Scale was detected between the two periods [76]. Inpatient mortality and postoperative complication rates were reported to be statistically significantly increased after implementation of work hour restrictions

[77, 78]. In a study of neurotrauma patients, there was a statistically significant 23% increase in complication following implementation of the ACGME work hour restrictions compared to a period prior to work hour restrictions—a difference not seen in nonteaching hospitals during the same time periods [79].

Finally, there are reports of mixed results following implementation of ACGME work hour restrictions, including lower postoperative mortality but increased operative morbidity with coronary artery bypass grafting surgery [80]. Another study showed neurosurgical patients had decreased mortality that was not statistically significant and increased morbidity that was statistically significant [81]. There are also studies showing no difference in outcomes before and after work hour restrictions in mortality [82–84] and complication rates [84]. Resident workload does not appear to be associated with differences in patient outcomes [46]. A study of ICU patient outcomes before and after work hour restrictions found a decrease in inpatient mortality after the work hour restrictions in both academic and nonacademic hospitals, suggesting to the authors that this was an effect of improvement in care rather than an effect of the work hour restrictions [85]. One systematic review of the literature concerning the impact of resident duty hour restrictions on surgery patient care found no evidence of improved outcomes [86], and another reported 28 studies with no difference in patient outcomes, with only 4 studies showing patient outcome improvements and 2 studies showing increased complications [87].

Because work hour restrictions are being applied to residents in training who will be the next generation of physicians, the long-term patient safety implications of the impacts on resident training must be considered as much as the short-term safety implications for the patients currently cared for by the residents. A systematic review of the literature concerning work hour restrictions found 2 studies showing improvement in resident education, 12 studies showing worsening resident education, and 27 studies showing no change in resident education [87]. More specifically related to head trauma, a study of neurosurgery residents demonstrated a statisti-

cally significant 16% decrease in board examination scores and 7% decrease in number of abstracts presented at national meetings following the implementation of the 2003 ACGME resident work hour restrictions, suggesting a negative impact on resident training [88]. Even if the studies definitively showed an improvement in patient care or resident education with the work hour restrictions, there is evidence of lack of buy-in among residents that would make universal compliance difficult. In a survey of residents performed more than one decade into ACGME work hour restrictions, only 33% of residents reported that they were comfortable with signing out unfinished work to the resident on the next shift, and 81% reported that there are residents that exceed the work hour restrictions [89]. These residents cited professionalism as the driving force behind these attitudes and behaviors. A randomized study of work hour restriction schedules compared to a traditional resident work schedule showed a 130–200% increase in handoffs [90]. With this level of increase in handoffs, reluctance to pass off work and the attitude of staying beyond hour restrictions become significant problems. This same study showed decreased availability of residents at teaching conferences and decreased presence of interns during the day as well as significant safety concerns that led to early termination of 1 work hour restriction experimental group. However, residents do seem to grasp the complexity of the issue and the need to balance the negative aspects of each potential work hour schedule. The most common reason for errors reported by residents was the lack of adequate supervision at 20%, followed by excessive work hours at 19%, and then handoffs at 15% [91]. No schedule can eliminate all risks of adverse events.

The mixed results of studies show that the positive and negative effects of resident work hour restrictions are not clearly known. However, given the striking opinions of the public and patients supporting work hour restrictions, the restrictions are not going away. Clinicians caring for TBI patients must consider all of the potential negative effects of the work hour restrictions on patient care and develop strategies for reducing or eliminating these impacts to make sure only the potential benefits of the restrictions come through.

Conclusions

Modern TBI care is highly complex, and the environment of patient care in general is in a state of higher regulation, all of which lead to more fragmentation of care and the involvement of multiple physicians in care. The effectiveness and complexity of TBI guidelines give the trauma physicians more influence in the overall patient care and make close collaboration and better communication between the trauma physicians and the neurosurgeons a necessary component of care. Taking a team approach in which all caregivers, including the nurses, are included in regular communication about patient care plans will help maximize the benefits of ICU care while limiting the negative impacts of this highly unnatural environment. Resident work hour restrictions and shift changes necessary to provide 24-h patient coverage make handoffs much more important. Because handoffs are associated with errors in patient care, intentional management of the process should be implemented using guidelines developed through study results. Careful consideration of the factors that lead to the "Who's my doctor?" phenomenon will allow physicians to reduce the negative impacts of this confusing care environment.

References

1. Stein SC, Georgoff P, Meghan S, Mizra K, Sonnad SS. 150 years of treating severe traumatic brain injury: a systematic review of progress in mortality. J Neurotrauma. 2010;27(7):1343–53.
2. Gerber LM, Chiu YL, Carney N, Hartl R, Ghajar J. Marked reduction in mortality in patients with severe traumatic brain injury. J Neurosurg. 2013;119(6):1583–90.
3. Fakhry SM, Trask AL, Waller MA, Watts DD. Management of brain-injured patients by an evidence-based medicine protocol improves outcomes and decreases hospital charges. J Trauma. 2004;56(3):492–9; discussion 499–500.
4. Arabi YM, Haddad S, Tamim HM, Al-Dawood A, Al-Qahtani S, Ferayan A, et al. Mortality reduction after implementing a clinical practice guidelines-based management protocol for severe traumatic brain injury. J Crit Care. 2010;25(2):190–5.
5. Clayton TJ, Nelson RJ, Manara AR. Reduction in mortality from severe head injury following introduction of a protocol for intensive care management. Br J Anaesth. 2004;93(6):761–7.
6. Patel HC, Menon DK, Tebbs S, Hawker R, Hutchinson PJ, Kirkpatrick PJ. Specialist neurocritical care and outcome from head injury. Intensive Care Med. 2002;28(5):547–53.
7. Shi HY, Hwang SL, Lee KT, Lin CL. Temporal trends and volume-outcome associations after traumatic brain injury: a 12-year study in Taiwan. J Neurosurg. 2013;118(4):732–8.
8. Minei JP, Fabian TC, Guffey DM, Newgard CD, Bulger EM, Brasel KJ, et al. Increased trauma center volume is associated with improved survival after severe injury: results of a resuscitation outcomes consortium study. Ann Surg. 2014;260(3):456–64; discussion 464–455.
9. Tepas JJ III, Pracht EE, Orban BL, Flint LM. High-volume trauma centers have better outcomes treating traumatic brain injury. J Trauma Acute Care Surg. 2013;74(1):143–7; discussion 147–148.
10. Raj R, Bendel S, Reinikainen M, Hoppu S, Luoto T, Ala-Kokko T, et al. Traumatic brain injury patient volume and mortality in neurosurgical intensive care units: a Finnish nationwide study. Scand J Trauma Resusc Emerg Med. 2016;24(1):133.
11. Sasabuchi Y, Yasunaga H, Matsui H, Lefor AK, Horiguchi H, Fushimi K, et al. The volume-outcome relationship in critically ill patients in relation to the ICU-to-hospital bed ratio. Crit Care Med. 2015;43(6):1239–45.
12. MacKenzie EJ, Rivara FP, Jurkovich GJ, Nathens AB, Frey KP, Egleston BL, et al. A national evaluation of the effect of trauma-center care on mortality. N Engl J Med. 2006;354(4):366–78.
13. Lingsma HF, Roozenbeek B, Li B, Lu J, Weir J, Butcher I, et al. Large between-center differences in outcome after moderate and severe traumatic brain injury in the international mission on prognosis and clinical trial design in traumatic brain injury (impact) study. Neurosurgery. 2011;68(3):601–7; discussion 607–608.
14. Patel HC, Bouamra O, Woodford M, King AT, Yates DW, Lecky FE. Trends in head injury outcome from 1989 to 2003 and the effect of neurosurgical care: an observational study. Lancet. 2005;366(9496):1538–44.
15. Hartl R, Gerber LM, Iacono L, Ni Q, Lyons K, Ghajar J. Direct transport within an organized state trauma system reduces mortality in patients with severe traumatic brain injury. J Trauma. 2006;60(6):1250–6; discussion 1256.
16. Sampalis JS, Denis R, Frechette P, Brown R, Fleiszer D, Mulder D. Direct transport to tertiary trauma centers versus transfer from lower level facilities: impact on mortality and morbidity among patients with major

trauma. J Trauma. 1997;43(2):288–95; discussion 295–286.

17. Andriessen TM, Horn J, Franschman G, van der Naalt J, Haitsma I, Jacobs B, et al. Epidemiology, severity classification, and outcome of moderate and severe traumatic brain injury: a prospective multicenter study. J Neurotrauma. 2011;28(10):2019–31.

18. Wilson MH, Kolias AG, Hutchinson PJ. Neurotrauma—a multidisciplinary disease. Int J Clin Pract. 2014;68(1):5–7.

19. Ciesla DJ, Moore EE, Cothren CC, Johnson JL, Burch JM. Has the trauma surgeon become house staff for the surgical subspecialist? Am J Surg. 2006;192(6):732–7.

20. Ciesla DJ, Moore EE, Moore JB, Johnson JL, Cothren CC, Burch JM. The academic trauma center is a model for the future trauma and acute care surgeon. J Trauma. 2005;58(4):657–61; discussion 661–652.

21. Maas AI, Stocchetti N, Bullock R. Moderate and severe traumatic brain injury in adults. Lancet Neurol. 2008;7(8):728–41.

22. Roozenbeek B, Maas AI, Menon DK. Changing patterns in the epidemiology of traumatic brain injury. Nat Rev Neurol. 2013;9(4):231–6.

23. Pronovost PJ, Angus DC, Dorman T, Robinson KA, Dremsizov TT, Young TL. Physician staffing patterns and clinical outcomes in critically ill patients: a systematic review. JAMA. 2002;288(17):2151–62.

24. Wilcox ME, Chong CA, Niven DJ, Rubenfeld GD, Rowan KM, Wunsch H, et al. Do intensivist staffing patterns influence hospital mortality following ICU admission? A systematic review and meta-analyses. Crit Care Med. 2013;41(10):2253–74.

25. Wilcox ME, Harrison DA, Short A, Jonas M, Rowan KM. Comparing mortality among adult, general intensive care units in England with varying intensivist cover patterns: a retrospective cohort study. Crit Care. 2014;18(4):491.

26. Kerlin MP, Small DS, Cooney E, Fuchs BD, Bellini LM, Mikkelsen ME, et al. A randomized trial of nighttime physician staffing in an intensive care unit. N Engl J Med. 2013;368(23):2201–9.

27. Xie H, Kang J, Mills GH. Clinical review: the impact of noise on patients' sleep and the effectiveness of noise reduction strategies in intensive care units. Crit Care. 2009;13(2):208.

28. Bosma KJ, Ranieri VM. Filtering out the noise: evaluating the impact of noise and sound reduction strategies on sleep quality for ICU patients. Crit Care. 2009;13(3):151.

29. Alasad JA, Abu Tabar N, Ahmad MM. Patients' experience of being in intensive care units. J Crit Care. 2015;30(4):859.e857–11.

30. Rattray J, Johnston M, Wildsmith JA. The intensive care experience: development of the ICE questionnaire. J Adv Nurs. 2004;47(1):64–73.

31. Friese RS, Diaz-Arrastia R, McBride D, Frankel H, Gentilello LM. Quantity and quality of sleep in the surgical intensive care unit: are our patients sleeping? J Trauma. 2007;63(6):1210–4.

32. Pattison N. Psychological implications of admission to critical care. Br J Nurs. 2005;14(13):708–14.

33. Russell S. An exploratory study of patients' perceptions, memories and experiences of an intensive care unit. J Adv Nurs. 1999;29(4):783–91.

34. Roberts BL, Rickard CM, Rajbhandari D, Reynolds P. Patients' dreams in ICU: recall at two years post discharge and comparison to delirium status during ICU admission. A multicentre cohort study. Intensive Crit Care Nurs. 2006;22(5):264–73.

35. Lusk B, Lash AA. The stress response, psychoneuroimmunology, and stress among ICU patients. Dimens Crit Care Nurs. 2005;24(1):25–31.

36. Cochran J, Ganong LH. A comparison of nurses' and patients' perceptions of intensive care unit stressors. J Adv Nurs. 1989;14(12):1038–43.

37. Al-Qadheeb NS, Hoffmeister J, Roberts R, Shanahan K, Garpestad E, Devlin JW. Perceptions of nurses and physicians of their communication at night about intensive care patients' pain, agitation, and delirium. Am J Crit Care. 2013;22(5):e49–61.

38. Happ MB, Garrett K, Thomas DD, Tate J, George E, Houze M, et al. Nurse-patient communication interactions in the intensive care unit. Am J Crit Care. 2011;20(2):e28–40.

39. Alasad J, Ahmad M. Communication with critically ill patients. J Adv Nurs. 2005;50(4):356–62.

40. Sakr Y, Moreira CL, Rhodes A, Ferguson ND, Kleinpell R, Pickkers P, et al. The impact of hospital and ICU organizational factors on outcome in critically ill patients: results from the extended prevalence of infection in intensive care study. Crit Care Med. 2015;43(3):519–26.

41. Horwitz LI, Moin T, Krumholz HM, Wang L, Bradley EH. Consequences of inadequate sign-out for patient care. Arch Intern Med. 2008;168(16):1755–60.

42. Horwitz LI, Moin T, Krumholz HM, Wang L, Bradley EH. What are covering doctors told about their patients? Analysis of sign-out among internal medicine house staff. Qual Saf Health Care. 2009;18(4):248–55.

43. Arora V, Johnson J, Lovinger D, Humphrey HJ, Meltzer DO. Communication failures in patient sign-out and suggestions for improvement: a critical incident analysis. Qual Saf Health Care. 2005;14(6):401–7.

44. Borowitz SM, Waggoner-Fountain LA, Bass EJ, Sledd RM. Adequacy of information transferred at resident sign-out (in-hospital handover of care): a prospective survey. Qual Saf Health Care. 2008;17(1):6–10.

45. Solet DJ, Norvell JM, Rutan GH, Frankel RM. Lost in translation: challenges and opportunities in physician-to-physician communication during patient handoffs. Acad Med. 2005;80(12):1094–9.

46. Mueller SK, Call SA, McDonald FS, Halvorsen AJ, Schnipper JL, Hicks LS. Impact of resident workload and handoff training on patient outcomes. Am J Med. 2012;125(1):104–10.

47. Hasan H, Ali F, Barker P, Treat R, Peschman J, Mohorek M, et al. Evaluating handoffs in the con-

text of a communication framework. Surgery. 2017;161(3):861–8.

48. Bethune R, Campbell K, Rose A, Wassall R, Price C, Siese T, et al. Improving weekend handover between junior doctors on medical and surgical wards. BMJ Qual Improv Rep. 2014;2(2). pii: u483.w1045. https://doi.org/10.1136/bmjquality.u483.w1045.

49. Boyer M, Tappenden J, Peter M. Improving weekend out of hours surgical handover (WOOSH). BMJ Qual Improv Rep. 2016;5(1). pii: u209552.w4190. https://doi.org/10.1136/bmjquality.u209552.w4190.

50. Bradley A. Improving the quality of patient handover on a surgical ward. BMJ Qual Improv Rep. 2014;3(1). pii: u201797.w1958. https://doi.org/10.1136/bmjquality.u201797.w1958.

51. Culwick C, Devine C, Coombs C. Improving surgical weekend handover. BMJ Qual Improv Rep. 2014;3(1): u203298.w1533. https://doi.org/10.1136/bmjquality.u203298.w1533.

52. Din N, Ghaderi S, O'Connell R, Johnson T. Strengthening surgical handover: developing and evaluating the effectiveness of a handover tool to improve patient safety. BMJ Qual Improv Rep. 2012;1(1). pii: u492.w164. https://doi.org/10.1136/bmjquality.u492.w164.

53. Jardine AG, Page T, Bethune R, Mourant P, Deol P, Bowden C, et al. Bring on the weekend—improving the quality of junior doctor weekend handover. BMJ Qual Improv Rep. 2014;2(2). pii: u202379.w1297. https://doi.org/10.1136/bmjquality.u202379.w1297.

54. Karayiannis P, Warnock J. Improving handover of acute orthopaedic admissions. BMJ Qual Improv Rep. 2015;4(1). pii: u209209.w3901. https://doi.org/10.1136/bmjquality.u209209.w3901.

55 Michael E, Patel C. Improving medical handover at the weekend: a quality improvement project. BMJ Qual Improv Rep. 2015;4(1). pii: u207153.w2899. https://doi.org/10.1136/bmjquality.u207153.w2899.

56. Till A, Sall H, Wilkinson J. Safe handover: safe patients—the electronic handover system. BMJ Qual Improv Rep. 2014;2(2). pii: u202926.w1359. https://doi.org/10.1136/bmjquality.u202926.w1359.

57. Freemantle N, Richardson M, Wood J, Ray D, Khosla S, Shahian D, et al. Weekend hospitalization and additional risk of death: an analysis of inpatient data. J R Soc Med. 2012;105(2):74–84.

58. Segall N, Bonifacio AS, Schroeder RA, Barbeito A, Rogers D, Thornlow DK, et al. Can we make postoperative patient handovers safer? A systematic review of the literature. Anesth Analg. 2012;115(1):102–15.

59. Asch DA, Parker RM. The Libby Zion case. One step forward or two steps backward? N Engl J Med. 1988;318(12):771–5.

60. Drolet BC, Khokhar MT, Fischer SA. The 2011 duty-hour requirements—a survey of residency program directors. N Engl J Med. 2013;368(8):694–7.

61. Kesselheim JC, Cassel CK. Service: an essential component of graduate medical education. N Engl J Med. 2013;368(6):500–1.

62. Fletcher KE, Parekh V, Halasyamani L, Kaufman SR, Schapira M, Ertl K, et al. Work hour rules and contributors to patient care mistakes: a focus group study with internal medicine residents. J Hosp Med. 2008;3(3):228–37.

63. Drolet BC, Spalluto LB, Fischer SA. Residents' perspectives on ACGME regulation of supervision and duty hours—a national survey. N Engl J Med. 2010;363(23):e34.

64. Antiel RM, Van Arendonk KJ, Reed DA, Terhune KP, Tarpley JL, Porterfield JR, et al. Surgical training, duty-hour restrictions, and implications for meeting the accreditation council for graduate medical education core competencies: views of surgical interns compared with program directors. Arch Surg. 2012;147(6):536–41.

65. Drolet BC, Christopher DA, Fischer SA. Residents' response to duty-hour regulations—a follow-up national survey. N Engl J Med. 2012;366(24):e35.

66. Fletcher KE, Wiest FC, Halasyamani L, Lin J, Nelson V, Kaufman SR, et al. How do hospitalized patients feel about resident work hours, fatigue, and discontinuity of care? J Gen Intern Med. 2008;23(5):623–8.

67. Drolet BC, Hyman CH, Ghaderi KF, Rodriguez-Srednicki J, Thompson JM, Fischer SA. Hospitalized patients' perceptions of resident fatigue, duty hours, and continuity of care. J Grad Med Educ. 2014;6(4):658–63.

68. Blum AB, Raiszadeh F, Shea S, Mermin D, Lurie P, Landrigan CP, et al. US public opinion regarding proposed limits on resident physician work hours. BMC Med. 2010;8:33.

69. Mercuri JJ, Okey NE, Karia RJ, Gross RH, Zuckerman JD. Resident physician duty-hour requirements: what does the public think? J Am Acad Orthop Surg. 2016;24(11):789–95.

70. Lockley SW, Cronin JW, Evans EE, Cade BE, Lee CJ, Landrigan CP, et al. Effect of reducing interns' weekly work hours on sleep and attentional failures. N Engl J Med. 2004;351(18):1829–37.

71. Landrigan CP, Rothschild JM, Cronin JW, Kaushal R, Burdick E, Katz JT, et al. Effect of reducing interns' work hours on serious medical errors in intensive care units. N Engl J Med. 2004;351(18):1838–48.

72. Parthasarathy S, Hettiger K, Budhiraja R, Sullivan B. Sleep and well-being of ICU housestaff. Chest. 2007;131(6):1685–93.

73. Jamal MH, Doi SA, Rousseau M, Edwards M, Rao C, Barendregt JJ, et al. Systematic review and meta-analysis of the effect of North American working hours restrictions on mortality and morbidity in surgical patients. Br J Surg. 2012;99(3):336–44.

74. Morrison CA, Wyatt MM, Carrick MM. Impact of the 80-hour work week on mortality and morbidity in trauma patients: an analysis of the national trauma data bank. J Surg Res. 2009;154(1):157–62.

75. Poulose BK, Ray WA, Arbogast PG, Needleman J, Buerhaus PI, Griffin MR, et al. Resident work hour limits and patient safety. Ann Surg. 2005;241(6):847–56; discussion 856–860.

76. Parshuram CS, Amaral AC, Ferguson ND, Baker GR, Etchells EE, Flintoft V, et al. Patient safety, resident well-being and continuity of care with different resident duty schedules in the intensive care unit: a randomized trial. CMAJ. 2015;187(5):321–9.

77. Businger AP, Laffer U, Kaderli R. Resident work hour restrictions do not improve patient safety in surgery: a critical appraisal based on 7 years of experience in Switzerland. Patient Saf Surg. 2012;6(1):17.

78. Kaderli R, Businger A, Oesch A, Stefenelli U, Laffer U. Morbidity in surgery: impact of the 50-hour workweek limitation in Switzerland. Swiss Med Wkly. 2012;142:w13506.

79. Hoh BL, Neal DW, Kleinhenz DT, Hoh DJ, Mocco J, Barker FG II. Higher complications and no improvement in mortality in the ACGME resident duty-hour restriction era: an analysis of more than 107,000 neurosurgical trauma patients in the nationwide inpatient sample database. Neurosurgery. 2012;70(6):1369–81; discussion 1381–1362.

80. Gopaldas RR, Chu D, Dao TK, Huh J, LeMaire SA, Coselli JS, et al. Impact of ACGME work-hour restrictions on the outcomes of coronary artery bypass grafting in a cohort of 600,000 patients. J Surg Res. 2010;163(2):201–9.

81. Dumont TM, Rughani AI, Penar PL, Horgan MA, Tranmer BI, Jewell RP. Increased rate of complications on a neurological surgery service after implementation of the accreditation council for graduate medical education work-hour restriction. J Neurosurg. 2012;116(3):483–6.

82. Volpp KG, Rosen AK, Rosenbaum PR, Romano PS, Even-Shoshan O, Wang Y, et al. Mortality among hospitalized Medicare beneficiaries in the first 2 years following ACGME resident duty hour reform. JAMA. 2007;298(9):975–83.

83. Afessa B, Kennedy CC, Klarich KW, Aksamit TR, Kolars JC, Hubmayr RD. Introduction of a 14-hour work shift model for housestaff in the medical ICU. Chest. 2005;128(6):3910–5.

84. de Virgilio C, Yaghoubian A, Lewis RJ, Stabile BE, Putnam BA. The 80-hour resident workweek does not adversely affect patient outcomes or resident education. Curr Surg. 2006;63(6):435–9; discussion 440.

85. Prasad M, Iwashyna TJ, Christie JD, Kramer AA, Silber JH, Volpp KG, et al. Effect of work-hours regulations on intensive care unit mortality in United States teaching hospitals. Crit Care Med. 2009;37(9):2564–9.

86. Ahmed N, Devitt KS, Keshet I, Spicer J, Imrie K, Feldman L, et al. A systematic review of the effects of resident duty hour restrictions in surgery: impact on resident wellness, training, and patient outcomes. Ann Surg. 2014;259(6):1041–53.

87. Moonesinghe SR, Lowery J, Shahi N, Millen A, Beard JD. Impact of reduction in working hours for doctors in training on postgraduate medical education and patients' outcomes: systematic review. BMJ. 2011;342:d1580.

88. Jagannathan J, Vates GE, Pouratian N, Sheehan JP, Patrie J, Grady MS, et al. Impact of the accreditation council for graduate medical education work-hour regulations on neurosurgical resident education and productivity. J Neurosurg. 2009;110(5):820–7.

89. Coverdill JE, Alseidi A, Borgstrom DC, Dent DL, Dumire RD, Fryer J, et al. Professionalism in the twilight zone: a multicenter, mixed-methods study of shift transition dynamics in surgical residencies. Acad Med 2016;91(11 Association of American Medical Colleges Learn Serve Lead: Proceedings of the 55th Annual Research in Medical Education Sessions):S31–6.

90. Desai SV, Feldman L, Brown L, Dezube R, Yeh HC, Punjabi N, et al. Effect of the 2011 vs 2003 duty hour regulation-compliant models on sleep duration, trainee education, and continuity of patient care among internal medicine house staff: a randomized trial. JAMA Intern Med. 2013;173(8):649–55.

91. Jagsi R, Kitch BT, Weinstein DF, Campbell EG, Hutter M, Weissman JS. Residents report on adverse events and their causes. Arch Intern Med. 2005;165(22):2607–13.

Index